Gynecologic Decision Making

Gynecologic Decision Making

ROGER P. SMITH, M.D.

Professor and Vice Chairman
Program Director
Ambulatory Care Director
Department of Obstetrics and Gynecology
University of Missouri, Kansas City
Attending Physician, Truman Medical Center
Kansas City, Missouri

W.B. SAUNDERS COMPANY
A Harcourt Health Sciences Company
Philadelphia   London   New York   St. Louis   Sydney   Toronto

W.B. SAUNDERS COMPANY
A Harcourt Health Sciences Company

The Curtis Center
Independence Square West
Philadelphia, Pennsylvania 19106

Library of Congress Cataloging-in-Publication Data

Smith, Roger P. (Roger Perry)
  Gynecologic decision making / Roger P. Smith -- 1st ed.
     p. cm.
  ISBN 0-7216-8761-X
  1. Gynecology—Decision making.   I. Title.

  RG103.7.S656   2001
  618.1—dc21
                                                    00-049268

GYNECOLOGIC DECISION MAKING   ISBN 0–7216–8761–X

Printed in the United States of America

Last digit is the print number: 9   8   7   6   5   4   3   2   1

Preface

While no one believes that the practice of medicine can or should be reduced to the level of a "cook book," many clinical situations and conditions lend themselves to the application of decision algorithms. As the health care of women has received greater emphasis, more and more clinicians are faced with the diagnosis and management of "female" problems that once were the province of the specialist. In addition, the evolving complexity, depth of understanding of pathophysiology, and the breadth of therapeutic options available now make the visual algorithm an attractive tool for the gynecologist in practice or in training. The intent of this text, therefore, is to provide practical strategies for the diagnosis and management of problems that are either unique or particularly common in the care of women. These algorithms are based on clinical experience, bolstered by published studies and standard texts. Where differences or alternatives exist, these have been supplied to provide balance and to reaffirm that no one method of management should ever be construed as absolute. In all cases, the intervention of a caring, concerned, and thoughtful professional is required to reach the optimum approach for the individual patient.

Roger P. Smith, M.D.

NOTICE

Contents

Gynecologic Decision Making

Abnormal Menstrual Periods

INTRODUCTION

While the occurrence of periodic menstruation has variable connotations for most women, abnormalities in the interval or character are almost uniformly distressing. To evaluate these symptoms it is important to ensure that both patient and provider have agreed on the character of the disturbance. Once the exact nature of the disturbance is understood, a possible diagnosis may be established.

❶ The first aspect of the menstrual disturbance that needs to be ascertained is the presence or absence of rhythmicity. When there is background regularity but a change in the character of flow, the evaluation is directed differently from when the fundamental timing of periods is affected.

❷ Periods that have little or no pattern of timing should be differentiated from those with an altered, but predictable, pattern. When the bleeding pattern is one of prolonged interval, processes that suppress ovulation should be considered. These include those that result in anovulation as well as those that result in oligo-ovulation.

❸ Vaginal bleeding that has a variable or cryptic rhythm may arise as a result of a dysfunction of ovulation or nonmenstrual bleeding superimposed on a background of otherwise unaltered menstrual cycles. Bleeding that is heavy is most often due to uterine pathology such as fibroids or polyps. Endometritis, endometrial hyperplasia, or cancer may also present in this way. Reproductive-age women who have, or might have, been pregnant may have retained products of conception.

❹ Vaginal bleeding that has a variable or cryptic rhythm but is of normal character suggests irregular or oligo-ovulation.

❺ Menses that retain their rhythm but have an altered character generally do not reflect alterations in the hypothalamic–pituitary–ovarian axis. The character of the bleeding abnormality may help to separate some of the pathologies that should be considered.

❻ Processes that affect the cervix or the uterine lining may result in intermenstrual bleeding that is light and easily distinguished from the normal menstrual cycle. This bleeding is different from the heavier bleeding that may obscure the background cycles that is referred to in No. 3. Some causes are iatrogenic, such as use of the intrauterine contraceptive device (IUCD) or oral contraceptives, and are easily identified and treated. Others may require additional evaluations, including imaging or biopsy, to establish the diagnosis.

❼ Light but regular periods may be caused by chronic disease (renal failure) or by the influence of exogenous steroids (contraceptives).

❽ Bleeding that is regular but heavy constitutes menorrhagia, the evaluation of which is discussed separately.

REFERENCES

American College of Obstetricians and Gynecologists. Dysfunctional Uterine Bleeding. ACOG Technical Bulletin 134. Washington, DC: ACOG, 1989.

Cowan BD, Morrison JC. Management of abnormal genital bleeding in girls and women. N Engl J Med 1991;324:1710.

Field CS. Dysfunctional uterine bleeding. Prim Care 1988;15:561.

Fraiser IS. Treatment of ovulatory and anovulatory dysfunctional uterine bleeding with oral progestogens. Aust NZ J Obstet Gynaecol 1990;30:353.

Neese RE. Managing abnormal vaginal bleeding. Postgrad Med 1991;89:205.

Smith RP. Gynecology in Primary Care. Baltimore: Williams & Wilkins, 1997, pp 25–48.

Smith RP. Gynecology in Primary Care. Baltimore: Williams & Wilkins, 1997, pp 375–388.

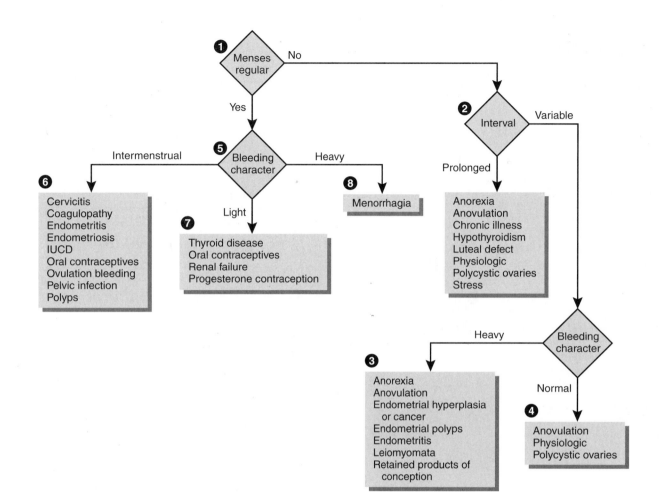

1 Menses regular

No → **2** Interval

Yes ↓

Variable →

5 Bleeding character

Prolonged ↓

Intermenstrual →

Heavy →

Light ↓

6
Cervicitis
Coagulopathy
Endometritis
Endometriosis
IUCD
Oral contraceptives
Ovulation bleeding
Pelvic infection
Polyps

7
Thyroid disease
Oral contraceptives
Renal failure
Progesterone contraception

8 Menorrhagia

Anorexia
Anovulation
Chronic illness
Hypothyroidism
Luteal defect
Physiologic
Polycystic ovaries
Stress

Bleeding character

Heavy →

Normal ↓

3
Anorexia
Anovulation
Endometrial hyperplasia
  or cancer
Endometrial polyps
Endometritis
Leiomyomata
Retained products of
  conception

4
Anovulation
Physiologic
Polycystic ovaries

Abnormal Pap Smear

Atypical Glandular Cells of Undetermined Significance

INTRODUCTION

Atypical glandular cells of undetermined significance (AGCUS) is one of the most confusing categories of the Bethesda system of reporting cellular cytology. It includes a range of findings, from benign reactive changes in endocervical or endometrial cells to adenocarcinoma. Under normal conditions, this finding should account for 0.2% to 0.4% of all Pap smears.

❶ One important aspect of the Bethesda system of cytologic smear interpretation is the adequacy and limitations of the sample. When the specimen is reported to be inadequate, limited by inflammatory changes or drying artifact, or limited by the degree of cellularity (number of cells available for study), the test should be repeated.

❷ If the specimen submitted was adequate for interpretation, management may be guided by any additional comments rendered by the pathologist. The Bethesda system was designed to make the evaluation of Pap smears more like a con-

sultation, and this should be exploited when possible.

❸ Under some circumstances, the pathologist may be able to suggest the origin of the cells seen. This will help to guide further evaluations. If the pathologist suggests the cells are inflammatory and endocervical in origin, the evaluation will be different from that when a tubal origin is possible.

❹ The patient's history and physical examination should be reviewed in an effort to find any risk factors that may be present. Has the patient been exposed to teratogens, or been treated for cervical or uterine abnormalities in the past? Is she at risk for endometrial hyperplasia or carcinoma? The answers to such questions can guide further management.

❺ If no risk factors are present, an increased frequency of Pap smears should be maintained until the abnormality is resolved or further diagnosis is established.

❻ When the patient is at increased risk for glandular (endometrial or endocervical) abnormalities, additional test such as sonohysterography, hysteroscopy, laparoscopy, or cone biopsy should be considered.

REFERENCES

American College of Obstetricians and Gynecologists. Cervical Cytology: Evaluation and Management of Abnormalities. ACOG Technical Bulletin 183. Washington, DC: ACOG, 1993.

Bose J, Kannan V, Kline TS. Abnormal endocervical cells: Really abnormal? Really endocervical? Am J Clin Pathol 1994;101:708.

Goff BA, Atanasoff P, Brown E, et al. Endocervical glandular atypia in Papanicolaou smears. Obstet Gynecol 1992;79:101.

Higgins RV, Hall JB, McGee JA, et al. Appraisal of the modalities used to evaluate an initial abnormal Papanicolaou smear. Obstet Gynecol 1994;84(2):174–178.

Smith RP. Gynecology in Primary Care. Baltimore: Williams & Wilkins, 1997, pp 305–318.

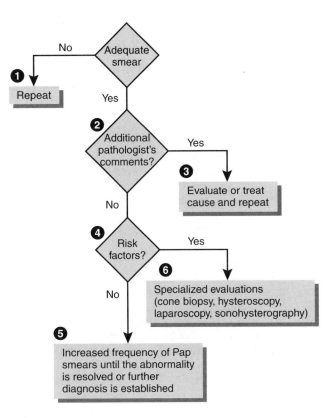

Abnormal Pap Smear

Atypical Squamous Cells of Undetermined Significance

INTRODUCTION

The *atypical squamous cells of undetermined significance (ASCUS)* diagnosis was developed to describe squamous cell changes that are more severe than reactive changes, but not as marked as those found in squamous intraepithelial lesions (SIL). This designation is not equivalent to the previous "squamous atypias" or "class II" Pap smears, which accounted for almost 20% of all smears and were associated with cervical changes that ranged from benign inflammation to premalignant lesions. ASCUS should occur in approximately 3% to 5% of all Pap smears.

❶ Patients who are at high risk by virtue of history (previous abnormal Pap smears, history of human papillomavirus or human immunodeficiency virus infection) or behavior (multiple sexual partners, smoking) should probably be managed by proceeding directly to colposcopic examination. These patients should also be followed more closely even after their Pap smear has returned to normal.

❷ When the cytologic diagnosis is ASCUS with no additional qualifiers or explanations provided by the pathologist, many suggest that watchful waiting is sufficient. Roughly 60% or more of patients will experience a spontaneous return to normal if their Pap smears are closely followed. If the Pap smear remains normal for three or four samplings taken at 6-month intervals, a return to routine annual screening is appropriate.

❸ One benefit of the Bethesda system of cytologic smear interpretation is that it allows assessment of other characteristics of the sample. When inflammation is present, the patient should be evaluated for the possibility of a vaginal or cervical infection and treatment instituted. Even in the face of a normal examination, empiric therapy followed in 8 to 12 weeks by a repeat Pap smear may be appropriate.

❹ Patients who are postmenopausal and have a diagnosis of ASCUS will often benefit from estrogen therapy. This may be topical or systemic, based on the other needs of the patient. Vaginal and cervical atrophy may take up to 6 months to reverse even on adequate therapy.

❺ If two consecutive Pap smears show cellular changes indicative of ASCUS, an evaluation by colposcopy is indicated.

REFERENCES

Higgins RV, Hall JB, McGee JA, et al. Appraisal of the modalities used to evaluate an initial abnormal Papanicolaou smear. Obstet Gynecol 1994;84(2):174–178.

Kurman RJ, Henson DE, Herbst AL, et al. Interim guidelines for management of abnormal cervical cytology. The 1992 National Cancer Institute Workshop. JAMA 1994;271(23):1866–1869.

Montz FJ, Bradley JM, Fowler JM, Nguyen L. Natural history of the minimally abnormal Papanicolaou smear. Obstet Gynecol 1992;80:385–388.

Smith RP. Gynecology in Primary Care. Baltimore: Williams & Wilkins, 1997, pp 305–318.

Toon PG, Arrand JR, Wilson LP, Sharp DS. Human papillomavirus infection of the uterine cervix of women without cytological signs of neoplasia. Br Med J 1986;293:1261–1264.

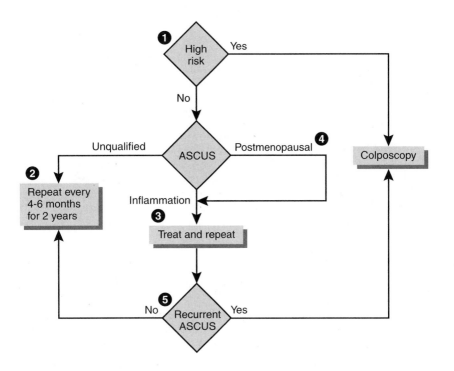

Abnormal Pap Smear

High-Grade Squamous Intraepithelial Lesions

INTRODUCTION

High-grade squamous intraepithelial lesions (HSILs) include cervical intraepithelial neoplasia (CIN) types II and III, as well as carcinoma in situ (CIS). They should account for less than 2% of Pap smears. These changes require careful further evaluation to establish a diagnosis and plan the appropriate treatments.

❶ The mainstay of the diagnosis and treatment of HSILs is colposcopy. On colposcopic examination vascular changes leading to mosaicism and punctation may be seen. Findings at the time of colposcopy can guide biopsies or additional therapy. Often, when pathologists report an HSIL, they will also indicate whether they believe the lesion to be of low or high grade. Low-grade lesions include those associated with human papillomavirus (HPV). Even if this is suspected clinically, colposcopy is still indicated.

❷ Colposcopy is considered adequate if all of the transformation zone is seen and the full extent of any lesions present can be demarcated. Endocervical curettage should be included in the evaluation.

❸ When inflammation is present, the patient should be evaluated for the possibility of a vaginal or cervical infection and treatment instituted. Even in the face of a normal examination, empiric therapy followed in 8 to 12 weeks by a repeat Pap smear may be appropriate. Patients who are postmenopausal will often benefit from estrogen therapy. This may be topical or systemic, based on the other needs of the patient. Vaginal and cervical atrophy may take up to 6 months to reverse even with adequate therapy.

❹ If the colposcopic examination is adequate, no lesion is seen, and there are no abnormalities found on the endocervical curettage, close follow-up with Pap smears every 4 to 6 months is adequate.

❺ High-grade lesions include those associated with significant atypia, and early and advanced cancer. Even if frank cancer is suspected clinically, colposcopy, biopsy (to establish histologic confirmation), and staging are still indicated. When the character and extent of the cervical lesion (that is compatible with the cytologic findings) can be established, therapy may proceed.

❻ When colposcopy is inadequate or the full extent of any lesions present cannot be seen, diagnostic conization of the cervix is required to establish the diagnosis. Based on the findings at diagnostic conization, additional therapy (if needed) may be planned.

❼ Significant lesions should be treated. When the full extent of the lesion can be seen, ablative therapies (cryosurgery, hot cautery, laser ablation, large loop excision of the transformation zone (LLETZ)/loop electrosurgical excision procedure (LEEP)) are appropriate. Conization of the cervix may be either diagnostic or therapeutic, or both.

REFERENCES

American College of Obstetricians and Gynecologists. Cervical Cytology: Evaluation and Management of Abnormalities. ACOG Technical Bulletin 183. Washington, DC: ACOG, 1993.

Brinton LA, Hamman RF, Huggins GH, et al. Sexual and reproductive risk factors for invasive squamous cell cervical cancer. J Natl Cancer Inst 1987;79:23–30.

Carmichael JA, Maskens PD. Cervical intraepithelial neoplasia: examination, treatment and follow-up: review. Obstet Gynecol Surg 1985;40:545–552.

Kurman RJ, Henson DE, Herbst AL, et al. Interim guidelines for management of abnormal cervical cytology. The 1992 National Cancer Institute Workshop. JAMA 1994;271(23):1866–1869.

Nasiell K, Roger V, Nasiell M. Behavior of mild cervical dysplasia during long-term follow-up. Obstet Gynecol 1986;67:665–669.

Smith RP. Gynecology in Primary Care. Baltimore: Williams & Wilkins, 1997, pp 305–318.

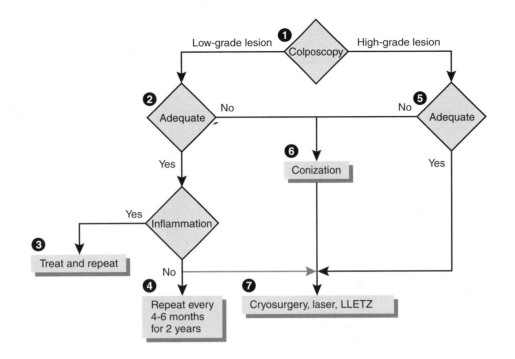

Abnormal Pap Smear

Low-Grade Squamous Intraepithelial Lesions

INTRODUCTION

Low-grade squamous intraepithelial lesions (LSILs) encompass changes associated with human papillomavirus (HPV), mild dysplasia, and cervical intraepithelial neoplasia type I (CIN I). They should account for less than 5% of Pap smears.

❶ Because most of the Pap smear abnormalities associated with LSILs are less sinister than those associated with HSILs, some latitude may be afforded these patients. When risk factors are present, or there is reason for concern, evaluation by colposcopy may be an appropriate first step. The risk and the degree of compliance that may be expected from the patient are both reasonable factors upon which to base evaluation strategies: patients who lack risk factors and are compliant may be followed with repeat Pap smears only; those at greater risk or those unwilling or unlikely to be able to cooperate with close follow-up should be evaluated by colposcopy.

❷ On colposcopic examination vascular changes leading to mosaicism and punctation may be seen. Findings at the time of colposcopy can guide biopsies or additional therapy. Low-grade lesions include those associated with HPV. Even if this is suspected clinically, colposcopy is still indicated.

❸ Colposcopy is considered adequate if all of the transformation zone is seen and the full extent of any lesions present can be demarcated. Endocervical curettage should be included in the evaluation.

❹ When inflammation is present, the patient should be evaluated for the possibility of a vaginal or cervical infection and treatment instituted. Even in the face of a normal examination, empiric therapy followed in 8 to 12 weeks by a repeat Pap smear may be appropriate. Patients who are postmenopausal will often benefit from estrogen therapy. This may be topical or systemic, based on the other needs of the patient. Vaginal and cervical atrophy may take up to 6 months to reverse even with adequate therapy.

❺ Increased frequency of Pap smears until the abnormality is resolved or further diagnosis is established is reasonable for selected patients with LSILs. (For a follow-up Pap smear to be "negative" it must have normal or benign findings, but also be "satisfactory for interpretation.")

❻ High-grade lesions include those associated with significant atypia, and early and advanced cancer. Even if frank cancer is suspected clinically, colposcopy, biopsy (to establish histologic confirmation), and staging are still indicated.

❼ When colposcopy is inadequate or the full extent of any lesions present cannot be seen, diagnostic conization of the cervix is required to establish the diagnosis. Based on the findings at diagnostic conization, additional therapy (if needed) may be planned. When the character and extent of the cervical lesion (that is compatible with cytologic findings) can be established, therapy may proceed.

❽ Significant lesions should should be treated. When the full extent of the lesion can be seen, ablative therapies (cryosurgery, hot cautery, laser ablation, large loop excision of the transformation zone (LLETZ), and the loop electrosurgical excision procedure (LEEP) are appropriate. Conization of the cervix may be either diagnostic, therapeutic, or both.

REFERENCES

American College of Obstetricians and Gynecologists. Cervical Cytology: Evaluation and Management of Abnormalities. ACOG Technical Bulletin 183. Washington, DC: ACOG, 1993.

Brinton LA, Hamman RF, Huggins GH, et al. Sexual and reproductive risk factors for invasive squamous cell cervical cancer. J Natl Cancer Inst 1987;79:23–30.

Carmichael JA, Maskens PD. Cervical intraepithelial neoplasia: examination, treatment and follow-up: review. Obstet Gynecol Surg 1985;40:545–552.

Kurman RJ, Henson DE, Herbst AL, et al. Interim guidelines for management of abnormal cervical cytology. The 1992 National Cancer Institute Workshop. JAMA 1994;271(23):1866–1869.

Nasiell K, Roger V, Nasiell M. Behavior of mild cervical dysplasia during long-term follow-up. Obstet Gynecol 1986;67:665–669.

Smith RP. Gynecology in Primary Care. Baltimore: Williams & Wilkins, 1997, pp 305–318.

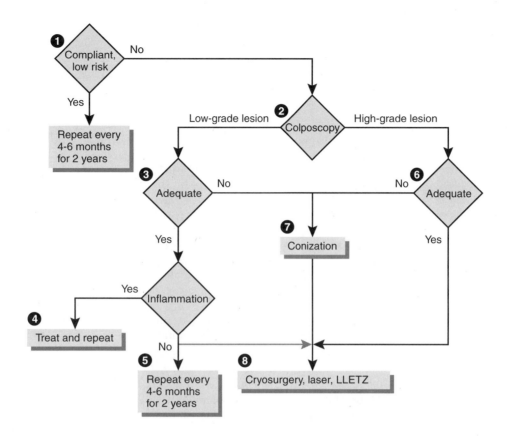

Abnormal Pap Smear

Management Principles

INTRODUCTION

The intent of the Bethesda system of reporting for cervical cytology is to make the report of cytologic findings more like a clinical consultation. This protocol is designed to encompass three elements: the adequacy of the specimen for interpretation, a general categorization of the findings (normal or abnormal), and a descriptive diagnosis.

❶ One of the first aspects of the Pap smear to be considered is the adequacy of the specimen. Under the Bethesda system this is included in every report. When the specimen is considered inadequate (ie, because of inadequate cellularity, drying artifact, or the presence of blood or inflammation), it must be repeated.

❷ When the cytologic smear is adequate, the smear may be repeated at intervals dictated by the clinical indications: low-risk patients who have had two or more normal smears at 1-year intervals may choose to have their Pap smears repeated at intervals up to 3 years; those at high risk or with a history of abnormal smears should continue to undergo the test at more frequent intervals. When a Pap smear is reported to be abnormal, the type and degree of abnormality should be specified by the pathologist or cytologist.

❸ The presence of benign reactive changes (atypical glandular cells of undetermined significance AGCUS) suggests the presence of infection or atrophy. Under most circumstances, the underlying cause should be identified and treated, and the cytology repeated.

❹ When atypical squamous cells of undetermined significance (ASCUS) are reported, the patient should be managed as shown separately.

❺ When low-grade squamous intraepithelial lesions (LSILs) are reported, the patient should be managed as shown separately.

❻ When high-grade squamous intraepithelial lesions (HSILs) are reported, the patient should be managed as shown separately.

❼ When carcinoma is identified on cervical cytology, careful pelvic examination with histologic confirmation is generally required. Colposcopy may be necessary to assist in directing the location for appropriate biopsies.

REFERENCES

Brinton LA, Hamman RF, Huggins GH, et al. Sexual and reproductive risk factors for invasive squamous cell cervical cancer. J Natl Cancer Inst 1987;79:23–30.

Higgins RV, Hall JB, McGee JA, et al. Appraisal of the modalities used to evaluate an initial abnormal Papanicolaou smear. Obstet Gynecol 1994;84(2):174–178.

Kurman RJ, Henson DE, Herbst AL, et al. Interim guidelines for management of abnormal cervical cytology. The 1992 National Cancer Institute Workshop. JAMA 1994;271(23):1866–1869.

Montz FJ, Bradley JM, Fowler JM, Nguyen L. Natural history of the minimally abnormal Papanicolaou smear. Obstet Gynecol 1992;80:385–388.

Sherlaw-Johnson C, Gallivan S, Jenkins D, Jones MH. Cytological screening and management of abnormalities in prevention of cervical cancer: an overview with stochastic modeling. J Clin Pathol 1994;47(5):430–435.

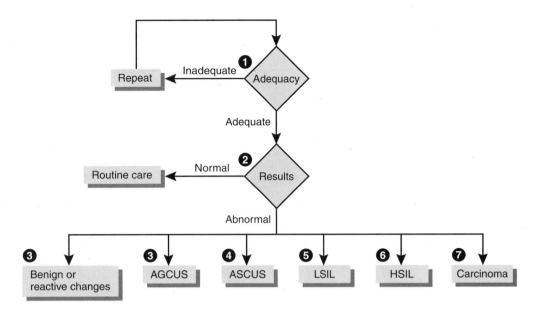

Abortion

INTRODUCTION

The failure of an early pregnancy is often signaled by abdominal cramping and vaginal bleeding. The differentiation among the various types of abortion helps to determine clinical management. In all forms of abortion, the mother's Rh status must be determined and Rh immune globulin given when indicated.

❶ Some abdominal cramping is common in early pregnancy. The uterus has periodic contractions from the time of conception onward. Multiparous patients may be better attuned to the presence of this activity or better appreciate its significance, though the activity appears to occur equally in nulliparous and multiparous patients alike. Bleeding is more ominous in early pregnancy, though some visible blood loss may occur during the implantation process.

❷ The first step in the evaluation of cramping and bleeding in early pregnancy is sterile speculum and bimanual examinations. These examinations should focus on the source of bleeding, the state of the cervix, and the presence of tissue.

❸ When it can be determined that tissue has been passed and the cervix is found to be closed with minimal or no bleeding, the diagnosis of *complete abortion* may be tentatively established. Care must be taken in deciding if tissue is actually present or has been passed. An organized clot may easily be mistaken for products of conception. In general, a clot will have a homogenous, liver-like character, while products of conception will be gray-tan and have the appearance of a bloody wash cloth. Watchful waiting, with or without uterotonic agents, is appropriate. Additional management is discussed separately.

❹ When the cervix is closed and there has been no passage of tissue, the diagnosis of *threatened abortion* is applied. The management of these patients is discussed separately.

❺ When the cervix is open, the patient may be experiencing either an inevitable or an incomplete abortion based on the presence of tissue at the os. In either case, the outcome is the uniform loss of the pregnancy. In multiparous patients, some dilation of the external cervical os may be normal. It is the presence of dilation of the inner os that is used to make the diagnosis. Management is similar to that discussed under Incomplete Abortion.

❻ The diagnosis of *incomplete abortion* is rendered when some, but not all, of the products of conception have been expelled. The management of incomplete abortion is discussed separately.

REFERENCES

American College of Obstetricians and Gynecologists. Early Pregnancy Loss. ACOG Technical Bulletin 212. Washington, DC: ACOG, 1995.

Batzofin JH, Fielding WI, Friedman EA. Effect of vaginal bleeding in early pregnancy on outcome. Obstet Gynecol 1984;63:515.

Goldstein SR. Embryonic death in early pregnancy: a new look at the first trimester. Obstet Gynecol 84:294, 1994.

Mackenzie WE, Holmes DS, Newton JR. Spontaneous abortion rate in ultrasonographically viable pregnancies. Obstet Gynecol 1988;71:81.

Poland BJ, Miller JR, Jones DC, Trimble BK. Reproductive counseling in patients who have had a spontaneous abortion. Am J Obstet Gynecol 1977;127:685–691.

Smith RP. Gynecology in Primary Care. Baltimore: Williams & Wilkins, 1997, p 99.

Thom DH, Nelson LM, Vaughan TL. Spontaneous abortion and subsequent adverse birth outcomes. Am J Obstet Gynecol 1992;166:111.

Warburton D, Fraser FC. Spontaneous abortion risks in man: data from reproductive histories collected in a medical genetics unit. Am J Human Genet 1964;16:1–25.

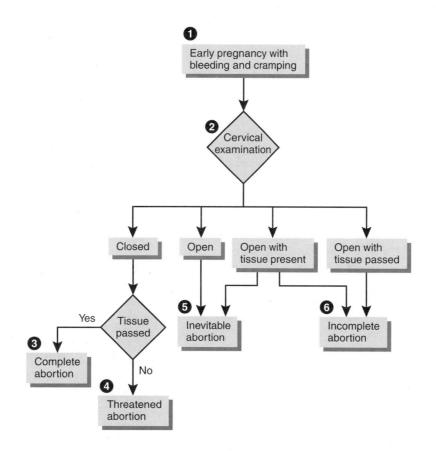

Abortion

Incomplete

INTRODUCTION

Incomplete abortion is the spontaneous passage of some, but not all, of the products of conception. It is associated with uniform pregnancy loss. If not treated, continuing bleeding and possible uterine or pelvic infection may result. In all forms of abortion, the mother's Rh status must be determined and Rh immune globulin given when indicated.

1 Some abdominal cramping is common in early pregnancy. The uterus has periodic contractions from the time of conception onward. Multiparous patients may be better attuned to the presence of this activity or better appreciate its significance, though the activity appears to occur equally for nulliparous and multiparous patients alike. Bleeding is more ominous in early pregnancy, though some visible blood loss may occur during the implantation process.

2 The first step in the evaluation of cramping and bleeding in early pregnancy is sterile speculum and bimanual examinations. These examinations should focus on the source of bleeding, the state of the cervix, and the presence of tissue.

3 When products of conception are present at a dilated cervix, the pregnancy is doomed. Gentle traction on the tissue at the os may be successful in removing the gestational sac intact. If bleeding is minimal, the patient may be managed as a complete abortion. When complete removal cannot be confirmed, the patient is managed as an incomplete abortion.

4 When some tissue has been passed, but there is reason to believe that additional tissue remains, the diagnosis of incomplete abortion is rendered.

5 To assist in the management of the patient with an incomplete abortion, transvaginal ultrasonography may be used to assess the contents of the uterus. Clinical suspicion, or continued moderate bleeding with a persistently dilated cervix may be sufficient to direct management without the use of ultrasonography.

6 The management of an incomplete abortion generally begins with the administration of oxytocin. This is frequently sufficient to prompt the passage of the remaining tissue and control blood loss. Even when curettage is planned, the use of oxytocin can result in reduced blood loss and provide temporization while plans are finalized and the patient is prepared for uterine evacuation.

7 If oxytocin therapy results in the passage of the remaining tissue, the bleeding slows or stops, and the cervix begins to close, the patient may be treated as a complete abortion.

8 In the majority of cases of incomplete abortion, active evacuation of the uterus will be required. This may be accomplished by either suction or sharp curettage, carried out under paracervical block with sedation or a regional anesthetic, or under a light general anesthesia based on the needs of the individual patient.

REFERENCES

American College of Obstetricians and Gynecologists. Early Pregnancy Loss. ACOG Technical Bulletin 212. Washington, DC: ACOG, 1995.

Smith RP. Gynecology in Primary Care. Baltimore: Williams & Wilkins, 1997, p 99.

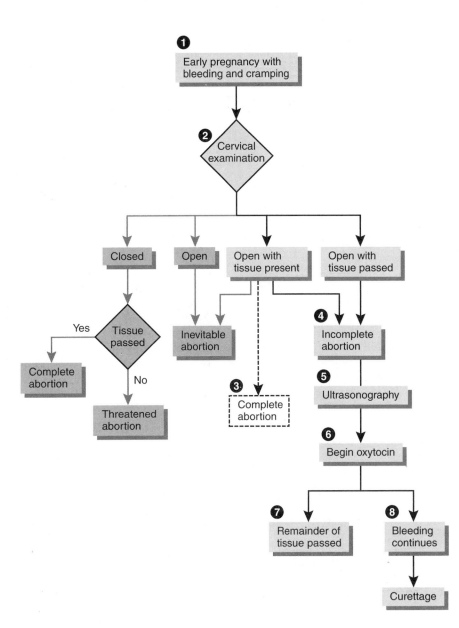

Abortion

Missed

INTRODUCTION

A missed abortion is a pregnancy that has failed but has not undergone the normal processes that result in the loss of the products of conception. This may result from a number of possible causes, but is most often associated with major chromosomal abnormalities. A missed abortion may be signaled by abdominal cramping and vaginal bleeding, or abnormalities of normal uterine growth. In all forms of abortion, the mother's Rh status must be determined and Rh immune globulin given when indicated.

❶ Some abdominal cramping is common in early pregnancy. The uterus has periodic contractions from the time of conception onward. Multiparous patients may be better attuned to the presence of this activity or better appreciate its significance, though the activity appears to occur equally for nulliparous and multiparous patients alike. Bleeding is more ominous in early pregnancy, though some visible blood loss may occur during the implantation process. None of the findings are unique to patients with missed abortions.

❷ The first step in the evaluation of cramping and bleeding in early pregnancy is sterile speculum and bimanual examinations. These examinations should focus on the source of bleeding, the state of the cervix, and the presence of tissue.

❸ When the cervix is closed, no tissue has been passed, and bleeding is minimal, the patient may be experiencing either a missed abortion or a threatened abortion with a pregnancy that is still viable. Without further information, the distinction between these two cannot be made.

❹ Until a differentiation can be made, the diagnosis of threatened abortion is generally a more appropriate one.

❺ Frequently, the only symptoms of missed abortion are abnormalities of uterine growth, most commonly a uterus that fails to grow at the expected rate. This may be noted when the uterus fails to become palpable above the symphysis around the 12th week of pregnancy, or when screening ultrasound studies fail to identify fetal parts when expected.

❻ When a threatened or missed abortion is suspected, ultrasound studies and serial determinations of maternal serum beta-human chorionic gonadotropin (β-hCG) levels may be helpful in establishing the diagnosis. A missed abortion or ectopic pregnancy should be suggested by an absence of a gestational sac on ultrasonography when the β-hCG level is greater than 2500 mIU/ml.

❼ Serial measurements of maternal serum β-hCG can be very helpful in the management of patients with abnormalities of early pregnancy. These measurements should generally be obtained at intervals of between 48 and 72 hours. These values are expected to roughly double during this time.

❽ When an appropriate rise in serum β-hCG can be documented, the diagnosis of threatened abortion may be established and continued prenatal care with close follow-up maintained.

❾ When the serum concentration of β-hCG does not double in 48 to 72 hours, an abnormality of pregnancy is assured. The possibility of an ectopic pregnancy must be considered and is discussed elsewhere.

❿ Once an ectopic pregnancy can be ruled out, the focus shifts to the evacuation of the products of conception. This may be done by a scheduled procedure carried out under controlled conditions in the subsequent several days. Evacuation may be carried out by suction or sharp curettage, under local, regional, or general anesthesia based on the needs of the patient, availability of services, and local custom.

REFERENCES

American College of Obstetricians and Gynecologists. Early Pregnancy Loss. ACOG Technical Bulletin 212. Washington, DC: ACOG, 1995.

Bromley B, Harlow BL, Laboda LA, Benacerraf BR. Small sac size in the first trimester: a predictor of poor fetal outcome. Radiology 178:375, 1991.

Goldstein SR. Embryonic death in early pregnancy: a new look at the first trimester. Obstet Gynecol 84:294, 1994.

Smith RP. Gynecology in Primary Care. Baltimore: Williams & Wilkins, 1997, p 99.

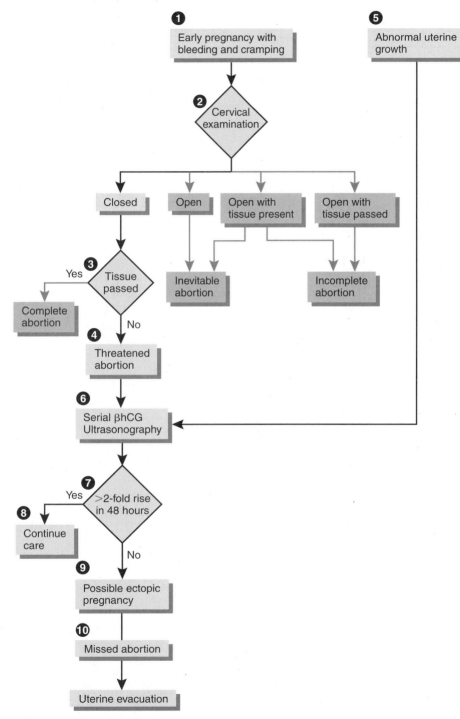

Abortion

Recurrent

INTRODUCTION

The term *recurrent abortion* is applied when a woman has had two consecutive, or three total, first-trimester spontaneous pregnancy losses. This affects 0.4% to 0.8% of women.

❶ When the losses have been early in gestation, there is a greater likelihood of a chromosomal abnormality as the cause.

❷ Five percent of couples who experience recurrent abortion will have a detectable parental chromosomal abnormality. Most chromosomal abnormalities result from disorders of meiosis in gamete formation or in mitosis after fertilization. Because these abnormalities may originate in either gamete, both parents must be evaluated.

❸ When pregnancy losses occur in mid or late pregnancy, a maternal cause is more likely. Attention should focus on the possibilities of uterine anomalies, immunologic factors, and endocrinopathies.

❹ The possibility of uterine anomalies must be explored through ultrasound studies and/or hysteroscopy. Anomalies that can result in pregnancy loss include fibroids, an incompetent cervix, intrauterine synechiae, and developmental abnormalities such as a septum or duplication. Uterine anomalies are found in 15% to 25% of women with recurrent abortion.

❺ The possibility of immunologic factors as a cause of recurrent losses should be evaluated. Examples include the presence of the lupus anticoagulant.

❻ Endocrinopathy (such as hypothyroidism) may account for recurrent pregnancy losses. Significant endocrine disturbances are likely to result in infertility, but more subtle abnormalities should be considered when losses occur.

REFERENCES

American College of Obstetricians and Gynecologists. Early Pregnancy Loss. ACOG Technical Bulletin 212. Washington, DC: ACOG, 1995.

Byrne JLB, Ward K. Genetic factors in recurrent abortion. Clin Obstet Gynecol 1994;37:693–704.

Harger JH, Archer DF, Marchese SG, et al. Etiology of recurrent pregnancy losses and outcome of subsequent pregnancies. Obstet Gynecol 62:574, 1983.

Hatasaka HH. Recurrent miscarriage: epidemiologic factors, definitions, and incidence. Clin Obstet Gynecol 1994;37:625–634.

Scott JR. Recurrent miscarriage: overview and recommendations. Clin Obstet Gynecol 1994;37:768–773.

Smith RP. Gynecology in Primary Care. Baltimore: Williams & Wilkins, 1997, pp 99–124.

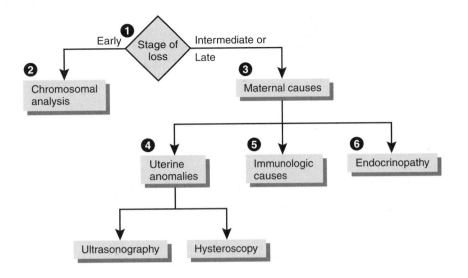

Abortion

Spontaneous (Complete)

INTRODUCTION

Complete abortion is the spontaneously passage of all of the products of conception. When it can be confirmed, supportive management is all that is required. In all forms of abortion, the mother's Rh status must be determined and Rh immune globulin given when indicated.

❶ Some abdominal cramping is common in early pregnancy. The uterus has periodic contractions from the time of conception onward. Multiparous patients may be better attuned to the presence of this activity or better appreciate its significance, though the activity appears to occur equally for nulliparous and multiparous patients alike. Bleeding is more ominous in early pregnancy, though some visible blood loss may occur during the implantation process.

❷ The first step in the evaluation of cramping and bleeding in early pregnancy is sterile speculum and bimanual examinations. These examinations should focus on the source of bleeding, the state of the cervix, and the presence of tissue.

❸ When it can be determined that tissue has been passed and the cervix is found to be closed with minimal or no bleeding, the diagnosis of complete abortion may be established. Care must be taken in deciding if tissue is present. An organized clot may easily be mistaken for products of conception. In general, a clot will have a homogenous, liver-like character, while products of conception will be gray-tan and have the appearance of a bloody wash cloth. Watchful waiting, with or without uterotonic agents, is appropriate when the diagnosis of complete abortion has been made.

❹ When products of conception are present at a dilated cervix, the pregnancy is doomed. Gentle traction on the tissue at the os may be successful in removing the gestational sac intact. If bleeding is minimal, the patient may be managed as a complete abortion. When complete removal cannot be confirmed, the patient is managed as an incomplete abortion.

❺ Patients should be counseled to seek care if there is a significant increase in bleeding, abdominal pain or cramping, or fever or chills. These symptoms suggest the possibility of an unrecognized incomplete abortion. The management of incomplete abortion is discussed separately.

❻ An important part of the management of patients who experience spontaneous pregnancy loss is support and counseling. These patients should be reassured that the process was one over which they had no control: Their actions could neither cause nor prevent the loss. Patients who experience two or more spontaneous losses should be considered for further evaluation or recurrent pregnancy loss (recurrent abortion).

REFERENCES

Hogue CJR. Impact of abortion on subsequent fecundity. Clin Obstet Gynaecol 1986;13:95.

Mackenzie WE, Holmes DS, Newton JR. Spontaneous abortion rate in ultrasonographically viable pregnancies. Obstet Gynecol 1988;71:81.

Poland BJ, Miller JR, Jones DC, Trimble BK. Reproductive counseling in patients who have had a spontaneous abortion. Am J Obstet Gynecol 1977;127:685–691.

Smith RP. Gynecology in Primary Care. Baltimore: Williams & Wilkins, 1997, p 99.

Thom DH, Nelson LM, Vaughan TL. Spontaneous abortion and subsequent adverse birth outcomes. Am J Obstet Gynecol 1992;166:111.

Warburton D, Fraser FC. Spontaneous abortion risks in man: data from reproductive histories collected in a medical genetics unit. Am J Human Genet 1964;16:1–25.

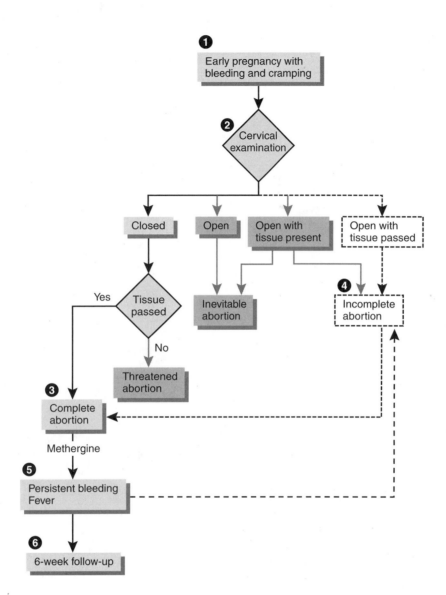

Abortion

Threatened

INTRODUCTION

The diagnosis of threatened abortion is rendered any time the success of a pregnancy seems in jeopardy. In all forms of abortion, the mother's Rh status must be determined and Rh immune globulin given when indicated.

❶ Some abdominal cramping is common in early pregnancy. The uterus has periodic contractions from the time of conception onward. Multiparous patients may be better attuned to the presence of this activity or better appreciate its significance, though the activity appears to occur equally for nulliparous and multiparous patients alike. Bleeding is more ominous in early pregnancy, though some visible blood loss may occur during the implantation process.

❷ The first step in the evaluation of cramping and bleeding in early pregnancy is sterile speculum and bimanual examinations. These examinations should focus on the source of bleeding, the state of the cervix, and the presence of tissue.

❸ If the cervix is open, the diagnosis of threatened abortion cannot be rendered; instead, the patient must be experiencing an inevitable or incomplete loss. Until a differentiation between a threatened and a missed abortion can be made, the diagnosis of threatened abortion is generally the most appropriate one.

❹ When a threatened abortion is suspected, ultrasound studies and serial determinations of maternal serum beta-human chorionic gonadotropin (β-hCG) levels may be helpful in establishing the diagnosis. A missed abortion or ectopic pregnancy should be suggested by an absence of a gestational sac on ultrasonography when the β-hCG is greater than 2500 mIU/ml.

❺ Serial measurements of maternal serum β-hCG can be very helpful in the management of patients with abnormalities of early pregnancy. These measurements should generally be obtained at intervals of between 48 and 72 hours. These values are expected to roughly double during this time.

❻ When an appropriate rise in serum β-hCG can be documented, the diagnosis of threatened abortion may be finally established and continued prenatal care with close follow-up maintained. Many suggest the use of a follow-up ultrasound evaluation to assess fetal development and to provide reassurance. The cost effectiveness of this remains controversial.

❼ When the serum concentration of β-hCG does not double in 28 to 72 hours, an abnormality of pregnancy is assured. The possibility of an ectopic pregnancy or missed abortion must be considered and are discussed elsewhere.

REFERENCES

American College of Obstetricians and Gynecologists. Early Pregnancy Loss. ACOG Technical Bulletin 212. Washington, DC: ACOG, 1995.

Batzofin JH, Fielding WI, Friedman EA. Effect of vaginal bleeding in early pregnancy on outcome. Obstet Gynecol 1984;63:515.

Boklage CE. Survival probability of human conceptions from fertilization to term. Int J Fertil 1990;35:75–94.

Funderburk SJ, Guthrie D, Meldrum D. Outcome of pregnancies complicated by early vaginal bleeding. Br J Obstet Gynecol 1980;87:100.

Smith RP. Gynecology in Primary Care. Baltimore: Williams & Wilkins, 1997, p 99.

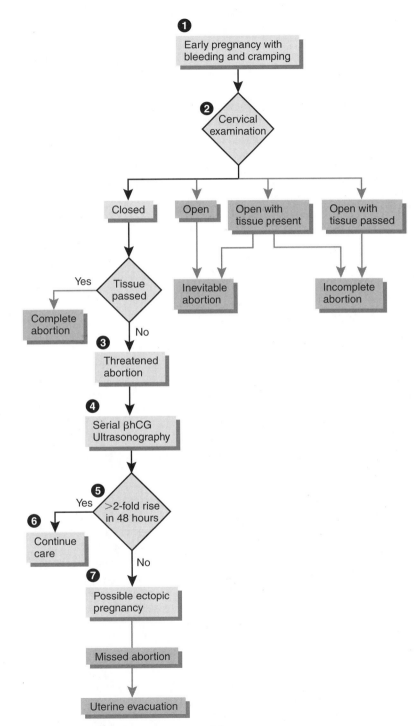

❶ Early pregnancy with bleeding and cramping

❷ Cervical examination

Closed

Open

Open with tissue present

Open with tissue passed

Yes — Tissue passed

Complete abortion

Inevitable abortion

Incomplete abortion

No

❸ Threatened abortion

❹ Serial βhCG Ultrasonography

❺ >2-fold rise in 48 hours

Yes

❻ Continue care

No

❼ Possible ectopic pregnancy

Missed abortion

Uterine evacuation

Acne

INTRODUCTION

Production of sebum in response to androgens can lead to oily skin, clogged hair follicles, folliculitis, and acne. Inflammation of the sebaceous glands can result in comedones, papules, inflammatory pustules, and scarring. While the incidence of acne is equal for males and females, and males tend to have the more severe form, societal pressures often result in a greater concern and impact for women, often exceeding that dictated by medical considerations. It is often a reason to either choose or discontinue the use of oral contraceptives. Acne may also provide an opportunity for both the patient and the care giver to discuss other issues, including lifestyle and contraception.

❶ Acne is often seen as a part of the rite of passage that is puberty. Virtually 100% of teens experience some manifestation, though only 15% seek medical advice. When acne persists into the twenties or beyond it becomes a greater concern. New-onset acne after the age of 20 is generally associated with environmental exposure or elevations in androgens.

❷ Exposure to oils, grease, or tar can result in acne. These may take the form of oil-based cosmetics, cleansing creams, or moisturizers. The warmth and excessive oils generated by occlusion by holding hands, telephones, or sports equipment against the skin may also contribute. If these factors are present they should be minimized or eliminated.

❸ Exposure to androgenic steroids, either topically or systemically, may cause the development of acne. The androgenic potential of some oral contraceptive formulations may be responsible in some patients. Other medications such as iodides or bromides, lithium, and phenytoins may also stimulate the development of acne.

❹ Patients with late-onset acne without other cause should be suspected of having excess androgen even in the absence of masculinization or hirsutism. When signs of masculinization are absent, elevations in the adrenal androgens dehydroepiandrosterone (DHA) and dehydroepiandrosterone sulfate (DHEAS) may be present and should be evaluated. Mild elevations may be treated with low-dose oral contraceptives, glucocorticoid suppression, spironolactone, or cyproterone acetate. Empiric treatment with these agents may be justified in some cases.

❺ The first line of therapy for adolescent patients is hygienic measures such as gentle surface cleansing with a mild soap and water once or twice a day and the avoidance of oils such as cosmetics and sunscreens. Frequent hand washing and keeping the fingernails clipped short (to reduce scratching, trauma, and secondary infection) is also advisable. For mild cases, this is often adequate.

❻ If simple hygienic measures are insufficient, topical drying agents or antibiotics may be added. Benzoyl peroxide (5% to 10%) may be applied at bedtime to help dry the skin. Topical erythromycin or clindamycin (2% solution) may be applied to reduce infection and inflammation. Topical therapy will generally take 4 weeks or longer to show an effect. Some skin redness is common with the use of drying agents; this will generally improve with use.

❼ Before systemic therapy or more aggressive topical therapy is considered, the patient's risk and desire for pregnancy must be assessed. Many of the agents used for more difficult cases of acne carry teratogenic risks. If the patient is using reliable contraception or she or her partner is sterile, a systemic antibiotic such as tetracycline or erythromycin (both 250 mg po qid for 7 to 10 days, then tapering to lowest effective dose) may be used. Topical treatment with retinoic acid (0.025% cream applied at bedtime) or isotretinoin (0.5 to 1.0 mg/kg/day, in two doses, for 12 to 16 weeks) may be added. The latter is associated with significant potential side effects and is generally reserved for resistant cases. Transient flaring of lesions at the start of treatment with retinoic acid is common, and the patient should be warned of this occurrence.

❽ Patients who want to become pregnant but have persistent acne must continue conservative management to avoid risk to their fetus from the medications used in resistant cases. Those who are willing to delay pregnancy should be considered for low-dose oral contraceptive therapy using a formulation with low androgenic potential. This may be sufficient to provide both contraception and relief of symptoms. If necessary, additional agents may be added once satisfactory contraception has been established. Oral contraception should be used for at least 1 month before and after isotretinoin therapy.

REFERENCES

Leyden JJ. Retinoids in acne. J Am Acad Dermatol 1988;19:164–168.

McClintoch JH, Arpey CJ, Whitaker DC. Dermatologic disease common to women. In Ling FW, Laube DW, Nolan TE, et al (eds): Primary Care in Gynecology. Baltimore: Williams & Wilkins, 1996, pp 369–394.

Shalita AR, Leyden JE Jr, Pochi PE, et al. Acne vulgaris. J Am Acad Dermatol 1987;16:410–412.

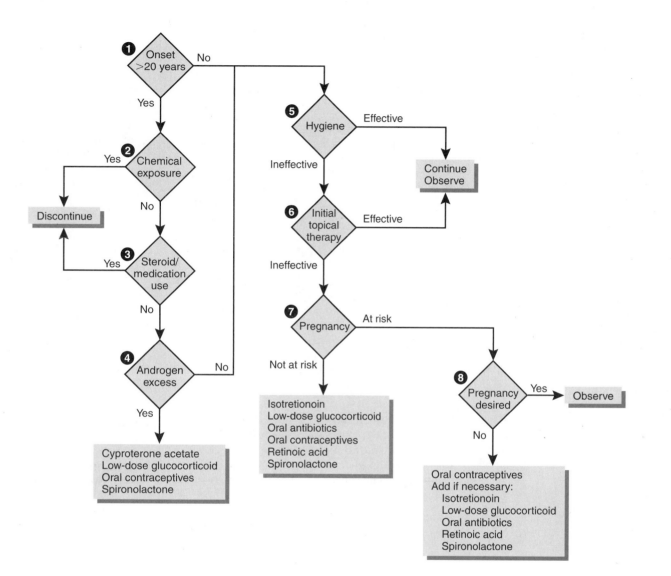

Actinomyces Infection

INTRODUCTION

Infection by the indolent, anaerobic, gram-positive filamentous bacterium *Actinomyces israelii* is uncommon and is most often associated with the use of an intrauterine contraceptive device (IUD) or chronic pelvic inflammatory disease. This slow-growing partially acid-fast bacterium forms small masses of organisms and inflammatory debris referred to as "sulfur granules." Colonization occurs in up to 5% of IUD users.

❶ Infection by *A. israelii* is most often asymptomatic. The diagnosis may be suspected on Pap smear, though only 40% of those with a suggestive Pap smear are actually colonized. Statistically, these women do have a three- to four-fold increase in their risk of pelvic inflammatory disease, though a causal relationship is difficult to prove. Though rarely symptomatic, infections thought to involve this organism require aggressive and prolonged therapy with penicillin or tetracycline (with other agents as needed).

❷ Infection by *A. israelii* is almost unheard of in non-IUD wearers but the presence of an IUD alters therapy.

❸ If a non-IUD user is suspected of having an infection and has other risk factors for pelvic infection, empiric antibiotic therapy is indicated. This most often takes the form of penicillin G or tetracycline for 10 to 14 or more days. Much of the older literature suggests 4 to 6 weeks of parenteral treatment and up to 6 months of oral therapy, though recent evidence has shifted this to a shorter course.

❹ When an IUD is present in an asymptomatic patient, empiric therapy is probably warranted. *Actinomyces* species are difficult to culture and take up to a week to grow under anaerobic conditions. As a result, a culture is optional and should not impede therapy.

❺ A cytologic specimen (Pap smear) may be used to assess the results of therapy if desired. If this suggests continued colonization, the IUD should be removed and a new cycle of antibiotic therapy begun.

❻ An optional method of treatment consists of simply removing the IUD. For the majority of patients, this is curative and no further therapy is needed. If a follow-up Pap smear suggests continuing colonization, penicillin or tetracycline therapy may be started. This method does require the institution of a different form of contraception for the duration of treatment. There is no evidence that low-risk women should be denied use of an IUD because of past episodes of asymptomatic colonization.

REFERENCES

Braby H, Dougherty CM, Mickal A. Actinomycosis of the female genital tract. Obstet Gynecol 1964;23:580.

Dougherty CM, Pastorek JG II. Sexually transmitted diseases and miscellaneous pelvic infections. In Sciarra JJ (ed): Gynecology and Obstetrics. Philadelphia: JB Lippincott, 1997;(1)41:19.

Droegemueller W. Infections of the upper genital tract. In Mishell DR, Stenchever MA, Droegemueller W, Herbst AL (eds): Comprehensive Gynecology, 3rd ed. St Louis: CV Mosby, 1997, p 677.

Eschenbach DA. Acute pelvic inflammatory disease. In Sciarra JJ (ed): Gynecology and Obstetrics. Philadelphia: JB Lippincott, 1992;(1)44:5.

Smith RP. Gynecology in Primary Care. Baltimore: Williams & Wilkins, 1997, p 216.

Valicenti JF, Pappa AA, Graberc D, et al. Detection and prevalence of IUD-associated Actinomyces colonization and related morbidity. JAMA 1982;247:1149.

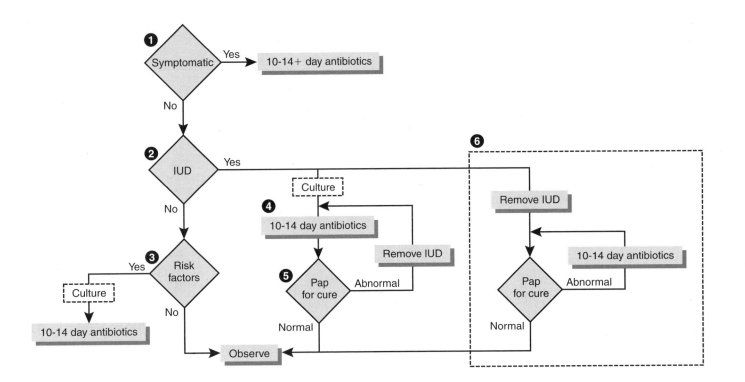

Adnexal Torsion

INTRODUCTION

Adnexal torsion refers to the twisting of part or all of the adnexa on its mesentery, resulting in tissue ischemia and frank infarction. This usually involves the ovary, but may include the fallopian tube as well. In most cases, an abnormality of the adnexa predisposes to the torsion (50% to 60% will have an ovarian tumor or cyst). Torsion accounts for about 2% to 3% of gynecologic surgical emergencies. The average age of patients with torsion is the mid-twenties, though it can occur in postmenopausal women with benign tumors and is more likely during pregnancy (20% of torsion cases).

❶ The most common presenting signs and symptoms of adnexal torsion are pain (generally abrupt, intense, and unilateral), nausea and vomiting (60% to 70%), and a unilateral palpable (tender) mass (90% of patients). The presence of one or more of these in a reproductive-age woman should suggest the possibility of torsion, though a large number of other pathologies may present in a similar manner. Often the patient will relate the onset of symptoms to an abrupt change in position or will have had similar intermittent symptoms for some time before presentation.

❷ The acuity and severity of symptoms associated with adnexal torsion often results in a surgical abdomen at the time of initial evaluation. These patients must be acutely stabilized and surgically explored regardless of the working diagnosis. The preoperative diagnosis of tubal torsion is made in only about 20% of cases, while the diagnosis of ovarian or adnexal torsion is more easily established before surgery. If a torsion is confirmed at the time of surgery, the intraoperative management may proceed as in step 8.

❸ For patients with less acute symptoms, ultrasonography (abdominal or transvaginal) may be a useful adjunct in establishing the diagnosis. If the adnexa appear normal, the possibility of torsion is greatly reduced, but not eliminated. Torsion of normal adnexa is most common during pregnancy (ovary) or childhood (fallopian tube). Dermoid tumors are the most commonly reported tumors to undergo torsion, though the relative risk is greater with parovarian cysts, solid benign tumors, and serous cysts.

❹ The most common finding (by imaging or pelvic examination) is an 8- to 12-cm tender, cystic structure. When the mass is of this size, surgical exploration to address both the possible torsion and the underlying adnexal enlargement will be required. The use of 5 cm as a threshold is arbitrary and will vary with location and individual circumstances.

❺ If Doppler flow studies are available, they may be used to suggest torsion, though the inability to document blood flow is not the same as a true absence of flow.

❻ Patients will mild symptoms and normal or slight adnexal enlargement (and normal blood flow, if assessed) may be managed by conservative means. If symptoms fail to improve or worsen, surgical exploration, often by laparoscopy, should be pursued. A low-grade fever and leukocytosis suggest necrosis.

❼ Because the majority of women suspected of having adnexal torsion are of reproductive age, every effort should be made to be conservative in the surgical therapy chosen. Laparoscopy or minilaparotomy is generally sufficient to establish a diagnosis and accomplish any procedures required. Conservation of the adnexa is possible in approximately 75% of cases.

❽ If the adnexa are frankly gangrenous, excision may be the only option. Care should be taken in reaching this decision as the venous congestion and cyanosis of partial venous obstruction may look similar.

❾ Recent studies suggest that even in the face of significant torsion, untwisting of the adnexa is safe and allows for conservation of the ovary. If a return of blood flow seems to be apparent clinically, through intraoperative Doppler studies or the use of intravenous fluorescein (viewed with an ultraviolet light), the adnexa may be left in place.

❿ In 75% of cases, conservation of the ovary is possible, but any predisposing pathology must be dealt with before completion of the surgical procedure. Simple cyst excision is commonly sufficient. Many authors advocate the placement of a suture to stabilize the ovary to prevent future torsion. Up to 10% of patients will have an episode involving the opposite adnexa, suggesting that if stabilization is used, it should be used on both sides.

REFERENCES

Bayer AI, Wiskind AK. Adnexal torsion: Can the adnexa be saved? Am J Obstet Gynecol 1994;171:1506–1511.

Bider D, Maschiach S, Dulitzky M, et al. Clinical, surgical and pathologic findings of adnexal torsion in pregnant and nonpregnant women. Surg Gynecol Obstet 1991;173:363.

Gordon JD, Hopkins KL, Jeffrey RB, Giudice LC. Adnexal torsion: color Doppler diagnosis and laparoscopic treatment. Fertil Steril 1994;61:383.

Hibbard LT. Adnexal torsion. Am J Obstet Gynecol 1985;152:456.

Nichols DH, Julian PJ. Torsion of the adnexa. Clin Obstet Gynecol 1985;28:375.

Oelsner G, Bider D, Goldenberg M, et al. Long-term follow-up of the twisted ischemic adnexa managed by detorsion. Fertil Steril 1993;60:976.

Zweizig S, Perron J, Grubb D, Mishell DR Jr. Conservative management of adnexal torsion. Am J Obstet Gynecol 1993;168:1791.

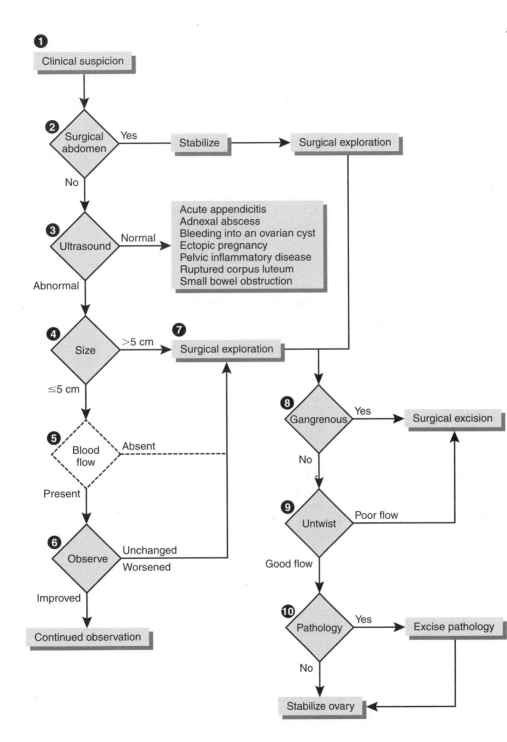

① Clinical suspicion

② Surgical abdomen — Yes → Stabilize → Surgical exploration

No

③ Ultrasound — Normal →
Acute appendicitis
Adnexal abscess
Bleeding into an ovarian cyst
Ectopic pregnancy
Pelvic inflammatory disease
Ruptured corpus luteum
Small bowel obstruction

Abnormal

④ Size — >5 cm → ⑦ Surgical exploration

≤5 cm

⑤ Blood flow — Absent

Present

⑥ Observe — Unchanged / Worsened

Improved

Continued observation

⑧ Gangrenous — Yes → Surgical excision

No

⑨ Untwist — Poor flow

Good flow

⑩ Pathology — Yes → Excise pathology

No

Stabilize ovary

Amenorrhea

Postpartum

INTRODUCTION

The return of menstrual function following a pregnancy is sometimes unpredictable. Typical non-breastfeeding mothers experience a return of menses in 7 to 16 weeks. Delays beyond this point or patient concern should prompt a clinical enquiry.

❶ The first step in the evaluation of any patient with postpartum amenorrhea is a serum or urinary pregnancy test. Pregnancy (intended or otherwise) is the most common cause of secondary amenorrhea at any time (outside of menopause).

❷ Because many forms of contraception affect the return of menstrual function, the contraceptive method the patient has chosen (if any) should be established.

❸ Of mothers who breastfeed fully, only 18% resume ovulation by 3 months and only 20% to 43% do so by 6 months after delivery. In one Australian study, 64% of breastfeeding women had ovulated and 70% had menstruated by 12 months, leaving 30% amenorrheic. Even sporadic nursing may significantly delay the return of menses. Unless the patient is actively seeking another pregnancy, reassurance and observation is all that is required.

❹ Patients who choose a long-acting progestin contraceptive agent (depomedroxyprogesterone ace-tate (DMPA) or levonorgestrel rods) frequently experience amenorrhea. Amenorrhea is more common when these agents are begun in the immediate postpartum period than when begun remote from pregnancy. Amenorrhea rates of 70% or greater are common with DMPA, with lower rates found in patients who use contraceptive rods.

❺ The use of low-dose combination oral contraceptives may result in amenorrhea at any point in a woman's life. Increasing the relative strength of the estrogen component will generally result in a resumption of menses. After several cycles, the dose may be reduced again if desired.

❻ If the patient is using a barrier or no method of contraction and is not pregnant, she should be evaluated as a case of secondary amenorrhea. A progestin withdrawal (challenge test) will help to suggest additional potential diagnoses.

❼ When the progestin challenge produces bleeding, anovulation is suggested and the patient should be further evaluated in the manner discussed for secondary amenorrhea.

❽ When no bleeding results from progestin withdrawal, consideration must be given to uterine and outflow tract abnormalities or the possibility of pituitary damage during delivery (Sheehan syndrome). Uterine or cervical scarring following curettage, cesarean delivery, or cervical injury may all result in a lack of menstrual flow.

REFERENCES

American College of Obstetricians and Gynecologists. Amenorrhea. ACOG Technical Bulletin 128. Washington, DC: ACOG, 1989.

Balogh SA, Cole LP. Contraceptive services for the postpartum and postabortion woman. In Sciarra JJ (ed): Gynecology and Obstetrics. Philadelphia: Lippincott–Raven, 1994;(6)15:1–11.

Chetterton RT Jr. Physiology of lactation and fertility regulation. In Sciarra JJ (ed): Gynecology and Obstetrics. Philadelphia: Lippincott–Raven, 1994;(6)35:1–9.

Lewis PR, Brown JB, Renfree MB, Short RV. The resumption of ovulation and menstruation in a well-nourished population of women breastfeeding for an extended period of time. Fertil Steril 1991;55:529.

McNeilly AS. Lactational amenorrhea. Endocrinol Metab Clin North Am 1993;22:59.

Rivera R, Kennedy KI, Ortiz E, et al. Breastfeeding and the return to ovulation in Durango, Mexico. Fertil Steril 1988;49:780.

Smith RP. Gynecology in Primary Care. Baltimore: Williams & Wilkins, 1997, p 405.

Speroff L, Glass RH, Kase NG. Clinical Gynecologic Endocrinology and Infertility, 5th ed. Baltimore: Williams & Wilkins, 1994, pp 401–456.

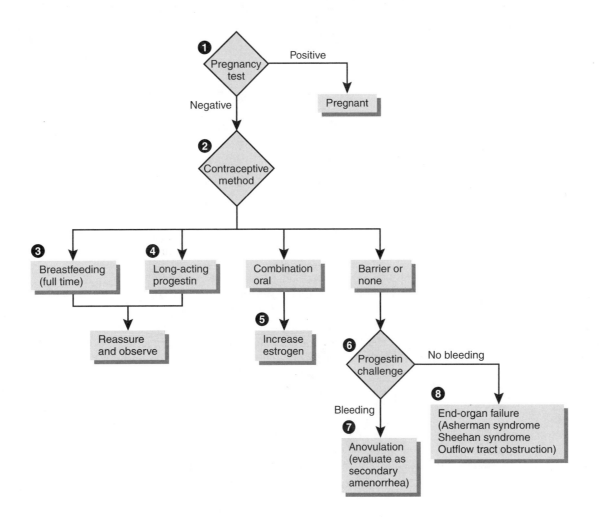

Amenorrhea

Primary: Chromosomal Analysis

INTRODUCTION

Primary amenorrhea is the absence of normal menstruation in a patient without previously established cycles. This diagnosis is generally applied when there are no periods by age 14 with no secondary sex changes, no periods by age 16 regardless of secondary sex changes, or no periods by 2 years after the start of secondary sex changes. The evaluation of primary amenorrhea may be based on developmental characteristics or the primary evaluation of chromosomes. Because roughly one third of patients with primary amenorrhea have a chromosomal abnormality, some authors suggest a different algorithm based on an initial assessment of chromatin.

❶ When the evaluation of primary amenorrhea is to be based on chromosomal analysis, it begins with a buccal smear to detect the presence of two X chromosomes as indicated by the presence of a Barr body. A buccal smear will be positive in genotypic females, but negative in females with only one X chromosome or in genotypic males. Results may be mixed when mosaicism is present. Because only about a third of patients with a mosaicism involving a Y chromosome will show signs of virilization, a chromosomal analysis should be considered even when the patient is phenotypically normal.

❷ When a Barr body is not detected, the presence of a Y chromosome must be sought by quinacrine mustard staining, immunologic detection of the H-Y antigen, or other method. If present, testicular feminization (androgen insensitivity syndrome), pure gonadal dysgenesis, or mosaicism (XX XY) may be responsible.

❸ When the buccal smear is negative and there is no Y chromosome present, gonadal dysgenesis or mosaicism (XO or XO XX) must be suspected.

❹ When the buccal smear shows the presence of a Barr body, a trial of progestin withdrawal can help to differentiate a large group of possible causes. This step presumes that a pelvic examination has been performed and no gross anomalies have been detected. It should be noted that in pure gonadal dysgenesis and XX/XY mosaicism, a uterus will be present.

❺ When no withdrawal bleeding occurs following the progestin challenge, a measurement of serum follicle stimulating hormone (FSH) should be performed. Elevation of the FSH is found in patients with gonadal dysgenesis or ovarian failure.

❻ When the FSH is normal or low, hypogonadotropic hypogonadism or central nervous system tumor or trauma should be suspected.

❼ Progestin withdrawal is expected to cause bleeding in patients with congenital adrenogenital syndrome or feminizing ovarian tumor.

REFERENCES

American College of Obstetricians and Gynecologists. Amenorrhea. Technical Bulletin 128, Washington, DC: ACOG, 1989.

Smith RP. Gynecology in Primary Care. Baltimore: Williams & Wilkins, 1997, p 405.

Speroff L, Glass RH, Kase NG. Clinical Gynecologic Endocrinology and Infertility, 5th ed. Baltimore: Williams & Wilkins, 1994, pp 401–456.

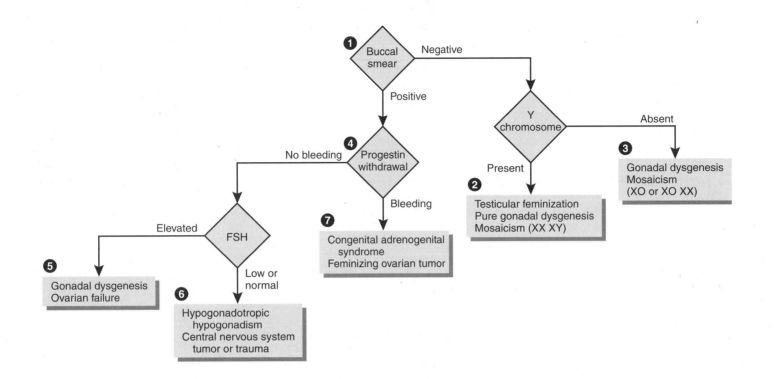

Amenorrhea

Primary: Developmental Analysis

INTRODUCTION

Primary amenorrhea is the absence of normal menstruation in a patient without previously established cycles. This diagnosis is generally applied when there are no periods by age 14 with no secondary sex changes, no periods by age 16 regardless of secondary sex changes, or no periods by 2 years after the start of secondary sex changes. The evaluation of primary amenorrhea may be based on developmental characteristics or the primary evaluation of chromosomes. Menstruation and fertility may be restored for many of these patients if there are no structural or chromosomal conditions that preclude the possibility (uterine agenesis, androgen insensitivity syndrome, gonadal dysgenesis).

❶ When the evaluation of primary amenorrhea is to be based on developmental milestones, the assessment begins with breast development. Breast development requires and documents the presence of estrogen. (It is presumed that a pregnancy test has been performed and is negative.)

❷ If breast development is not documented, the presence of a uterus must be determined. In most cases, this may be accomplished by simple pelvic or rectal examination. This can also identify outflow tract anomalies such as an imperforate hymen. When greater uncertainty exists, pelvic ultrasonography or even laparoscopy may be required.

❸ If there is no breast development and the uterus appears to be absent, a karyotype must be per-

formed. If the karyotype shows the patient to be 46 XX then congenital absence of the uterus or agonadism must be suspected. If the karyotype shows the patient to be 46 XY, an enzyme deficiency (e.g., 17 α-hydroxylase deficiency) or agonadism may be the cause. These conditions are rarely encountered in clinical practice.

❹ If there is no breast development and the uterus appears to be present, measurement of serum follicle stimulating hormone (FSH) should be made. This is elevated in patients with gonadal dysgenisis (in its many forms) and normal in patients with hypogonadotropic hypogonadism. This latter group includes patients with normal constitutional delays.

❺ When breast development is exhibited, the production of estrogen may be presumed but the presence of a uterus must still be determined. In most cases, this may be accomplished by simple pelvic or rectal examination. This can also identify outflow tract anomalies such as an imperforate hymen. When greater uncertainty exists, pelvic ultrasonography or even laparoscopy may be required.

❻ If a uterus appears to be absent, measurement of serum testosterone may establish the diagnosis. Testosterone levels will be normal in patients with congenital absence of the uterus but elevated in patients with androgen insensitivity syndrome.

❼ The most common clinical presentation is the patient with partial breast development and a uterus.

The next step for these patients is the measurement of serum prolactin (PRL) levels. If these are elevated, computed tomography or magnetic resonance imaging of the pituitary and surrounding tissues must be performed.

❽ If the serum prolactin levels are normal, a progestin challenge (withdrawal) should be the next step. This can confirm the presence of a normal, responsive outflow tract.

❾ If bleeding is produced, measurement of serum luteinizing hormone (LH) can differentiate between patients with hypothalamic dysfunction (normal levels) and patients with polycystic ovarian disease (elevated levels).

❿ Failure of progestins to cause withdrawal bleeding suggests ovarian or hypothalamic failure. These may be distinguished by elevated levels of FSH in patients with ovarian failure and normal or low levels in patients with hypothalamic or pituitary dysfunction.

REFERENCES

American College of Obstetricians and Gynecologists. Amenorrhea. Technical Bulletin 128, Washington, DC: ACOG, 1989.

Smith RP. Gynecology in Primary Care. Baltimore: Williams & Wilkins, 1997, p 405.

Speroff L, Glass RH, Kase NG. Clinical Gynecologic Endocrinology and Infertility, 5th ed. Baltimore: Williams & Wilkins, 1994, pp 401–456.

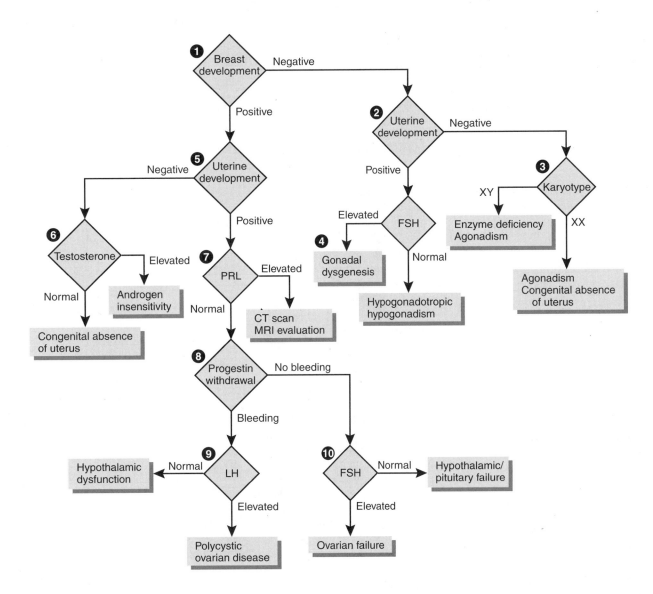

Amenorrhea

Secondary

INTRODUCTION

Secondary amenorrhea is the absence of normal menstruation in a patient with previously established cycles. It may be due to physiologic or pathologic causes and deserves prompt investigation and treatment where indicated. In many cases, secondary amenorrhea may be associated with symptoms that suggest the cause. Treatment is aimed at restoring or inducing ovulation if pregnancy is desired.

❶ The first step in the evaluation of any patient with secondary amenorrhea is a serum or urinary pregnancy test. Pregnancy (intended or otherwise) is the most common cause of secondary amenorrhea outside of menopause. Not only will a pregnancy test potentially render a diagnosis, it will protect the pregnancy from risks associated with other tests.

❷ When the pregnancy test is negative, a progestin withdrawal test should be performed. To be valid, sufficient progestin for a sufficient duration is required. This may take many forms but a common regimen is medroxyprogesterone acetate given at a dose of 10 mg/day for 10 days.

❸ If withdrawal bleeding occurs, the presumptive diagnosis of anovulation may be made. This diagnosis, however, dose not establish the cause of ovulatory failure and further evaluation is indicated.

❹ When withdrawal bleeding is not produced following a progestin challenge, a review of the patient's history is necessary to determine the next step. If the patient has had a dilatation and curettage, an infected abortion, or postpartum curettage, uterine scarring (Asherman syndrome) must be considered. Adding estrogen and repeating the progestin challenge may clinically test this possibility. Withdrawal bleeding confirms the ability of the uterus and endometrium to react to hormonal stimulation. If the patient has no history to suggest these possibilities, anovulation may be presumed and the evaluation continued.

❺ If no bleeding is provoked by the combination of estrogen and progestin, uterine scarring or an outflow tract obstruction is probable. Physical examination and diagnostic hysteroscopy will establish the diagnosis.

❻ The patient with presumed anovulation should next have her serum prolactin (PRL) level, follicle stimulating hormone (FSH) level, and thyroid function tested. The results of these three tests will often establish the cause for the ovulatory failure.

❼ If the prolactin level is elevated, the possibility of a drug-induced rise should be considered. Drugs to consider are most often those that affect dopamine or serotonin. Other causes of elevated prolactin such as chest wall irritation (herpes zoster, nipple stimulation or disease, etc.), hypothyroidism, sarcoidosis, lupus erythematosis, cirrhosis, or hepatic disease should be considered. If a drug is suspected, withdrawal of the medication may result in the return of menses.

❽ If the FSH level is normal or low, or the prolactin level is high without obvious cause, computed tomography or magnetic resonance imaging of the pituitary and surrounding structures must be carried out to evaluate for the possibility of a mass lesion.

❾ Mass lesions or other abnormalities that may be identified through imaging and that are associated with amenorrhea include adenoma, craniopharyngioma, Sheehan syndrome, tuberculosis, sarcoid, and the empty sella syndrome.

❿ When no mass lesions or other abnormalities are identified through imaging, the possibilities of anorexia or nutritional deprivation, overtraining (athletes), psychological stress, or the effects of drugs or medications must be considered as causes for the amenorrhea.

⓫ An elevated FSH level suggests ovarian failure, but like the diagnosis of anovulation, does not identify the cause. Natural failure (menopause, premature or otherwise) is most common but the possibility of Savage syndrome (gonadotropin-resistant ovary syndrome), exposure to toxins (including alkylating chemotherapy), surgical damage, or autoimmune disease should be considered as well. Women who have ovarian failure below age 30 should have a karyotype performed.

⓬ Abnormalities of thyroid function, most notably hypothyroidism, may account for the loss of menstrual function. Correction of the underlying problem often results in the prompt return of periods and fertility.

REFERENCES

American College of Obstetricians and Gynecologists. Amenorrhea. Technical Bulletin 128, Washington, DC: ACOG, 1989.

Smith RP. Gynecology in Primary Care. Baltimore: Williams & Wilkins, 1997, p 405.

Speroff L, Glass RH, Kase NG. Clinical Gynecologic Endocrinology and Infertility, 5th ed. Baltimore: Williams & Wilkins, 1994, pp 401–456.

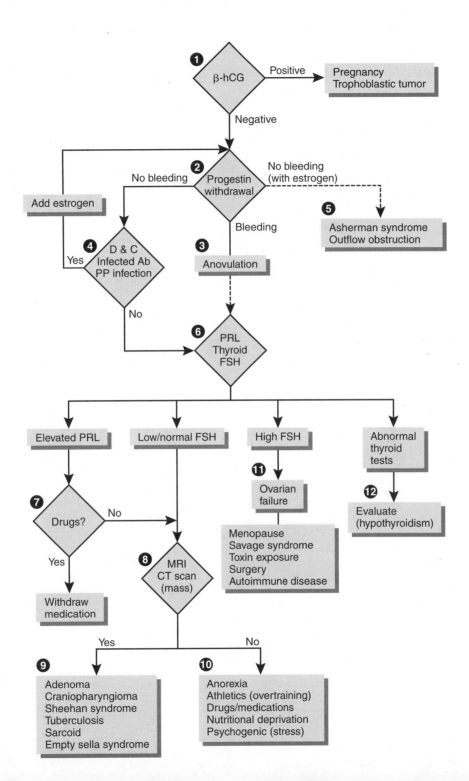

Anemia

INTRODUCTION

Because of continuing menstrual blood loss, women normally have a lower average hemoglobin than do men. When anemia occurs in women, it is most often due to menstrual loss, but this cannot be presumed until other causes have been considered.

❶ When anemia is present, measurement of mean corpuscular volume and reticulocyte count is appropriate. The mean corpuscular volume may be used to broadly separate possible causes.

❷ When the mean corpuscular volume is low, iron deficiency, disturbances in other minerals (copper or zinc), abnormalities of hemoglobin formation (thalassemia), and chronic disease must be considered. Serum iron studies, a peripheral blood smear, and hemoglobin electrophoresis will differentiate these possible causes.

❸ When the mean corpuscular volume is normal, hemorrhagic loss or hemolysis must be considered. Hemorrhagic losses may be subtle and include losses due to excessive amount, duration, or frequency of menstruation and losses via the gastrointestinal tract.

❹ Congenital causes for hemolytic anemias include thalassemia and sickle cell disease. Less common congenital metabolic diseases may also result in hemolytic anemias.

❺ Acquired processes such as artificial heart valves, chronic disease (hepatic or renal), drug use or abuse, immune diseases, and endocrine disease (adrenal or thyroid) may result in anemia with a normal MCV.

❻ Folate or B_{12} deficiencies, hepatic disease, and hypothyroidism may all result in an elevated mean corpuscular volume. These may be assessed by peripheral blood smear and the measurement of B_{12} and red blood cell folate levels.

REFERENCES

Millman RS, Ault KA. Hematology in Clinical Practice. A Guide to Diagnosis and Management. New York: McGraw–Hill, 1995.

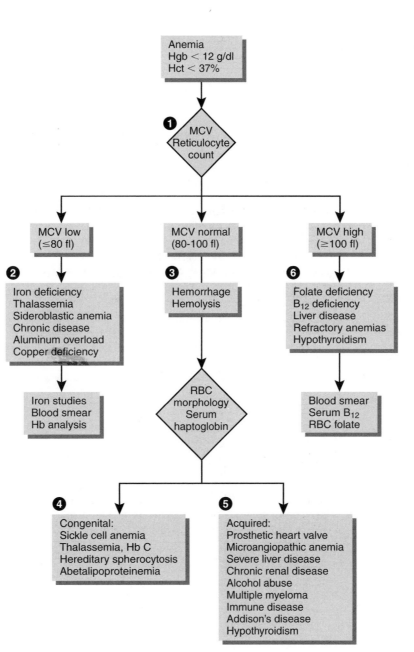

Anemia
Hgb < 12 g/dl
Hct < 37%

1 MCV
Reticulocyte
count

MCV low
(≤80 fl)

MCV normal
(80-100 fl)

MCV high
(≥100 fl)

2
Iron deficiency
Thalassemia
Sideroblastic anemia
Chronic disease
Aluminum overload
Copper deficiency

3
Hemorrhage
Hemolysis

6
Folate deficiency
B_{12} deficiency
Liver disease
Refractory anemias
Hypothyroidism

Iron studies
Blood smear
Hb analysis

RBC
morphology
Serum
haptoglobin

Blood smear
Serum B_{12}
RBC folate

4
Congenital:
Sickle cell anemia
Thalassemia, Hb C
Hereditary spherocytosis
Abetalipoproteinemia

5
Acquired:
Prosthetic heart valve
Microangiopathic anemia
Severe liver disease
Chronic renal disease
Alcohol abuse
Multiple myeloma
Immune disease
Addison's disease
Hypothyroidism

Anorectal and Rectovaginal Fistulae

INTRODUCTION

Rectovaginal fistulae most often are the result of obstetric trauma, while anorectal and perineal fistulae may be the result of underlying pathologies. Foul vaginal discharge, with marked vaginal and vulvar irritation, fecal incontinence, and soiling, along with the passage of fecal matter or gas from the vagina, are pathognomonic. Anorectal abscess results from infection of an anal gland in the intermuscular space. Roughly 50% of patients treated with external drainage of these abscesses will develop fistula-in-ano and require additional therapy.

❶ The location of the fistula can suggest both the cause and the most appropriate approach to treatment.

❷ Most patients with a rectovaginal fistula will have a history of episiotomy or obstetric trauma. When that history is proximate to the onset of symptoms, additional evaluations for pathology are unnecessary.

❸ Stool softeners and observation should initially be used to treat rectovaginal fistulae that result from obstetric trauma. Some small fistulae will heal spontaneously. In cases of recurrent fistulae, fecal diversion by colostomy may be required. Once adequate time has elapsed to allow inflammation to resolve, surgical treatment is appropriate.

❹ Fistulae that are not associated with vaginal delivery may result from surgical trauma, irradiation, or malignancy. Rarely, a pelvic or perirectal abscess may spontaneously drain, resulting in a fistula, but these more frequently drain into the rectum and do not result in fistula formation. Physical examination, anoscopy, sigmoidoscopy, and pelvic imaging through computed tomography, ultrasonography, or magnetic resonance imaging should be brought to bear to identify complicating or causal pathology. A combined abdominal and perineal or vaginal approach to surgical correction may be required.

❺ Inersphincteric (or high intermuscular) abscesses or fistulae may be difficult to diagnose. These patients have dull pain that is made worse with defecation. Physical examination can be normal. An examination under anesthesia may be required to establish the diagnosis and determine the optimal approach to repair.

❻ Fistulae that communicate with the perineum or perianal area may have rectal openings that are difficult to identify. Goodsall's rule states: When the external opening lies anterior to the midtransverse plane, the internal opening is located radially; when the external opening lies posterior to the plane, the internal opening will be found in the posterior midline. Anterior external openings that are greater than 3 cm from the anal verge usually have their internal openings located in the posterior midline.

❼ When anoscopic and proctoscopic examinations are normal, simple unroofing of the fistulous tract is generally curative.

❽ Anoscopic and proctoscopic examinations are directed toward identifying possible causative pathologies. Thirty-five percent of patients with Crohn's disease will develop perineal fistulas. In up to 10% of these patients, the first indication of disease may be the development of the fistula. When the disease is inactive or mild, simple fistulectomy may be curative. Unfortunately, for some patients colectomy or proctectomy may be required.

REFERENCES

American College of Obstetricians and Gynecologists. Genitourinary Fistulas. ACOG Technical Bulletin 83. Washington, DC: ACOG, 1985.

Bassford T. Treatment of common anorectal disorders (review). Am Fam Phys 1992;45(4):1787–1794.

Hancock BD. ABC of colorectal diseases. Anal fissures and fistulas (review). BMJ 1992;304(6831):904–907.

Smith RP, Ling FW. Procedures in Women's Health Care. Baltimore: Williams & Wilkins, 1997, pp 153–158, 163–166, 175–182, 201–203.

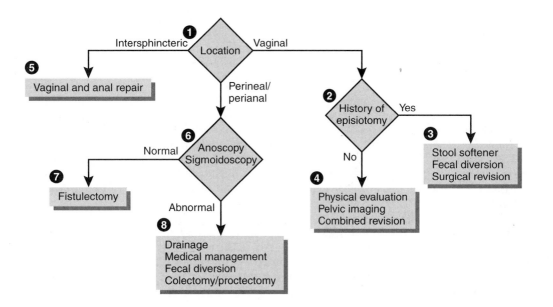

Assisted Reproduction

INTRODUCTION

Roughly 10% to 15% of infertile couples will require or benefit from assisted reproductive technologies. The treatment of an infertile couple is based on identifying the impediment to fertility and overcoming or bypassing it to achieve pregnancy. A number of techniques are available to accomplish this end. Most are less exotic than their acronyms would suggest. Among infertile couples seeking treatment, 85% to 90% can be treated with conventional medical and surgical procedures, and will not require assisted reproductive technologies such as in vitro fertilization. Success of treatment is dependent to a great extent on the identified cause of infertility, as some problems are more easily overcome than others.

❶ Methods of circumventing male-factor infertility are varied and are somewhat specialized in their application. Technologies such as intracellular sperm injection (ICSI) may allow fertility with as few as one sperm per oocyte. When low sperm counts are present, greater effectiveness may be made of those available through the use of the first portion of the ejaculate, coupled with artificial insemination. A slight improvement in success rates for subfertile men may be obtained by the use of washed and centrifuged samples that are then placed directly into the uterine cavity.

❷ When ovulation disorders are encountered, ovulation induction or control may be used to enhance the likelihood of pregnancy. The use of donor oocytes may be appropriate when complete ovarian failure or absence is present.

❸ Tubal-factor infertility may be addressed by either surgical repair of the damage or by bypassing the tubes completely through in vitro fertilization and embryo transfer (IVF/ET). Success rates for surgical repair, including the reversal of previous sterilization procedure, is highly variable.

❹ In a small number of patients, no specific cause of infertility will be evident. For these patients, in vitro fertilization, zygote intrafallopian transfer (ZIFT), or surrogate parenting should be considered. Adoption is always an option to be considered, though may couples view it as less desirable than biologic parenting.

REFERENCES

American College of Obstetricians and Gynecologists. Infertility. ACOG Technical Bulletin 125. Washington, DC: ACOG, 1989.

American College of Obstetricians and Gynecologists. New Reproductive Technologies. ACOG Technical Bulletin 140. Washington, DC: ACOG, 1990.

Office of Technology Assessment. Infertility: Medical and Social Choices. Washington, DC: Congress of the United States, 1988:25.

Smith RP. Gynecology in Primary Care. Baltimore: Williams & Wilkins, 1997, pp 339–358.

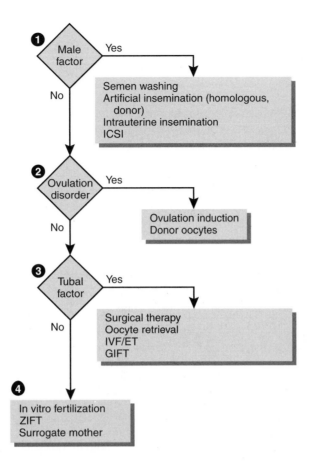

❶ Male factor — Yes → Semen washing
Artificial insemination (homologous, donor)
Intrauterine insemination
ICSI

No ↓

❷ Ovulation disorder — Yes → Ovulation induction
Donor oocytes

No ↓

❸ Tubal factor — Yes → Surgical therapy
Oocyte retrieval
IVF/ET
GIFT

No ↓

❹ In vitro fertilization
ZIFT
Surrogate mother

Bartholin Gland Cysts

INTRODUCTION

Approximately 2% of adult women develop infection or enlargement of one or both Bartholin glands. Because 85% of Bartholin gland infections occur during the reproductive years, any swelling or enlargement in women before menarche or after menopause must presumed to be of other origin until proven otherwise.

❶ The successful treatment of Bartholin gland cysts and abscess is predicated on establishing a correct diagnosis. Cystic masses that are located in the anterior portion of the vulva must be suspected to be Skene gland abscess or cysts. Occasionally, a suburethral cyst or urethral diverticulum may be sufficiently displaced laterally to be confused with a Skene duct process. These require specialized evaluation and care.

❷ Cystic masses that are located in the posterior portion of the vulva or perineum may be mucinous or inclusion cysts. These are most likely when there is an old scar, such as that from an episiotomy, present. These are generally asymptomatic. Unroofing the lesion or excision with careful closure will be curative.

❸ The amount of time mass has been present can differentiate between quiescent cysts and acute abscesses.

❹ Acute inflammation of the Bartholin gland duct can result in stenosis or chronic obstruction, leading to cyst formation. The resulting cysts are often small and asymptomatic.

❺ When Bartholin gland cysts remain asymptomatic and do not change over time, continued observation is warranted.

❻ Occasionally, even small stable Bartholin gland cysts may cause discomfort while sitting or insertional dyspareunia. When small (<1 to 2 cm), excision may be appropriate. Larger cysts are often best treated by surgical marsupialization.

❼ Acutely occurring Bartholin gland cysts should be suspected to be due to inflammation. Redness, surrounding edema, and exquisite tenderness are the hallmarks of infection and abscess formation. When symptoms are mild and the cyst small, symptomatic therapies such as sitz baths and analgesic may be sufficient. Warm to hot sitz baths provide relief and promote drainage. Spontaneous drainage will generally occur in 1 to 4 days. Many prefer to add systemic antibiosis as well. Broad-spectrum antibiotics such as ampicillin (500 mg po qid) should be considered if cellulitis is present.

❽ Simple drainage is associated with reoccurrence, therefore, placement of a Word catheter or packing with iodoform gauze, or surgical marsupialization of the gland, is desirable. Excision of the gland is often difficult and is associated with significant risk of morbidity, including intraoperative hemorrhage, hematoma formation, secondary infection, scar formation, and dyspareunia. For these reasons, excision is not generally recommended except for the smallest of cysts.

REFERENCES

Aghajanian A, Bernstein L, Grimes DA. Bartholin's duct abscess and cyst: a case-control study. South Med J 1994;87:26–29.

Cheetham DR. Bartholin's cyst: marsupialization or aspiration? Am J Obstet Gynecol 1985;152:569–570.

Smith RP. Gynecology in Primary Care. Baltimore: Williams & Wilkins, 1997, pp 603–632.

Wells EC. Simple operation of the vulva. In Sciarra JJ (ed): Gynecology and Obstetrics. Philadelphia: JB Lippincott, 1997;(1)11:6.

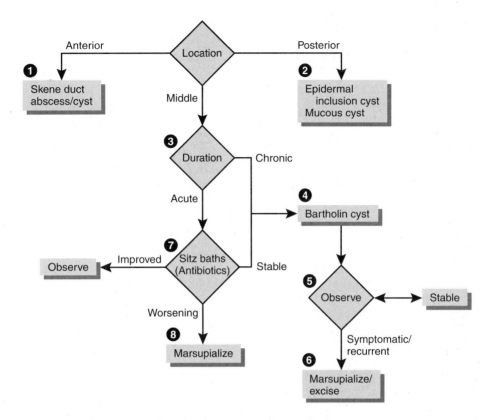

Bleeding in Pregnancy

INTRODUCTION

The failure of an early pregnancy is often signaled by abdominal cramping and vaginal bleeding. A more dangerous cause of vaginal bleeding is the ectopic implantation of the pregnancy. Failure to diagnosis an ectopic pregnancy in a timely manner can be associated with significant risk, including death. The prognosis for the pregnancy itself is almost uniformly bad. Ectopic implantation occurs in between 10 and 15 of every 1000 pregnancies, but varies with age, race, and location (highest in Jamaica and Vietnam).

❶ The first consideration in the evaluation of vaginal bleeding in early pregnancy is the establishment of a possible source. Bleeding that results from cervical or vaginal sources does not imply a risk to the pregnancy or an abnormality of implantation.

❷ When the bleeding can be established to be from the uterus and the cervical os is closed, the patient may be experiencing a threatened abortion, missed abortion, or ectopic pregnancy. Transvaginal ultrasound studies can be of great assistance in making the differentiation.

❸ When fetal parts can be seen inside the uterus, the diagnosis of threatened abortion is established and the patient may be managed as discussed separately.

❹ If fetal parts cannot be identified, it may be because either the pregnancy is not sufficiently advanced or there is an ectopic implantation. If the maternal serum beta-human chorionic gonadotropin (β-hCG) is greater than 3000 mIU/ml fetal parts should be identified; their absence strongly suggests an ectopic pregnancy. With improved ultrasonography equipment and increased operator skill, this threshold level may be reduced to 2500 mIU/ml. The combination of ultrasonography and sensitive measurements of serum β-hCG have generally replaced culdocentesis in the diagnosis of ectopic pregnancy.

❺ When serum β-hCG is below the threshold for ultrasound detection of the pregnancy, the quantitative serum β-hCG should be measured again in 48 to 72 hours. Failure of this level to double suggest a significant abnormality of pregnancy requiring further evaluation. The management of suspected ectopic pregnancy is discussed separately.

❻ When an appropriate rise in β-hCG is documented, follow-up ultrasound studies should be considered. In rare circumstances, an ectopic pregnancy may be associated with early, normal hormone rises.

REFERENCES

American College of Obstetricians and Gynecologists. Early Pregnancy Loss. ACOG Technical Bulletin 212. Washington, DC: ACOG, 1995.

Batzofin JH, Fielding WI, Friedman EA. Effect of vaginal bleeding in early pregnancy on outcome. Obstet Gynecol 1984;63:515.

Goldstein SR. Embryonic death in early pregnancy: a new look at the first trimester. Obstet Gynecol 84:294, 1994.

Mackenzie WE, Holmes DS, Newton JR. Spontaneous abortion rate in ultrasonographically viable pregnancies. Obstet Gynecol 1988;71:81.

Smith RP. Gynecology in Primary Care. Baltimore: Williams & Wilkins, 1997, p 99.

Warburton D, Fraser FC. Spontaneous abortion risks in man: data from reproductive histories collected in a medical genetics unit. Am J Hum Genet 1964;16:1–25.

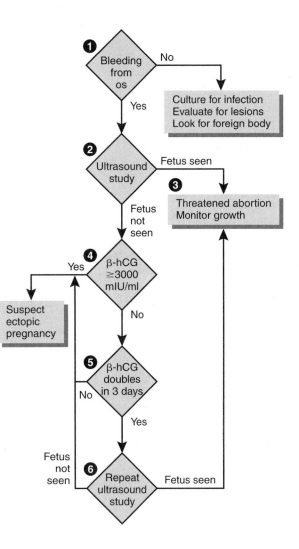

❶ Bleeding from os — No → Culture for infection / Evaluate for lesions / Look for foreign body

Yes ↓

❷ Ultrasound study — Fetus seen → **❸ Threatened abortion / Monitor growth**

Fetus not seen ↓

❹ β-hCG ≥3000 mIU/ml — Yes → Suspect ectopic pregnancy

No ↓

❺ β-hCG doubles in 3 days — No → (to β-hCG ≥3000)

Yes ↓

❻ Repeat ultrasound study — Fetus not seen / Fetus seen → Threatened abortion / Monitor growth

Breast

Cancer Screening Strategies

INTRODUCTION

Breast cancer is the most common malignancy of women, accounting for almost one third of all women's malignancies. With roughly 185,000 new cases per year, and approximately 46,000 breast cancer deaths per year in the United States, breast cancer is still the most common cause of death in women in their forties. Roughly one new case of breast cancer is diagnosed every 3 minutes and every 11 minutes there is a breast cancer death. Breast cancer accounts for approximately 18% of cancer deaths and results in about the same number of deaths per year as auto accidents. Widespread use of mammography has been credited with reducing the mortality rate of breast cancer by up to 30%.

❶ Screening for breast cancer may be based on patient concerns, symptoms, the presence of risk factors, or health maintenance principles.

❷ If imaging (mammography) has recently been performed and was negative, the diagnosis may be established based on the clinical examination, fine-needle aspiration, or other modality. When a recent study was abnormal (but not indicative of malignancy) histologic confirmation through core or open biopsy is almost always required.

❸ When screening is to be based on patient concerns or general health maintenance principles, the presence of risk factors (most notably a family history of a first-degree relative with breast cancer) modifies the normal recommendations.

❹ When risk factors are present, most recommend that annual screening begin 5 years before that age of the earliest occurrence of breast cancer in the family.

❺ It has been estimated that breast cancer mortality could be reduced by as much as one half if all women over the age of 40 were screened annually. Roughly 35% of breast cancers are found by an abnormal mammogram, without a palpable mass present. Mammography can identify small lesions (1 to 2 mm), calcifications, or other changes suspicious for malignancy roughly 2 years before a lesion is clinically palpable. Ten-year disease-free survival for these lesions is 90% to 95%. The average lesion found on breast self-examination is 2.5 cm, and half of these patients have nodal involvement. For these patients, 10-year survival falls to between 50% and 70%.

REFERENCES

American College of Obstetricians and Gynecologists. Carcinoma of the Breast. ACOG Technical Bulletin 158. Washington, DC: ACOG, 1991.

Butler JA, Vargas HI, Worthen N, Wilson SE. Accuracy of combined clinical-mammographic-cytologic diagnosis of dominant breast masses: a prospective study. Arch Surg 1990;125:893.

Fletcher SW, Black W, Harris R, et al. Report of the International Workshop on Screening for Breast Cancer. Bethesda, MD: National Cancer Institute, 1993.

Harris JR, Lippman ME, Veronesi U, Willett W. Breast cancer. New Engl J Med 1992;327:319–328, 390–398, 473–480.

Marchant DJ, Sutton SM. Use of mammography—United States 1990. MMWR 1990;39:621.

Medical News and Perspectives: Breast cancer screening guidelines agreed on by AMA, other medically related organizations. JAMA 1989;262:1155.

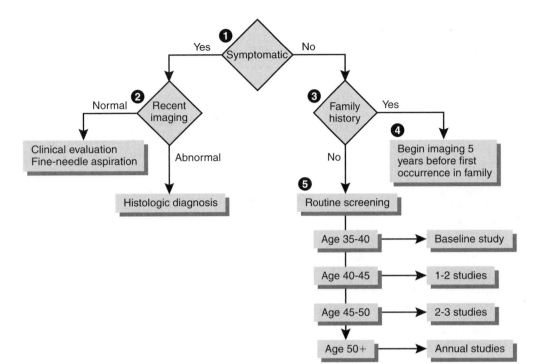

Breast

Management of Fibrocystic Breast Change

INTRODUCTION

Fibrocystic changes appear in three steps: proliferation of stroma produces the induration and tenderness experienced by these patients; marked proliferation of the ducts and alveolar cells occurs, adenosis ensues, and cysts are formed; and in the late stages, the cysts enlarge and pain generally decreases. Proliferative changes may be extensive (though usually benign) in any of the involved tissues. The cause, or causes, of fibrocystic change are unknown, but are postulated to arise from an exaggerated response to hormones.

1 Fibrocystic change is estimated to occur in one third to three quarters of all women. Fibrocystic change produces symptoms in roughly half of these women. While it is most common between ages 30 and 50 years, 10% of women under the age of 21 will have some degree of change. Effective treatment of fibrocystic change is difficult and is based mainly of the character and severity of symptoms experienced by the individual patient. When the patient experiences specific complaints, therapy may be governed by, and be specific for, those complaints.

2 When symptoms are acute, the underlying diagnosis must be carefully reconsidered because most patients with fibrocystic change experience some degree of manifestations on an almost continuous basis. These symptoms may wax and wane, often becoming worse around the time of menses, but there is often a baseline awareness present at all times.

3 Acute worsening of symptoms can often be treated with simple support, analgesics, and cold compresses or topical ice therapy.

4 As with the initial evaluation of symptoms, if specific complaints predominate, therapies targeted toward these characteristics may be formulated. Most often the difficulties encountered are more diffuse in both location and character. In general, therapies begin with simple interventions with few side effects and progress to more intense interventions with inherently greater expense and risk.

5 Firm support, such as a well-fitting brassiere worn day and night (with a specially designed sports bra when physical activity or sports are to be performed), analgesics, and reassurance provide the first line of therapy for most patients. For many, this will suffice.

6 Premenstrual restriction of salt or fluids and the reduction of caffeine and tobacco may provide relief for some patients. This is based on the proposed role of fluid storage and a suggested tie to methylxanthine intake.

7 Diuretics (such as spironolactone or hydrochlorothiazide given prior to periods) may be useful for some patients. Many lay publications advocate vitamin B_6 or E, iodine (kelp tablets), evening primrose oil, or diuretic teas for mastalgia or fibrocystic change. Most of these lack rigorous trials and in some cases, such as diuretic teas, many contain caffeine or other agents that may actually worsen symptoms.

8 Oral contraceptives or supplemental progestin use are all advocated and are successful in 50% to 70% of patients. If oral contraceptive therapy is chosen, a monophasic formulation is better tolerated than are the multiphasic types.

9 For patients with severe symptoms, danazol, bromocriptine, tamoxifen, or gonadotropin-releasing hormone (GnRH) agonists may be needed, but like the simpler modalities, success is not guaranteed and side effects with these agents are more significant.

10 Rarely, patients with intractable pain refractory to medical management require subcutaneous mastectomy.

REFERENCES

American College of Obstetricians and Gynecologists. Nonmalignant Conditions of the Breast. ACOG Technical Bulletin 156. Washington, DC: ACOG, 1991.

Boyle CA, Berkowitz GS, LiVolsi VA, et al. Caffeine consumption and fibrocystic breast disease: A case control epidemiologic study. J Natl Cancer Inst 1984;72:1015.

Donegan WL. Evaluation of a palpable breast mass. N Engl J Med 1992;327:937–942.

Ferguson CM, Powel RW. Breast masses in young women. Arch Surg 1989;124:1338–1341.

Seltzer MH, Skiles MS. Disease of the breast in young women. Surg Gynecol Obstet 1980;150:360.

Smith RP. Gynecology in Primary Care. Baltimore: Williams & Wilkins, 1997, pp 319–338.

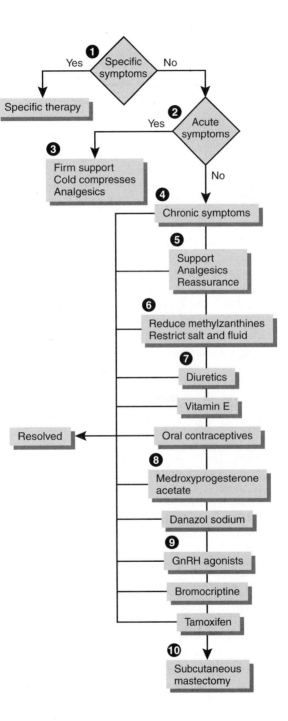

Breast

Mass

INTRODUCTION

Women with breast symptoms often exhibit justifiable anxiety out of a fear of breast cancer, increasing the urgency and significance of timely evaluation and treatment. Breast cancer is the most common female cancer and the leading cause of cancer death for women in their 40s. Roughly one in four women will require medical attention for some form of breast problem; often this takes the form of concerns over the presence of a palpable mass. Failure to diagnose breast cancer is one of the leading causes for an allegation of malpractice in the United States.

❶ The initial management of a palpable breast mass is based on the clinical impression. (Ultrasonography is useful in differentiating solid and cystic breast masses, but it has limited spacial resolution and is unable to differentiate benign and malignant tissues.) Masses that are cystic are less ominous than are solid masses, and the management strategies reflect this difference.

❷ When the mass is cystic in character, simple office aspiration of the mass using a 22-gauge needle and an appropriate syringe will generally provide both the diagnosis and needed therapy. Fluid aspirated from patients with fibrocystic change will customarily be straw colored. Fluid that is dark brown or green is found in cysts that have been present for a long time, but is equally innocuous. Bloody fluid requires further evaluation. Cytologic evaluation of the fluid obtained is of little value.

❸ Following aspiration of a cyst, the patient should be rechecked in 2 to 4 weeks. At this time the presence or absence of the cyst should be ascertained.

❹ If the cyst disappears completely, and does not reform by a 1-month follow-up examination, no further therapy is required. Some suggest mammography be performed to provide reassurance, and to look for occult or contralateral disease. This should be based on other clinical factors such as age and family history.

❺ If the mass fails to resolve or recurs, mammography should be performed to look for additional pathology in the same and opposite breasts before continuing to tissue diagnosis.

❻ For most patients in this group, tissue diagnosis should be established through excisional biopsy rather than fine-needle aspiration (FNA). If this establishes the presence of benign disease, routine follow-up may be scheduled. If a malignancy is present, the patient should be promptly referred for treatment.

❼ When a malignancy is clinically suspected many recommend that mammography be performed to document other occult lesions or lesions in the opposite breast before proceeding to plan diagnostic or therapeutic interventions. Diagnostic procedures such as FNA and incisional or excisional biopsies will all alter the architecture of the breast, making future mammography difficult or inaccurate. (Most radiologists suggest that a minimum of 1 month elapse before attempting mammography after FNA.)

❽ Despite clinical certainty of malignancy, a tissue diagnosis must be obtained. This may be obtained through FNA or incisional or excisional biopsies. The choice of technique will generally be driven by the size of the lesion, the experience and expertise of the clinician, and local custom. If FNA is chosen, it must be remembered that a negative or benign diagnosis is never sufficient to rule out a malignancy and must be followed by open biopsy. When FNA demonstrates malignancy, planning for definitive therapy may proceed.

❾ When the tissue diagnosis establishes benign disease, excisional biopsy is done to remove the mass (if not already performed). If mammography has not been performed, it should be considered as well.

❿ When a malignant tumor is present, a mammography to assist in planning and staging should be obtained (if not already performed). Prompt referral for definitive treatment is imperative.

REFERENCES

American College of Obstetricians and Gynecologists. Carcinoma of the Breast. ACOG Technical Bulletin 158. Washington, DC: ACOG, 1991.

Butler JA, Vargas HI, Worthen N, Wilson SE. Accuracy of combined clinical-mammographic-cytologic diagnosis of dominant breast masses: a prospecitve study. Arch Surg 1990;125:893–896.

Donegan WL. Evaluation of a palpable breast mass. N Engl J Med 1992;327:937–942.

Ferguson CM, Powel RW. Breast masses in young women. Arch Surg 1989;124:1338–1341.

Fletcher SW, Black W, Harris R, et al. Report of the International Workshop on Screening for Breast Cancer. Bethesda, MD: National Cancer Institute, 1993.

Harris JR, Lippman ME, Veronesi U, Willett W. Breast cancer. New Engl J Med 1992;327:319, 390, 473.

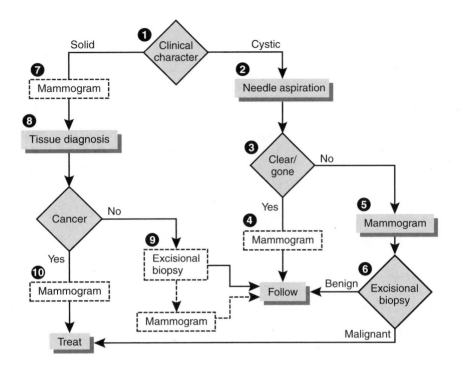

Breast

Mastitis and Abscess

INTRODUCTION

Mastitis is most common in nursing mothers 3 to 4 weeks after delivery. Infection comes from organisms carried in the nose and mouth of the nursing infant, most commonly *Staphylococcus aureus* and *Streptococcus* species. Pain, erythema, and fever mark the usual clinical presentation. Between 5% and 10% of patients will go on to abscess formation. Nonpregnant and postmenopausal women may also suffer from mastitis, accompanied by squamous metaplasia. This condition usually presents as a palpable, recurrent mass, accompanied by a multicolored discharge from the nipple or adjacent Montgomery follicle. When well established, ductal thickening may lead to nipple retraction.

❶ When the classic signs and symptoms of mastitis occur in a nursing mother, it is appropriate to make the empiric diagnosis of mastitis and proceed to formulation of a therapeutic plan. When mastitis is suspected in a non-nursing patient, other possibilities must be considered before the final diagnosis is established.

❷ The possibility of an abscess greatly modifies both the treatment and the risk of mastitis.

❸ Breast abscesses require prompt surgical drainage, usually under general anesthesia. Antibiotic therapy should be begun or maintained during and after surgical drainage. Close follow-up is indicated to evaluate the need for further surgical therapy.

❹ Patients with puerperal mastitis require aggressive antibiotic therapy with agents such as penicillin G or erythromycin (250–500 mg po qid, EES 400 po qid) for 10 days. First-generation oral cephalosporins (cephalexin 500 mg bid, cefaclor 250 mg tid) or amoxicillin/clavulanate (Augmentin, 250 mg tid) may also be used. Dicloxacillin may be required for penicillin-resistant strains or severe infections. Nursing or breast pumping should continue during therapy. If tenderness and fever do not respond promptly, abscess formation must be suspected.

REFERENCES

American College of Obstetricians and Gynecologists. Nonmalignant Conditions of the Breast. ACOG Technical Bulletin 156. Washington, DC: ACOG, 1991.

Brook L. Microbiology of non-puerperal breast abscesses. J Infect Dis 1988;157:377–379.

Seltzer MH, Skiles MS. Disease of the breast in young women. Surg Gynecol Obstet 1980;150:360.

Smith RP. Gynecology in Primary Care. Baltimore: Williams & Wilkins, 1997, p 319.

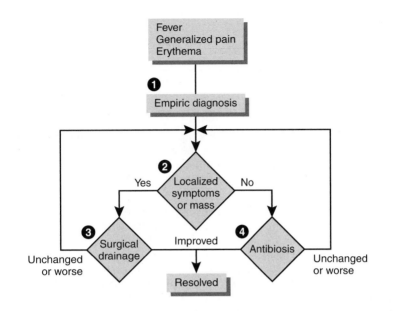

Breast

Nipple Discharge

INTRODUCTION

The evaluation of nipple discharge is based on the presence or absence of a palpable mass, the character of the discharge, and the presence of discharge from more than one duct.

❶ The causes of nipple discharge may quickly be segregated into those that cause bilateral secretions and those that are localized to one breast. This presumes that obvious causes such as cutaneous excoriation and acute mastitis have been excluded.

❷ The clinical character of bilateral discharge can often point to the underlying cause. Cytologic evaluation of the nipple discharge is associated with a false-negative rate of almost 20%, and is therefore of little value. When the fluid has a serous or milky appearance, a simple fat stain of the discharge will confirm the physiologic character of the discharge (milk). Purulent-appearing discharge should suggest an infection. Empiric therapy with antibiotics is often curative.

❸ When the fluid is serous or milky, a serum prolactin (PRL) level should be obtained. If this value is normal, physiologic causes (such as persistent nursing or nipple stimulation) are responsible and the patient may be reassured and followed. Elevated serum levels of PRL should be evaluated as discussed under Galactorrhea.

❹ Patients with unilateral nipple discharge should be carefully examined for the presence of an underlying mass. Care should be taken to examine the entire breast, including the areola and the contralateral breast.

❺ If a mass is present, many recommend that mammography be performed to document other occult lesions or lesions in the opposite breast before proceeding to plan diagnostic or therapeutic interventions. Diagnostic procedures such as fine-needle aspiration (FNA) and incisional or excisional biopsies will all alter the architecture of the breast, making future mammography difficult or inaccurate. (Most radiologists suggest that a minimum of 1 month elapse before attempting mammography after FNA.)

❻ A tissue diagnosis must be established prior to any treatment. This may be obtained through FNA or incisional or excisional biopsies. The choice of technique will generally be driven by the size of the lesion, the experience and expertise of the clinician, and local custom. If FNA is chosen, it must be remembered that a negative or benign diagnosis is never sufficient to rule out a malignancy and must be followed by open biopsy. When FNA demonstrates malignancy, planning for definitive therapy may proceed.

❼ When no gross lesion is found on clinical examination, mammography should be performed to look for occult or subclinical disease. If disease is found, a tissue diagnosis must be established

❽ If no lesions are seen on the mammographic studies, a careful examination to determine the exact source of the discharge must be done. If the discharge originates from more than one duct, a serum PRL level should be determined and the management carried out as outlined above (see No. 3).

❾ If the discharge arises from a single duct, duct radiography (ductogram) should be performed. The presence of mass will necessitate management as outlined above (see No. 6). If the radiograph is normal, reassurance and watchful waiting is appropriate.

REFERENCES

American College of Obstetricians and Gynecologists. Nonmalignant Conditions of the Breast. ACOG Technical Bulletin 156. Washington, DC: ACOG, 1991.

Devitt JE. Benign disorders of the breast in older women. Surg Gynecol Obstet 1986;162:340.

Isaacs JH. Other nipple discharge. Clin Obstet Gynecol 1994;37:898–902.

Seltzer MH, Skiles MS. Disease of the breast in young women. Surg Gynecol Obstet 1980;150:360.

Smith RP. Gynecology in Primary Care. Baltimore: Williams & Wilkins, 1997, pp. 319–338.

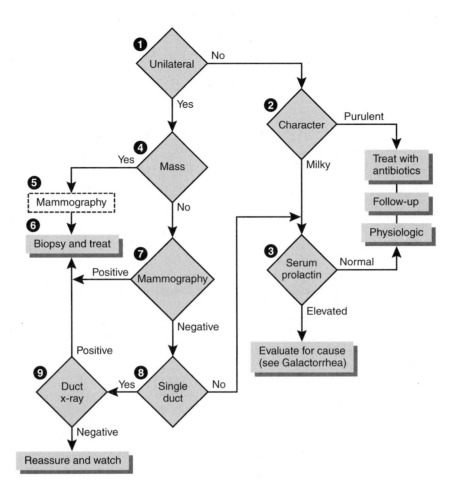

Breast

Pain (Mastalgia)

INTRODUCTION

Mastalgia (mastodynia) is the nonspecific term used for breast pain of any cause. Though patients are always concerned about the possibility, breast pain is a presenting complaint in less than 10% of patients with breast cancer. Mastalgia may be due to fibrocystic change, mastitis or breast abscess, trauma, or chest-wall abnormalities.

❶ The evaluation of breast pain begins with the simple dichotomy of symptoms that are unilateral and those that are bilateral. While some causes can account for either unilateral or bilateral symptoms, these are the exception rather than the rule.

❷ The presence or absence of evidence of inflammation should be evaluated. Inflammatory processes tend to be more acute in course and present a greater threat.

❸ Generalized unilateral pain, erythema over a portion of the breast (most often upper outer quadrant), and fever constitute the usual clinical presentation of mastitis (with or without abscess). When these signs are present in a nursing mother 3 to 4 weeks after delivery, empiric therapy should be begun immediately. Other sources include dorsal radiculitis and inflammatory changes in the costo-chondral junction (Tietze syndrome). Noncyclic pain is also common in sclerosing adenosis, chest-wall muscle spasms, costochondritis, neuritis, and referred pain, though these will generally lack signs of inflammation. Superficial inflammatory changes may be found in herpes zoster.

❹ When inflammation is absent and a mass is present, inflammatory carcinoma, trauma (with bruising, edema, and erythema) and galactocele should be considered. The evaluation of breast masses is discussed separately.

❺ When symptoms are bilateral, the presence or absence of nodularity can help to identify fibrocystic change. Fibrocystic changes most commonly present as cyclic, diffuse, bilateral pain and engorgement, with the worst symptoms occurring just prior to menses. The pain associated with fibrocystic change is diffuse, often with radiation to the shoulders or upper arms. On examination, scattered bilateral nodularity is typical. Well-localized breast pain may result from rapid expansion of a cyst, obstruction of a duct, trauma, or inflammation.

❻ When nodularity is not apparent the chest-wall causes must be ruled out before the nonspecific diagnosis of mastodynia is applied. The management of mastodynia is often similar to that of fibrocystic change (discussed separately).

REFERENCES

American College of Obstetricians and Gynecologists. Nonmalignant Conditions of the Breast. ACOG Technical Bulletin 156. Washington, DC: ACOG, 1991.

Boyle CA, Berkowitz GS, LiVolsi VA, et al. Caffeine consumption and fibrocystic breast disease: A case control epidemiologic study. J Natl Cancer Inst 1984;72:1015.

Ferguson CM, Powel RW. Breast masses in young women. Arch Surg 1989;124:1338–1341.

Seltzer MH, Skiles MS. Disease of the breast in young women. Surg Gynecol Obstet 1980;150:360.

Smith RP. Gynecology in Primary Care. Baltimore: Williams & Wilkins, 1997, p 319.

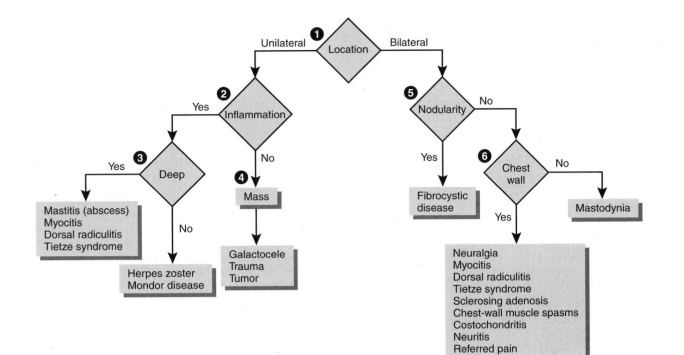

Mastitis (abscess)
Myocitis
Dorsal radiculitis
Tietze syndrome

Herpes zoster
Mondor disease

Galactocele
Trauma
Tumor

Fibrocystic
disease

Neuralgia
Myocitis
Dorsal radiculitis
Tietze syndrome
Sclerosing adenosis
Chest-wall muscle spasms
Costochondritis
Neuritis
Referred pain

Mastodynia

Cervical Cancer Staging

INTRODUCTION

The staging of cervical cancer is based on clinical findings and histologic confirmation. Chest roentgenography, intravenous pyelography, and computed tomography are used to assess extent of disease and to assign staging. Proper staging allows for the selection of the optimum therapeutic approach.

❶ Stage I cervical cancer is confined to the cervix (with any extension to the uterine body disregarded).

❷ When cervical carcinoma is clinically obvious, it is classified as stage IB. Therapy for this stage is generally hysterectomy (abdominal, vaginal, or radical), which is associated with a 78% 5-year survival rate.

❸ When cervical carcinoma is not clinically obvious, it is classified as stage IA. Stage IA is further subdivided based on histologic findings. When there is only minimal stromal invasion found on histologic examination, the stage is IA1. When there is invasion of greater than 5 mm or lateral spread of greater than 7 mm, the stage is IA2. Therapy for this stage is associated with a 90% 5-year survival rate.

❹ When cervical carcinoma has spread to the upper two thirds of the vagina or beyond the cervix, but not to the pelvic side wall, the stage is II.

❺ When parametrial invasion is absent, the stage is IIA. When parametrial involvement is present, the state is IIB. Stage II is treated by radical hysterectomy with lymph node disection or by radiation therapy. Therapy for this stage is associated with a 57% 5-year survival rate.

❻ When cervical cancer involves the lateral pelvic sidewall or the lower third of the vagina, it is classified as stage III. In stage III there is no cancer-free space evident on vaginal or rectal examination. Stage III disease is associated with only a 30% 5-year survival.

❼ If the extension of cervical cancer involves the lower third of the vagina but does not extend to full way to the sidewall, it is stage IIIA.

❽ If there is hydronephrosis present or extension of the cancer has resulted in a nonfunctional kidney, the cancer is stage IIIB.

❾ Stage IV cervical cancer has spread beyond the pelvis or has invaded the bladder or rectal mucosa. Stage IVA disease involves only adjacent organs, while stage IVB involves distant spread. Therapy for stage IV is palliative and 5-year survival is less than 10%.

REFERENCES

American College of Obstetricians and Gynecologists. Classification and Staging of Gynecologic Malignancies. ACOG Technical Bulletin 155. Washington, DC: ACOG, 1991.

Clement PB, Scully RE. Carcinoma of the cervix: Histologic types. Semin Oncol 1982;9:251.

Hacker NF, Berek JS, Lagasse LD. Carcinoma of the cervix associated with pregnancy. Obstet Gynecol 1982;59:735.

Leminen A, Paavonen J, Forss M, et al. Adenocarcinoma of the uterine cervix. Cancer 1990;65:53.

Weiss RS, Lucas WE. Adenocarcinoma of the cervix. Cancer 1986;57:1996.

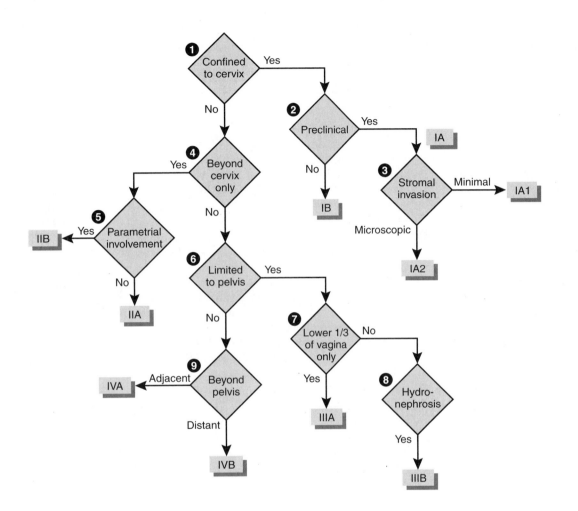

Cervical Cancer Treatment

Stage I

INTRODUCTION

Stage I cervical cancer (confined to the cervix, with any extension to the uterine body disregarded) can often be effectively treated while preserving fertility.

❶ The staging of cervical cancer is based on clinical findings and histologic confirmation. Chest roentgenography, intravenous pyelography, and computed tomography are used to assess extent of disease and to assign staging. Proper staging allows for the selection of the optimum therapeutic approach. (See Cervical Cancer Staging.)

❷ Stage IB cervical cancer must be treated in the same manner as stage IIA. As a result, those patients with clinically apparent disease (stage IIA) are considered separately.

❸ Stage IA disease is initially treated by cervical conization. This may be accomplished with a cold knife, electrosurgical device (loop electrosurgical excision procedure (LEEP)/large loop excision of the transformation zone (LLETZ)), or laser as long as a histologic specimen is available to assess the margins of resection and depth of invasion. When the margins of resection are involved, many oncologists recommend a radical hysterectomy with pelvic lymph node disection.

❹ Criteria for the diagnosis of microinvasion are not well formalized but generally involve the depth of invasion from the basement membrane, the pattern of invasion, and the presence of superficial invasion of vascular or lymphatic channels (vascular space invasion, VSI). Those patients with microscopic invasion (carcinoma in situ) are further managed based on depth. Those with early disease are managed conservatively with consideration of the patient's fertility plans.

❺ When the depth of invasion found on histologic specimen is 3 to 5 mm, or less than 3 mm with evidence of VSI, radical hysterectomy with pelvic lymph node disection is indicated. When invasion is less than 3 mm and there is no sign of vascular involvement, a simple hysterectomy may be considered.

❻ Patients with stage IA disease and only early signs of invasion who wish to preserve fertility may be followed by frequent Pap smears, while those who have completed their childbearing should be treated by simple hysterectomy. Ovarian preservation may be considered on an individual basis independent of the cervical cancer.

REFERENCES

American College of Obstetricians and Gynecologists. Classification and Staging of Gynecologic Malignancies. ACOG Technical Bulletin 155. Washington, DC: ACOG, 1991.

Clement PB, Scully RE. Carcinoma of the cervix: Histologic types. Semin Oncol 1982;9:251.

Hacker NF, Berek JS, Lagasse LD. Carcinoma of the cervix associated with pregnancy. Obstet Gynecol 1982;59:735.

Leminen A, Paavonen J, Forss M, et al. Adenocarcinoma of the uterine cervix. Cancer 1990;65:53.

Weiss RS, Lucas WE. Adenocarcinoma of the cervix. Cancer 1986;57:1996.

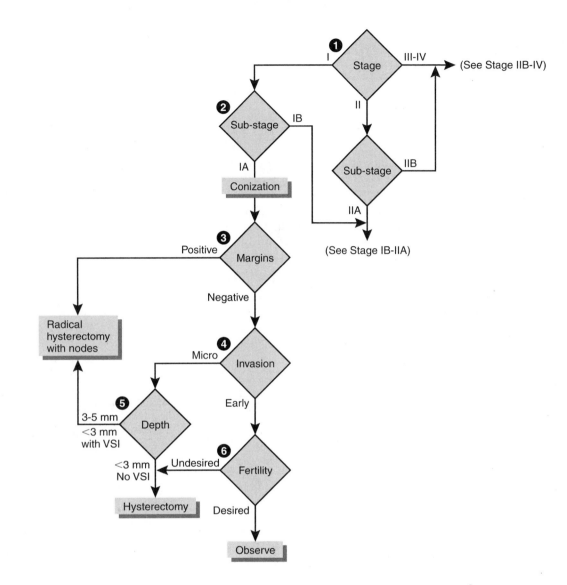

Cervical Cancer Treatment

Stages IB–IIA

INTRODUCTION

Stage IB and IIA cervical cancers are managed based on the size of the lesion and the presence or absence of nodal disease. Aggressive management can often be successful in controlling the malignancy.

❶ The staging of cervical cancer is based on clinical findings and histologic confirmation. Chest roentgenography, intravenous pyelography, and computed tomography are used to assess extent of disease and to assign staging. Proper staging allows for the selection of the optimum therapeutic approach. (See Cervical Cancer Staging.)

❷ Like stage I disease, the optimal treatment of stage II cervical cancer is based on the substage of disease present. Patients with parametrial involvement (stage IIB) are treated in the same way as patients with stage III and IV disease.

❸ When the lesion is greater than 4 mm in size, radiation therapy followed by radical hysterectomy and pelvic lymph node disection is the recommended course. Radiation therapy and surgery are complementary rather than competitive modalities, each improving the success of the other.

❹ Computed tomography, or more recently magnetic resonance imaging, is used to assess the pelvic and para-aortic lymph nodes in patients with lesions less than or equal to 4 mm in size.

❺ Patients thought to be free of nodal disease may be treated either by radiation therapy followed by close follow-up or by radical hysterectomy with disection of the pelvic and para-aortic lymph nodes. Success from these two modalities is similar, making the choice dependant on the availability of treatment resources and skills, the medical condition of the patient, and the patient's wishes. Both treatment modalities carry significant side effects.

❻ If surgical therapy is chosen, the histologic evaluation of the surgical specimen will determine the need for further therapy. If there are more than three positive lymph nodes, there is parametrial disease, the surgical margins contain disease, or there is macroscopic signs of nodal spread, pelvic radiation therapy is indicated.

❼ If nodal involvement is suspected on imaging studies, a staging laparotomy should be performed to accurately determine the extent of disease. Both radical hysterectomy followed by radiation therapy and pelvic radiation alone have been shown to be effective in these patients. The choice between these modalities is a matter of personal choice and the needs of the individual patient. Pelvic radiation therapy is generally provided as 180 rads per fraction given to a total of 4500 to 5000 rads.

REFERENCES

American College of Obstetricians and Gynecologists. Classification and Staging of Gynecologic Malignancies. ACOG Technical Bulletin 155. Washington, DC: ACOG, 1991.

Clement PB, Scully RE. Carcinoma of the cervix: Histologic types. Semin Oncol 1982;9:251.

Hacker NF, Berek JS, Lagasse LD. Carcinoma of the cervix associated with pregnancy. Obstet Gynecol 1982;59:735.

Leminen A, Paavonen J, Forss M, et al. Adenocarcinoma of the uterine cervix. Cancer 1990;65:53.

Weiss RS, Lucas WE. Adenocarcinoma of the cervix. Cancer 1986;57:1996.

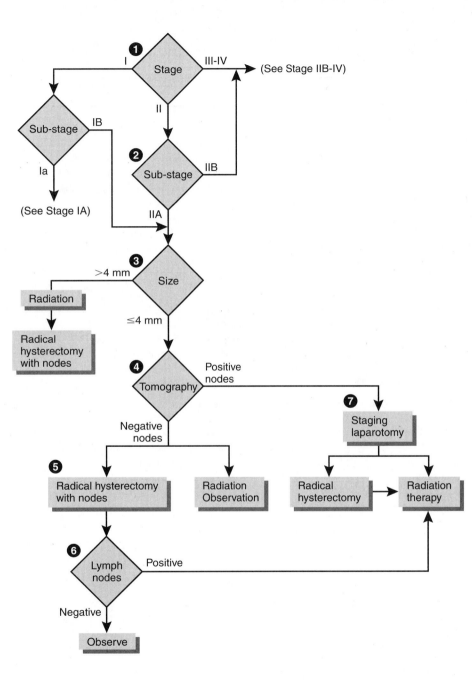

Cervical Cancer Treatment

Stages IIB–IV

INTRODUCTION

Advanced cervical cancer (stages IIB through IV) is most often managed by radiation therapy aimed at control of the disease, suppression, or palliation. In many cases, this may be supplemented by surgical management; in others it may be sufficient by itself.

❶ The staging of cervical cancer is based on clinical findings and histologic confirmation. Chest roentgenography, intravenous pyelography, and computed tomography are used to assess extent of disease and to assign staging. Proper staging allows for the selection of the optimum therapeutic approach. (See Cervical Cancer Staging.)

❷ Computed tomography, or more recently magnetic resonance imaging, is used to assess the pelvic and para-aortic lymph nodes in patients with advanced lesions. Patients not suspected of having nodal involvement are initially treated by pelvic radiation therapy.

❸ If the patient is suspected of having nodal involvement with her disease, a fine-needle biopsy of suspected nodes to confirm the diagnosis is indicated. This is often carried out under fluoroscopic control. If the biopsy does not find cancer, radiation therapy is the indicated therapy, while those with confirmed nodal involvement should receive a more extensive evaluation before the appropriate therapy can be determined.

❹ Patients with confirmed nodal disease must be assessed to determine the extent of disease spread. Scalene node biopsy is used for this purpose: Patients with cancer involvement in the scalene nodes have stage IVB disease and generally receive palliative radiation therapy based on their symptoms; those without scalene node involvement most often receive wide-field radiation therapy followed by a staging laparotomy.

❺ Patients without nodal involvement who receive radiation as their initial therapy should be evaluated after 2 months. Those with signs of recurrent or progressive disease must be restaged and surgically explored. Those who appear to have responded should undergo aortic node sampling (now often performed outside the peritoneal cavity by way of laparoscopy).

❻ If the aortic nodes sampled show no signs of involvement in the cancer, close follow-up with no further therapy is appropriate. If there are signs of nodal spread of the disease, a biopsy of the scalene nodes is used to assess distant spread. Often tomography of the chest is use to augment this evaluation.

REFERENCES

American College of Obstetricians and Gynecologists. Classification and Staging of Gynecologic Malignancies. ACOG Technical Bulletin 155. Washington, DC: ACOG, 1991.

Clement PB, Scully RE. Carcinoma of the cervix: Histologic types. Semin Oncol 1982;9:251.

Hacker NF, Berek JS, Lagasse LD. Carcinoma of the cervix associated with pregnancy. Obstet Gynecol 1982;59:735.

Leminen A, Paavonen J, Forss M, et al. Adenocarcinoma of the uterine cervix. Cancer 1990;65:53.

Weiss RS, Lucas WE. Adenocarcinoma of the cervix. Cancer 1986;57:1996.

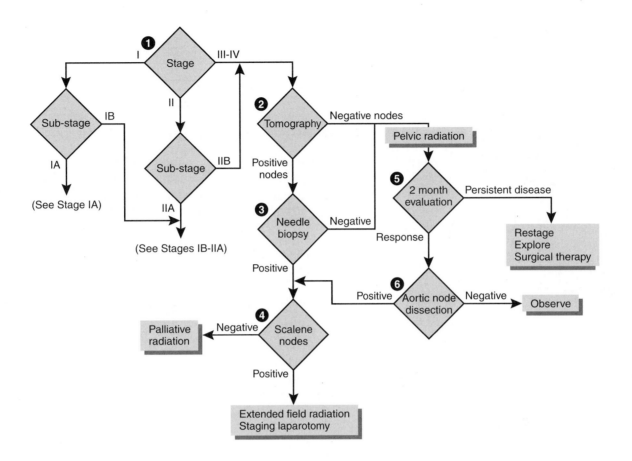

Cervical Eversion and Erosion

INTRODUCTION

The terms cervical eversion and erosion are often used interchangeably though they are actually very different in both etiology and significance: one represents a normal variant, the other a loss of the normal epithelial covering. Determining which is present is critical to determining the need for and direction of any treatment. Cervical eversion and erosion both present as red, roughened areas in or near the external cervical os. This must be differentiated from the friable changes associated with cervicitis. Unless frank infection is suspected, a Pap smear is appropriate although it may demonstrate inflammatory changes that result in a need to perform additional tests.

❶ The character of the lesion's border can help to differentiate these two entities. Smooth, regular borders are most typical of ectopy (cervical eversion).

❷ The character of the lesion's base is important as well. Ectopy (cervical eversion) most commonly has a red, velvety appearance while areas that have lost their overlying epithelial cover have a rough, raw appearance.

❸ Ectopy, or the outward migration of the squamocolumnar junction, may be physiologic or may occur in response to the effects of endogenous or exogenous estrogen (i.e., birth-control pills (BCPs), menarche, pregnancy). In utero exposure to diethylstilbestrol can also result in a turning outward of the junction.

❹ Processes that deprive the cervix of its normal epithelial surface can result in true erosion. Mechanical trauma, from tampon use, the string of an intrauterine device, a fingernail, or a sexual aid, may all result in the loss of a portion of epithelium. Infections such as herpesvirus and others can result in a similar loss. Other causes, including cervical cancer, are discussed separately under Cervical Lesions.

REFERENCES

Cain JM. Diagnosis and therapy of benign and preinvasive disease of the cervix. In Sciarra JJ (ed): Gynecology and Obstetrics. Philadelphia: JB Lippincott, 1997;(1)31:1.

Curry SL, Barclay DL. Benign disorders of the vulva and vagina. In DeCherney AH, Pernoll ML (eds): Current Obstetric & Gynecologic Diagnosis & Treatment, 8th ed. Norwalk, Connecticut: Appleton & Lange, 1994, p 689.

Droegemueller W. Benign gynecologic lesions. In Mishell DR, Stenchever MA, Droegemueller W, Herbst AL (eds): Comprehensive Gynecology, 3rd ed. St. Louis: CV Mosby, 1997, pp 479–483.

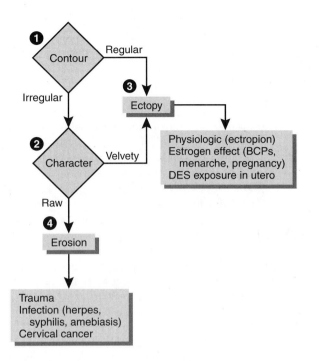

1 Contour

Regular

Irregular

3 Ectopy

Physiologic (ectropion)
Estrogen effect (BCPs,
    menarche, pregnancy)
DES exposure in utero

2 Character

Velvety

Raw

4 Erosion

Trauma
Infection (herpes,
    syphilis, amebiasis)
Cervical cancer

Cervical Lesions

INTRODUCTION

Inspection of the cervix is an important part of any pelvic examination and should always precede the performance of the Pap smear. Many of the lesions described in this algorithm should only be diagnosed by histologic evaluation of tissue obtained by biopsy. (The evaluation of cervical mass lesions is further discussed as a separate topic.)

❶ The character of the lesion seen can help to differentiate the cause. Lesions may be quickly classified as raised, flat, or depressed (punched out). Depressed lesions indicate the loss of surface epithelium. This may be a true loss (such as traumatic erosion) or an illusory loss (ectopy). Processes that undermine or destroy the surface layers, such as herpetic or syphilitic infections, may result in a depressed appearance of the surface. (Cervical ectopy and erosion are discussed separately.)

❷ Flat lesions of the cervix may be caused by human papillomavirus infection (condyloma) or by early hyperplastic or malignant changes in the surface epithelium.

❸ Raised cervical lesions may be present in several ways. The character of their contents may further classify those that appear to have a cystic nature.

❹ Clear cervical vesicles may be seen early in the course of herpetic infections. Inclusion cysts or nabothian cysts may also have a clear character to their appearance. Unusual conditions, such as pemphigus, may present in this manner.

❺ Inclusion or nabothian cysts may also have a bluish or opaque appearance. Cervical endometriosis will generally have an appearance that is similar to that seen with peritoneal implants, but may vary based on depth. Unusual conditions, such as cervicovaginitis emphysematosa, may present in this manner.

❻ Smooth, fleshy lesions are typical of endocervical polyps and prolapsing uterine fibroids that have not compromised their blood supply or become infected.

❼ Fungating, necrotic lesions must be suspected to be malignant, though cervical cancer may take many forms and appearances. Prolapsing polyps and fibroids may become infected and take on a malig-

nant appearance. Biopsy is always warranted to establish the diagnosis.

❽ Fungating, non-necrotic lesions may still be malignant in origin, making biopsy advisable. Prolapsing fibroids may have a fungating appearance before they become infected and take on a malignant appearance.

REFERENCES

Cain JM. Diagnosis and therapy of benign and preinvasive disease of the cervix. In Sciarra JJ (ed): Gynecology and Obstetrics. Philadelphia: JB Lippincott, 1997;(1)31:1.

Curry SL, Barclay DL. Benign disorders of the vulva and vagina. In DeCherney AH, Pernoll ML (eds): Current Obstetric & Gynecologic Diagnosis & Treatment, 8th ed. Norwalk, Connecticut: Appleton & Lange, 1994, p 689.

Droegemueller W. Benign gynecologic lesions. In Mishell DR, Stenchever MA, Droegemueller W, Herbst AL (eds): Comprehensive Gynecology, 3rd ed. St. Louis: CV Mosby, 1997, pp 479–483.

Goodman A, Hill EC. Premalignant and malignant disorders of the uterine cervix. In DeCherney AH, Pernoll ML (eds): Current Obstetric & Gynecologic Diagnosis & Treatment, 8th ed. Norwalk, Connecticut: Appleton & Lange, 1994, p 921.

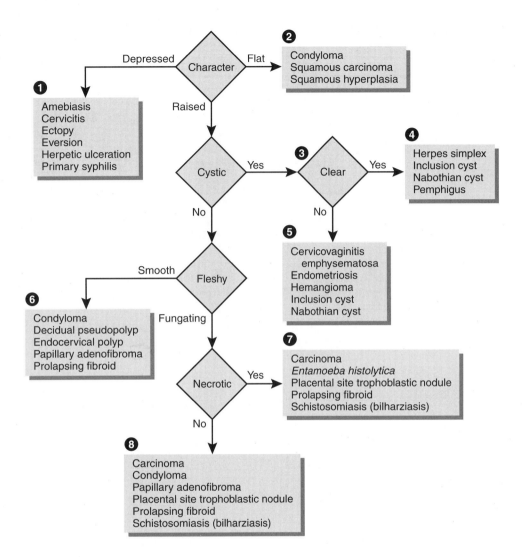

1
Amebiasis
Cervicitis
Ectopy
Eversion
Herpetic ulceration
Primary syphilis

Character
Depressed → (1)
Flat → (2)
Raised ↓

2
Condyloma
Squamous carcinoma
Squamous hyperplasia

Cystic
Yes → **Clear**
No ↓

Clear
Yes → (4)
No ↓

3

4
Herpes simplex
Inclusion cyst
Nabothian cyst
Pemphigus

5
Cervicovaginitis
  emphysematosa
Endometriosis
Hemangioma
Inclusion cyst
Nabothian cyst

Fleshy
Smooth → (6)
Fungating ↓

6
Condyloma
Decidual pseudopolyp
Endocervical polyp
Papillary adenofibroma
Prolapsing fibroid

7
Carcinoma
Entamoeba histolytica
Placental site trophoblastic nodule
Prolapsing fibroid
Schistosomiasis (bilharziasis)

Necrotic
Yes → (7)
No ↓

8
Carcinoma
Condyloma
Papillary adenofibroma
Placental site trophoblastic nodule
Prolapsing fibroid
Schistosomiasis (bilharziasis)

Cervical Mass

INTRODUCTION

Mass lesions found at the cervix may be of benign or malignant origin. The location and character of the mass may suggest a cause, but final diagnosis often rests on histologic examination of material obtained by biopsy.

❶ For small lesions, the site of origin may be apparent and can help to differentiate possible causes. Larger lesions may obscure their own origin. When this happens the lesion should be presumed to be of central origin. Those that appear to be eccentric in location are more likely to be cervical in origin. Cervical cancer, nabothian and inclusion cysts, hemangiomas, and infections (schistosomiasis or amebiasis) may all produce eccentric lesions.

❷ Masses, which appear to arise from the central portion of the cervix or the endocervical canal, should be inspected to determine the location of their base. Those that appear to be attached to the outer portion of the endocervical canal or the cervix itself often have a different cause than those that merely present at the cervical opening.

❸ Endocervical polyps and prolapsing uterine fibroids are the most common central masses that are found prolapsing through the external cervical os. Other, less common causes, such as papillary adenofibromas, and abnormalities of placental or decidual formation must also be considered.

❹ While cervical leiomyomas do occur, much more common sources of central, firmly attached mass lesions are the endocervical and cervical cancers. Obstruction of a cervical gland deep within the cervical stroma (nabothian cyst) may rarely mimic a central tumor. Biopsy is always appropriate.

REFERENCES

Duckman S, Suarez JR, Sese LQ. Giant cervical polyp. Am J Obstet Gynecol 1988;159:852.

Pradhan S, Chenoy R, O'Brien PMS. Dilatation and curettage in patients with cervical polyps: a retrospective analysis. Br J Obstet Gynaecol 1995;102:415.

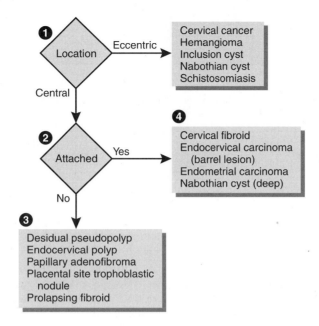

❶ Location
Eccentric →
- Cervical cancer
- Hemangioma
- Inclusion cyst
- Nabothian cyst
- Schistosomiasis

Central ↓

❷ Attached
Yes →

❹
- Cervical fibroid
- Endocervical carcinoma (barrel lesion)
- Endometrial carcinoma
- Nabothian cyst (deep)

No ↓

❸
- Desidual pseudopolyp
- Endocervical polyp
- Papillary adenofibroma
- Placental site trophoblastic nodule
- Prolapsing fibroid

Cervicitis

INTRODUCTION

Cervicitis is a common, though often undiagnosed, condition. Though technically always caused by infection, the true cause is often not clear; it may even result from cervical trauma, intrauterine contraceptive device or tampon use, or puerperal infection. Cervicitis is well recognized as a precursor of or risk factor for the development of pelvic inflammatory disease. Cervicitis may be diagnosed by finding mucopus (the presence of yellow or opaque endocervical mucus at the cervical os or present on a cervical swab) or by identifying 10 or more white blood cells per 400X power field of a Gram-stained smear.

❶ The cervical surface must be carefully cleared of vaginal material to properly see the presence of mucopus. When mucopus is present, a culture should be obtained immediately and treatment begun.

❷ *Chlamydia trachomatis* and *Neisseria gonorrhoeae* are the most common organisms causing cervicitis, and together they can be isolated in more than half of the women with the infection. Empiric treatment is appropriate any time mucopus is present and should be started before the results of the cervical culture are known. When chlamydia is found, doxycycline 100 mg po bid for 7 days, or azithromycin 1 g po (as a single dose) should be used. When gonorrhea is present, ceftriaxone 125 mg im, or a single dose of cefixime 400 mg po, ciprofloxacin 500 mg po, or ofloxacin 400 mg po, each combined with doxycycline 100 mg po bid for 7 days, may be used as effective treatment.

❸ Infection within columnar cervical epithelial cells often produces erythema, edema, and bleeding. When the cervix appears friable or bleeds easily upon wiping or while obtaining the cervical cytology specimen, cervicitis should be suspected and a culture taken. If the results of this culture are positive, therapy must be instituted.

❹ If the cervical culture is negative, empiric antibiotic treatment may still be appropriate based on the presence of risk factors. Uterine or vaginal infections, including herpesvirus, may also result in cervicitis. In the absence of these, direct treatment through cervicovaginal acidification or more aggressive therapies such as cautery and cryosurgery may be considered based on symptoms and the needs of the individual patient. (See also Cervical Eversion and Erosion, discussed separately.)

REFERENCES

American College of Obstetricians and Gynecologists. Antibiotics and Gynecologic Infections. ACOG Educational Bulletin 237. Washington, DC: ACOG, 1997.

Centers for Disease Control. Sexually transmitted diseases treatment guidelines. MMWR 42:56, 1993.

Curry SL, Barclay DL. Benign disorders of the vulva and vagina. In DeCherney AH, Pernoll ML (eds): Current Obstetric & Gynecologic Diagnosis & Treatment, 8th ed. Norwalk, Connecticut: Appleton & Lange, 1994, p 717.

Martin DH, Mroczkowski TF, Dalu ZA, et al. A controlled trial of a single dose of azithromycin for the treatment of chlamydial urethritis and cervicitis: the Azithromycin for Chlamydial Infections Study Group. N Engl J Med 1992;327:921–925.

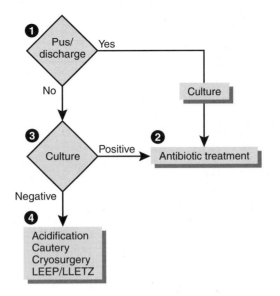

Clitoral Enlargement

INTRODUCTION

Enlargement of the clitoris is not only distressing, it may be the harbinger of significant endocrine disturbance or neoplasia.

❶ The causes of clitoromegaly differ according to the age of the patient. The differential diagnosis varies widely when the patient is a newborn, a youth, or a woman of reproductive age and beyond.

❷ Clitoromegaly at birth is most often caused by in utero exposure to androgens or androgenic substances. If progestational agents derived from testosterone (19-norprogestins) are given before 13 weeks of gestation, masculinization (with clitoral enlargement) may result. Agents such as danazol sodium given in doses of 800 mg/d during the first 10 to 12 weeks after conception have been reported to cause clitoral enlargement as well. The possibility of congenital adrenal hyperplasia must be considered because of the threat to life that it poses if the diagnosis is missed. Up to 60% of infants with a Y chromosome will show some degree of virilization.

❸ Clitoral enlargement that occurs in prepubertal girls may be due to late onset of 21-hydroxylase deficiency, exposure to exogenous anabolic or androgenic steroids, or, rarely, to tumors. The possibility of male pseudohermaphroditism should also be considered.

❹ When concern about enlargement of the clitoris exists, measurement of the clitoral index is useful. The clitoral index is defined as the vertical dimension times the horizontal dimension, in millimeters. The normal range is from 9 to 35 mm, with borderline values in the range of 36 to 99 mm. Values above 100 mm indicate severe hyperandrogenicity and should prompt aggressive evaluation and referral. Any time the diameter of the clitoris exceeds 12 mm it is considered abnormal. When the clitoral index is 35 mm or below, reassurance and observation are warranted.

❺ Clitoral indexes of 100 mm or greater are rare and almost invariably associated with markedly elevated levels of circulating testosterone (2 ng/ml or higher). These patients should be presumed to have an androgen-secreting tumor until proven otherwise. They should be evaluated in the same manner as a patient with frank virilization (discussed separately).

❻ When the clitoral index is in an intermediate range (36 to 99 mm) evidence for virilization should be sought. Hirsutism, acne, breast or voice changes, amenorrhea, and vaginal dryness should all suggest a markedly elevated level of androgens that should be aggressively evaluated.

❼ Patients with intermediate clitoral indexes and no other signs of virilization should be carefully questioned about the use of topical or systemic medications. Topically applied or ingested steroids, chronic irritation, or inflammation may all result in clitoral enlargement. When present, these factors should be re-evaluated and eliminated, if possible.

❽ Many processes can result in enlargement of the clitoris. Clitoral enlargement may be an early sign of ovarian hyperthecosis, polycystic ovary disease, or the presence of a luteoma of pregnancy. Late-onset 21-hydroxylase deficiency (LOHD) can result in symptoms of congenital adrenal hyperplasia occurring in the second or third decade of life. The incidence of LOHD varies with different races and populations and ranges from 0.1% to 3.7%. Cushing syndrome or adrenal tumors may present in much the same way. Neurofibromatosis and other forms of neoplasia, both primary and metastatic, should also be considered in the differential diagnosis.

REFERENCES

Rittmaster RS, Loriaux DL. Hirsuitism. Ann Intern Med 1987;106:95–107.

Tagitz GE, Kopher RA, Nagel TC, Okagaki T. The clitoral index: A bioassay of androgenic stimulation. Obstet Gyencol 1979;54:562–564.

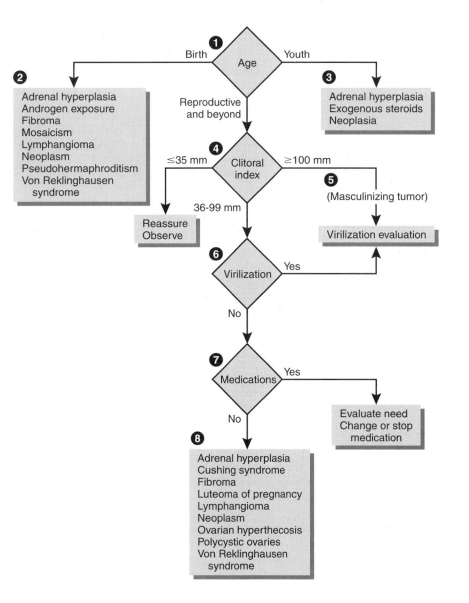

Contraception

Counseling Principles

INTRODUCTION

The choice of contraceptive methods can be daunting for some patients. Assisting them to choose the method or methods that are best for them is critical for effective contraception. Shown is one of many possible decision tree approaches to the choice of contraceptive methods. (Methods shown in gray have a relatively higher failure rate and should not be used if pregnancy prevention is a high priority.)

❶ One aspect of choosing contraceptive methods that must be considered is the couple's plans for future fertility. If the couple has decided that their family is complete (and have determined this with some degree of certainty) then a permanent method may be appropriate. When this decision has not been made or is equivocal, a temporary (reversible) method and should be used for as long as needed.

❷ If a permanent method is sought, the next decision to face the couple is which partner will have the procedure performed. This is most often a personal choice based on nonmedical factors. Female sterilization directly affects the person at risk for childbearing but is a major surgical procedure (the abdominal cavity is entered) and is associated with greater operative and postoperative risk. Male sterilization is routinely performed under local anesthesia and its efficacy may be verified easily (through follow-up semen analysis).

❸ If the decision is to use a reversible method of contraception, the next issue to address is who will be the responsible party; the man, the woman, or both.

❹ The list of male-driven contraception is limited to condoms and the poorly effective withdrawal method. When properly and consistently used, the male condom is associated with a failure rate of approximately 3% to 10%. Male condoms are used by approximately 15% to 20% of American couples.

❺ When both partners will share responsibility, abstinence (periodic or complete) or one of the various forms of natural family planning may be appropriate. To be effective, these methods require a high degree of motivation and regular, predictable menstrual cycles.

❻ When it will be the woman who takes responsibility, a useful method of separating the options available is by their dependence on use at the time of intercourse. Some methods (such a barriers and spermicides) require action at the time of intercourse, while others (such as hormonal methods and the intrauterine contraceptive device, IUCD) work independent of it.

❼ Female contraception that is based on actions at the time of intercourse include the barrier methods (diaphragm, vaginal condom), spermicides, and emergency contraceptive interventions. These latter options (discussed separately) are not generally recommended as a routine method of contraception, but patients should be aware of their existence and they should be readily available.

❽ Contraceptive interventions that occur outside the act of intercourse include the hormonal methods and the IUCD. Approximately 80% of American women of reproductive age are using, or have used, oral contraceptives (birth-control pills, BCPs), with approximately 25% to 35% of sexually active, fertile women using them at any given time. Roughly 5% of contraceptive users use a long-acting progestin as their contraceptive method (1% levonorgestrel rods, 4% depot medroxyprogesterone acetate). While only about 2% of women in United States use the IUCD, 60 million women worldwide use this method.

REFERENCES

American College of Obstetricians and Gynecologists. Managing the Anovulatory State: Hormonal Contraception. ACOG Technical Bulletin 198. Washington, DC: ACOG, 1994.

Castracane VD, Gimpel T, Goldzieher JW. When is it safe to switch from oral contraceptives to hormonal replacement therapy? Contraception 1995;52:371.

Grimes DA. Reversible contraception for the 1980s. JAMA 1986;255:69.

Smith RP. Gynecology in Primary Care. Baltimore: Williams & Wilkins, 1997, pp 209–236.

Speroff L, Darney PD. A Clinical Guide for Contraception, 2nd ed. Baltimore: Williams & Wilkins, 1996.

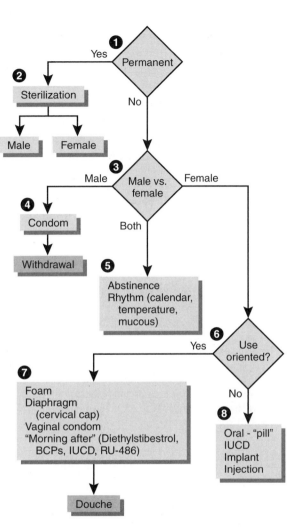

Contraception

Emergency Contraception

INTRODUCTION

To assist women who are at risk for unintended pregnancy because of contraceptive failure (e.g., condom rupture, displaced intrauterine contraceptive device (IUCD), or unprotected intercourse (e.g., unanticipated sexual activity, rape), emergency contraceptive options must be available. The patient must be warned not to have additional unprotected intercourse during the rest of the current cycle, as these techniques will not provide continuing contraception later in the cycle.

❶ The first step in counseling for the use of emergency contraception is the detection of an ongoing pregnancy. Because the situations under which this type of counseling must take place are stressful or even traumatic, the history about current contraception and even the possibility of an existing pregnancy may be unreliable. For this reason, a pregnancy test is always appropriate.

❷ If the sexual encounter was within 72 hours several hormonal therapies may be considered.

❸ Several hormonal therapies have been proposed and proven effective (as shown). The choice of method is often based on personal preference as all carry similar efficacy, though side effects are more common with some regimens (as shown). Efficacy is markedly reduced after 72 hours from exposure, or with multiple episodes of intercourse. Failure of hormonal interdiction is reported to be as low as 0.2 to 0.4 per 100 women treated.

❹ Insertion of a copper-bearing IUCD within 5 to 10 days after unprotected intercourse may offer some protection.

❺ If more than 10 days have elapsed since the act of unprotected intercourse, no interdiction is currently available. The anti-progesterone RU-486 holds promise as an effective "menstrual induction" agent. Studies from outside the United States show that this agent is safe and effective in inducing withdrawal bleeding ("menstruation") when taken at the time of anticipated menstruation or in the face of documented early pregnancy. The risk of pregnancy from a single act of unprotected intercourse is estimated to be approximately 7%.

REFERENCES

American College of Obstetricians and Gynecologists. Hormonal Contraception. ACOG Technical Bulletin 198. Washington, DC: ACOG, 1994.

Fasoli M, Parazzini F, Cecchetti G, et al. Post-coital contraception: an overview of published studies. Contraception 1989;39:459.

Glasier A, Thong KJ, Dewar M, et al. Mifepristone (RU486) compared with high-dose estrogen and progestogen for emergency popstcoital contraception. N Engl J Med 1992;327:1041.

Ho PC, Kwan MSW. A prospective randomized comparison of levonorgestrel with the Yuzpe regimen in post-coital contraception. Hum Reprod 1993;8:389.

Johnoson JH. Contraception: the morning after. Fam Plann Perspect 1984;16:266.

Speroff L, Darney PD. A Clinical Guide for Contraception. 2nd ed. Baltimore: Williams & Wilkins, 1996.

Van Santen MR, Haspels AA. A comparison of high-dose estrogens versus low-dose ethinylestradiol and norgestrel combination in postcoital interception: a study in 493 women. Fertil Steril 1985;43:206.

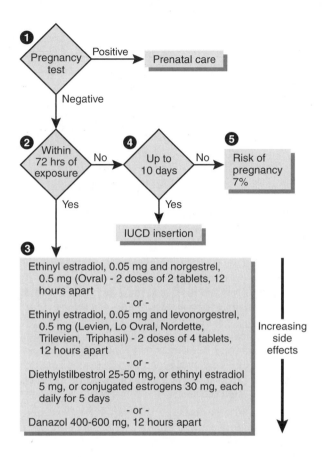

❶ Pregnancy test — Positive → Prenatal care

Negative

❷ Within 72 hrs of exposure — No → **❹** Up to 10 days — No → **❺** Risk of pregnancy 7%

Yes

Yes → IUCD insertion

❸

Ethinyl estradiol, 0.05 mg and norgestrel, 0.5 mg (Ovral) - 2 doses of 2 tablets, 12 hours apart

- or -

Ethinyl estradiol, 0.05 mg and levonorgestrel, 0.5 mg (Levien, Lo Ovral, Nordette, Trilevien, Triphasil) - 2 doses of 4 tablets, 12 hours apart

- or -

Diethylstilbestrol 25-50 mg, or ethinyl estradiol 5 mg, or conjugated estrogens 30 mg, each daily for 5 days

- or -

Danazol 400-600 mg, 12 hours apart

Increasing side effects

Cystocele / Urethrocele

INTRODUCTION

Loss of support for the anterior vagina, through rupture or attenuation of the pubovesical cervical fascia, can become manifest by descent or prolapse of the urethra (urethrocele) or bladder (cystocele). This loss of support may result in urinary, vaginal, or sexual symptoms or may be asymptomatic. Differentiating the source of the defect is vital to developing a treatment plan for those with symptoms.

❶ Often, the presumption of a cystocele or urethrocele is made based on symptoms of urinary incontinence. New-onset urinary incontinence should be presumed to be a urinary tract infection until proven otherwise. As a result, the evaluation of a patient suspected of having anterior vaginal wall support defects should begin with a urinalysis.

❷ If the urinalysis confirms infection, antibiotic therapy should be instituted. The diagnosis and treatment of urinary tract infections is discussed separately.

❸ Vaginal wall mobility is best demonstrated by having the patient strain or cough while observing the vaginal opening through the separated labia. When a urethrocele or cystocele is present, a downward movement and forward rotation of the vaginal wall toward the introitus will be demonstrated. When no mobility is demonstrated, other causes for the patient's symptoms must be considered. These might include detrusor instability, vaginal atrophy, or vulvar lesions.

❹ Careful inspection of the anterior vaginal wall should suggest the area of greatest mobility and loss of support. The use of gentle backward traction with a Sims speculum or the lower half of a Graves, Peterson, or other suitable speculum will facilitate visualizing the entire anterior vaginal wall while the patient strains.

❺ When only (or predominately) the apex of the vaginal wall appears to descend, the possibility of an anterior enterocele must be considered in addition to a simple cystocele. These are more common if the patient has had a hysterectomy, but can occur in any patient. Careful inspection and palpation may be sufficient to establish the diagnosis. This may be augmented by cystoscopy, which should be relatively normal (no distortion of the base of the bladder) when a cystocele is absent.

❻ When the outer third of the vagina prolapses, inspection for symmetry of the vaginal wall may suggest the presence of a Gartner's duct cyst or Skene's gland abnormality.

❼ If the distal third of the vagina appears to symmetrically protrude, a Q-tip test can differentiate between the loss of support for the urethra and midline distortions such as that found with urethral diverticula. To perform the test, a cotton-tipped applicator dipped in 2% lidocaine is placed in the urethra and anterior rotation with straining is measured. Rotation of greater than 30° is abnormal and confirms the loss of urethral support. Rotations of less than 30° may still suggest a urethrocele, but are generally not associated with symptoms.

❽ When the anterior vaginal wall defect appears to be concentrated in the mid-vagina or involves more than one area, a cystourethrocele is most likely. A Q-tip test may be performed, but is generally not necessary to make the diagnosis. Treatment of anterior vaginal wall prolapse should be based on the patient's overall need, the symptoms present, and the nature and extent of the defect. Therapeutic options include pessary support and surgical repair.

REFERENCES

American College of Obstetricians and Gynecologists. Pelvic Organ Prolapse. ACOG Technical Bulletin 214. Washington, DC: ACOG, 1995.

Federkiw DM, Sand PK, Retzky SS, Johnson DC. The cotton swab test. Receiver–operating characteristic curves. J Reprod Med 1995;40:42–46.

Kinn AC, Lindskog M. Estrogens and phenylpropanolamine in combination for stress urinary incontinence in postmenopausal women. Urology 1988;32:273–280.

Smith RP. Gynecology in Primary Care. Baltimore: Williams & Wilkins, 1997, p577–602.

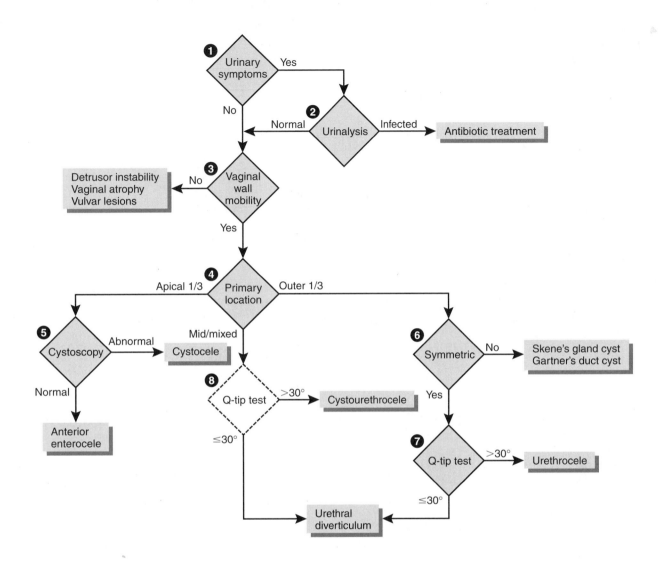

Depression (Unipolar)

INTRODUCTION

The management of depression is reasonably within the purview of the primary care setting. Indeed, the vast majority of antidepressant medications are prescribed by nonpsychiatrists.

There is roughly a 1 in 6 to 8 lifetime risk of developing a depressive disorder, and about 20 million Americans are affected each year. Depression affects twice as many women as men, making it an easily overlooked aspect of women's health care. It has been estimated that only 1 in 5 patients with depression are diagnosed and receive treatment. The diagnosis is established by a 2-week history of five or more of the following: depressed mood, loss of pleasure, weight loss, sleep changes, psychomotor changes, fatigue, feelings of worthlessness or guilt, inability to concentrate, or thoughts of death.

❶ On of the most important criteria in determining the appropriateness of the management of depression in the primary care setting is the presence of complications such as suicidal ideation or medical diseases that would complicate or interfere with therapy. When these are present, the patient should be referred to the care of a psychiatrist or other specialist with special training or experience in complicated cases.

❷ Once the decision to undertake the management of simple depression has been made, therapy should be instituted using a selective serotonin reuptake inhibitor (SSRI) or a serotonin norepinepherine reuptake inhibitor (SNRI). Other agents may be used as initial therapy, but these classes of medication have been associated with good success rates, minimal drug interactions, and tolerable side effect profiles. Once instituted, follow-up with the patient to look for side effects should occur in 1 to 2 weeks even though efficacy should not be evaluated until 6 weeks or longer into therapy.

❸ Because most of the commonly used antidepressant medications have a long half-life, effects will not be immediately apparent. As a result, after approximately 6 to 8 weeks of therapy the patient should be re-evaluated for efficacy.

❹ If the patient demonstrates good response to medical therapy (the most common situation), the current medication and dose should be continued and the patient rechecked in 6 more weeks (12 weeks of therapy). The patient should be maintained on therapy for a minimum of 4 to 6 months. When the decision is made to remove the patient from therapy, it should be withdrawn gradually and the patient observed for any recurrence of symptoms. Roughly 50% of patients diagnosed with a first episode of true depression will experience relapses. This number rises to 90% with three or more episodes.

❺ If the patient demonstrates fair response to medical therapy, the current medication may be continued and the dose adjusted. The patient should be rechecked in 6 more weeks (12 weeks of therapy) and the therapy modified or continued based on the response evident at that time.

❻ If inadequate response is demonstrated after 6 weeks of therapy, the patient should be changed to a drug from a different family or (in selected cases) or the original medication augmented with a second, complementary agent. These patients will need close follow-up and re-evaluation or referral.

REFERENCES

Association of Professors of Gynecology and Obstetrics. Depressive Disorders in Women: Diagnosis, Treatment, and Monitoring. Washington, DC: APGO, 1997.

American College of Obstetricians and Gynecologists. Depression in Women. ACOG Technical Bulletin 182. Washington, DC: ACOG, 1993.

Beck A. Depression Inventory. Philadelphia: Center for Cognitive Therapy, 1991.

McGrath E, Ketia GP, Strickland BR, Russo NF. Women and depression: risk factors and treatment issues. Washington, DC: American Psychological Association, 1990.

Notman MT. Depression in women. Psychoanalytic concepts. Psychiatr Clin North Am 1989;12:221–230.

Nurnberg HG. An overview of somatic treatments of psychotic depression during pregnancy and postpartum. Gen Hosp Psychiatry 1989;11:328.

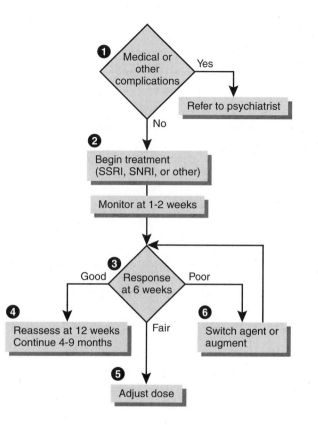

Dysmenorrhea

INTRODUCTION

The term "dysmenorrhea" literally means difficult flow. For 15% to 20% of reproductive-age women it means discomfort and time lost from school, home, and work on a regular basis. When a correct diagnosis is established, effective treatment with a high probability of success can be offered.

❶ The evaluation of patients with menstrual pain must begin with a careful history. A number of extragenital conditions can cause symptoms that occur or worsen at the time of menstruation, mimicking dysmenorrhea. Processes such as irritable bowel syndrome, myofascial and musculoskeletal disease, and somatization must be considered.

❷ A careful pelvic examination is carried out to identify the presence of pathologies associated with painful periods. Dysmenorrhea is classified by causation, not timing, and therefore the presence of a clinically identifiable process results in the diagnosis of secondary dysmenorrhea. Where no cause is clinically apparent, the diagnosis of primary dysmenorrhea is given.

❸ The treatment of patients with secondary dysmenorrhea generally begins with symptomatic treatment. This often takes the form of a nonsteroidal anti-inflammatory agent or other mild analgesic. These agents are given only at the time of menstrual flow and do not need to be started in advance of symptoms.

❹ Following the start of treatment, the patient should be reassessed after one to two cycles of therapy. If response is good, no change in treatment need be made. If the response is fair, a change in agent, the addition of a mild analgesic, or the modification of the menstrual periods themselves (with oral contraceptives, long-acting progestins, or gonadotropin-releasing hormone (GnRH) agonists) should be considered. When little response in evident, specific therapy for the underlying condition is required even though this may sometimes result in surgery (including hysterectomy).

❺ The mainstay of treatment for women with primary dysmenorrhea is nonsteroidal anti-inflammatory agents. These agents have the ability to block the synthesis, and in some cases the action, of prostaglandins (principally prostaglandin $F_{2\alpha}$).

❻ Following the start of treatment, the patient should be reassessed after one to two cycles of therapy. If response is good, no change in treatment need be made. If the response is fair, a change in strength or agent, the addition of a mild analgesic, or the modification of the menstrual periods themselves (with oral contraceptives, long-acting progestins, or GnRH agonists) should be considered. When the nonsteroidal agent is to be changed, a drug from a different chemical family is more likely to result in improved symtoms.

❼ Nonsteroidal anti-inflammatory agent therapy is so effective for patients with primary dysmenorrhea that if at least some improvement is not evident, the original diagnosis must be questioned. This should prompt a complete reassessment of the patient and may even prompt more invasive evaluations such as laparoscopy.

REFERENCES

American College of Obstetricians and Gynecologists. Dysmenorrhea. Technical Bulletin 68, Washington, DC: ACOG, 1983.

Dawood MY. Dysmenorrhea. Clin Obstet Gynecol 1990;33:168

Smith RP. Gynecology in Primary Care. Baltimore: Williams & Wilkins, 1997, p 389.

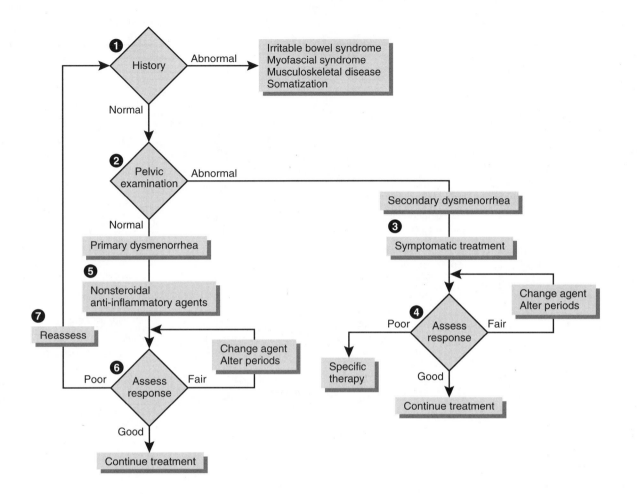

❶ History — Abnormal →
- Irritable bowel syndrome
- Myofascial syndrome
- Musculoskeletal disease
- Somatization

Normal ↓

❷ Pelvic examination — Abnormal → Secondary dysmenorrhea

Normal ↓

Primary dysmenorrhea

❸ Symptomatic treatment

❺ Nonsteroidal anti-inflammatory agents

❼ Reassess

Change agent / Alter periods

❻ Assess response
- Poor
- Fair → Change agent / Alter periods
- Good → Continue treatment

❹ Assess response
- Poor → Specific therapy
- Fair → Change agent / Alter periods
- Good → Continue treatment

Dyspareunia

Deep Thrust

INTRODUCTION

Deep-thrust dyspareunia is abdominal, pelvic, or vaginal pain that arises during sexual thrusting, especially with deep penetration. Roughly 15% of women experience deep pain with intercourse each year. Fortunately, in only 2% is the pain severe. Symptoms include an achelike pain, burning, a sense of fullness, or like something being bumped during deep sexual thrusting. Occasionally the pain is sharp and abrupt in character. The pain is often dependent on the type of sexual activity involved or the positions used. The pain experienced may either signal the presence of pathology or become a pathology in itself, resulting in sexual dysfunction and stress. In almost all cases, a diagnosis may be established, and effective therapeutic options offered.

❶ The evaluation of the patient with deep-thrust dyspareunia begins with a careful general and sexual history targeted to suggest the origin of the symptoms. This must include medical and emotional factors that may contribute to the symptoms present. Care must be taken to avoid labeling any dyspareunia as purely physical or only emotional in origin. Most often a mixture of factors will be present that cause or contribute to the problem.

❷ Pathology involving the urinary tract may result in pain during intercourse. Most represent chronic inflammatory processes, but acute infection may responsible for the abrupt onset of symptoms.

❸ A number of gastroenterologic conditions can present or be associated with pain during deep thrusting. A careful history will generally reveal symptoms that suggest the diagnosis.

❹ The possibility of musculoskeletal causes of pain during intercourse must not be overlooked. The physical activity associated with pelvic thrusting may easily uncover bone, joint, or neurologic pro-

cesses. Even such things as reduced range of hip motion may present in this way.

❺ When a gynecologic cause is suspected, a careful abdominal and pelvic examination is required. When seeking the cause of pain, it is not enough to identify portions of the examination that are uncomfortable, but the physician must ascertain whether the discomfort matches that experienced during intercourse.

❻ A pelvic mass such as uterine leiomyoma, ovarian mass, or endometriosis may be the source of discomfort when deep penetration occurs. Discomfort from these sources may be most noticeable in positions that result in direct impingement. Treatment ultimately centers around addressing the pathology present, though some improvement often results in modifying sexual positions to minimize the depth of penetration. Woman-astride positions allow the woman the most control of depth.

❼ Process that result in the loss of mobility of the pelvic organs can result in pain during deep penetration. Examples include the scarring caused by pelvic inflammatory disease (PID), endometriosis, or previous surgical procedures. Patients who have undergone radiation therapy in the past may experience scarring and fibrosis that result in painful intercourse.

❽ Pathologies of the vulva, vagina, and cervix may result in painful intercourse. Most processes that would result in deep-thrust pain will be readily diagnosed on careful pelvic examination. The sequellae of previous therapies such as shortening of the vagina following surgery or radiation therapy, or the presence of granulation tissue in a healing surgical wound may cause pain. When these examinations are normal, abnormalities of lubrication, muscle spasms (including vaginismus, dis-

cussed separately), or retroversion of the uterus may be responsible and are generally identifiable on examination.

❾ When the cause of dyspareunia is not apparent on physical examination, inquiry about the reproducibility of the symptoms should be explored. When the pain is produced only some sexual positions, the position involved may reveal a possible source: Pain during rear-entry positions suggests urethral or bladder pathologies; pain in male-superior positions is more typical of gastrointestinal, musculoskeletal, or gynecologic sources. Poor coital technique, abuse, and phobias must always be considered.

❿ Pain that is consistent and independent of positions with a normal pelvic examination should suggest conditions such as abuse (physical or sexual), depression, phobias, or vaginismus. A careful and sensitive exploration of these possibilities should be made. Some authors report rates of over 40% for intrapersonal causes and over 25% for interpersonal causes for coital pain.

REFERENCES

Fink P. Dyspareunia: current concepts. Med Asp Hum Sex 1972;6:28.

Fordney DS. Dyspareunia and vaginismus. Clin Obstet Gynecol 1978;21(1):205.

Fullerton W. Dyspareunia. Br Med J 1971;2:31.

Lamont JA. Female dyspareunia. Am J Obstet Gynecol 1980;136:282.

Steege JF. Dyspareunia and vaginismus. Clin Obstet Gynecol 1984;27(3):750–759.

Steege JF, Ling FW. Dyspareunia. A special type of chronic pelvic pain. Obstet Gynecol Clin North Am 1993;20(4):779–793.

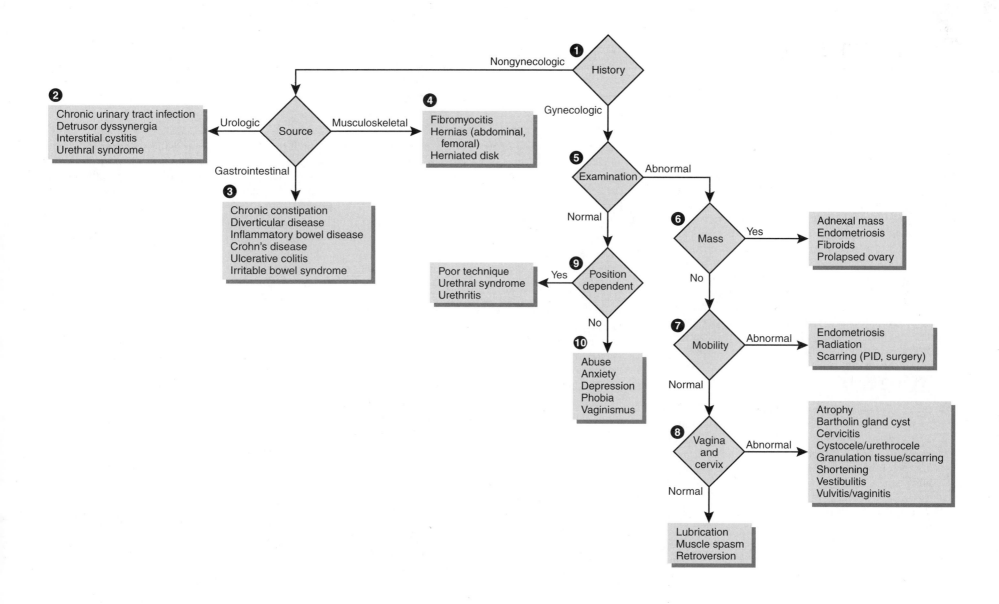

❶ History

Nongynecologic

❷
Chronic urinary tract infection
Detrusor dyssynergia
Interstitial cystitis
Urethral syndrome

Urologic — Source — Musculoskeletal

Gastrointestinal

❸
Chronic constipation
Diverticular disease
Inflammatory bowel disease
Crohn's disease
Ulcerative colitis
Irritable bowel syndrome

❹
Fibromyocitis
Hernias (abdominal, femoral)
Herniated disk

Gynecologic

❺ Examination

Abnormal

Normal

❻ Mass

Yes

❻
Adnexal mass
Endometriosis
Fibroids
Prolapsed ovary

No

❾ Position dependent

Yes

❾
Poor technique
Urethral syndrome
Urethritis

No

❿
Abuse
Anxiety
Depression
Phobia
Vaginismus

❼ Mobility

Abnormal

❼
Endometriosis
Radiation
Scarring (PID, surgery)

Normal

❽ Vagina and cervix

Abnormal

❽
Atrophy
Bartholin gland cyst
Cervicitis
Cystocele/urethrocele
Granulation tissue/scarring
Shortening
Vestibulitis
Vulvitis/vaginitis

Normal

Lubrication
Muscle spasm
Retroversion

91

Dyspareunia

Insertional

INTRODUCTION

Pain that occurs with sexual penetration is a symptom with a number of physical or psychological causes. The symptoms may be in the form of mild discomfort that may be tolerated, pain that completely prevents intromission, or anything in between. While the character may vary, the symptoms are generally attributed to the vaginal entrance or occur with initial penetration. Pain that is visceral or associated with deep thrusting is classified as deep-thrust dyspareunia (discussed separately). Dyspareunia is the most common self-reported sexual dysfunction encountered in office practice. It is estimated that virtually all women will experience discomfort with insertion on at least one occasion, but recurrent, distressing problems (true dyspareunia) occur in 4% to 40% of women, varying by age and study.

❶ When a patient reports sexual pain, it is important to determine the exact site of the pain, the duration and severity of symptoms, the frequency and circumstances of occurrence, and whether there were any precipitating factors. One method of differentiating some of the possible causes is to ascertain the reproducibility of the symptoms. Symptoms that are present only occasionally generally have a different source than when discomfort occurs with every attempt at coitus.

❷ Symptoms that are episodic and related to coital position suggest organic pathology and the position that creates the discomfort may even suggest the cause. Pain associated with rear-entry intromission may arise from urethral or urinary tract sources; pain during male-superior intercourse may be due to vulvar or rectal sources. Situational

pain that is unrelated to coital position may be caused by infection, poor lubrication or arousal, or prolonged sexual activity that exhausts the lubrication available. Poor coital technique must also be considered and explored.

❸ A careful examination may reveal the source of insertional pain. When no apparent pathology is present, a careful exploration of both psychological and physical factors must be made. Inadequate lubrication (due to inadequate arousal, phobia, or side effects of medications) and involuntary muscle spasms (vaginismus) are the most common causes. Studies indicate that up to 40% of cases have a functional or psychogenic cause. Urinary tract causes and infections of the Skene's glands may not be apparent on examination but should be sought.

❹ Abnormalities that may cause insertional discomfort may be found in the structures of the external genitalia, the vagina and vaginal opening, or the supporting and adjacent structures. Some pathologies may be manifested in more than one of these locations.

❺ Spasms in the supporting muscles of the vagina may be apparent during pelvic examination. Scarring from previous surgery, episiotomies, or cancer therapy may be present. Patients with significant gastrointestinal pathologies, such as inflammatory bowel disease, may have tenderness near the vaginal opening or along the outer portion of the posterior vaginal wall.

❻ Vulvar disease and a number of conditions that affect the vaginal vestibule may cause insertional pain. Many of these conditions will be apparent through the patient's history and are readily observ-

able during pelvic examination. Less obvious may be factors such as atrophy associated with breast-feeding. Vulvar pathologies may be further evaluated through colposcopic examination or biopsy.

❼ Vaginal atrophy, infection, or scarring from previous surgery are the most common sources of insertional pain that can be readily identified on pelvic examination. Examination must include the entire vaginal opening and barrel, and the quality of pelvic support should be evaluated. The presence of lesions in or just under the vaginal wall must be sought.

REFERENCES

Bachmann GA. Superficial dyspareunia and vestibulitis. In Sciarra JJ (ed): Gynecology and Obstetrics. Philadelphia: JB Lippincott, 1998;(1)77:1.

Fink P. Dyspareunia: current concepts. Med Asp Hum Sex 1972;6:28.

Fordney DS. Dyspareunia and vaginismus. Clin Obstet Gynecol 1978;21(1):205.

Friedrich EG, Jr. Vulvar vestibulitis syndrome. J Reprod Med 1987;32:110–114.

Fullerton W. Dyspareunia. Br Med J 1971;2:31.

Lamont JA. Dyspareunia and vaginismus. In Sciarra JJ (ed): Gynecology and Obstetrics, Philadelphia: JB Lippincott, 1998;(6)102:2.

Pecknam EM, Maki DG, Patterson JJ, et al. Focal vulvitis: a characteristic syndrome and cause of dyspareunia. Am J Obstet Gynecol 1986;154:855.

Steege JF. Dyspareunia and vaginismus. Clin Obstet Gynecol 1984;27(3):750.

Steege JF, Ling FW. Dyspareunia. A special type of chronic pelvic pain. Obstet Gynecol Clin North Am 1993;20(4):779.

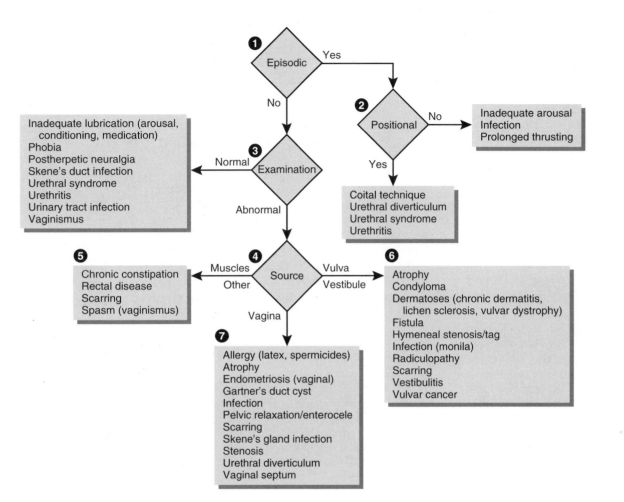

1 Episodic

Yes

No

2 Positional

No → Inadequate arousal
Infection
Prolonged thrusting

Yes

Coital technique
Urethral diverticulum
Urethral syndrome
Urethritis

3 Examination

Normal →
Inadequate lubrication (arousal,
   conditioning, medication)
Phobia
Postherpetic neuralgia
Skene's duct infection
Urethral syndrome
Urethritis
Urinary tract infection
Vaginismus

Abnormal

4 Source

Muscles / Other →
5
Chronic constipation
Rectal disease
Scarring
Spasm (vaginismus)

Vulva / Vestibule →
6
Atrophy
Condyloma
Dermatoses (chronic dermatitis,
   lichen sclerosis, vulvar dystrophy)
Fistula
Hymeneal stenosis/tag
Infection (monila)
Radiculopathy
Scarring
Vestibulitis
Vulvar cancer

Vagina

7
Allergy (latex, spermicides)
Atrophy
Endometriosis (vaginal)
Gartner's duct cyst
Infection
Pelvic relaxation/enterocele
Scarring
Skene's gland infection
Stenosis
Urethral diverticulum
Vaginal septum

Dysuria

INTRODUCTION

Painful urination is most often encountered in the context of acute urinary tract infections. This symptom is nonspecific and may arise from may sources. As with most symptoms, successful resolution of the symptom is tied to the identification of the underlying cause.

❶ Symptoms of discomfort or pain during voiding may stem from processes internal or external to the urinary tract. A careful history will often suggest whether the distress is experienced in the area of the vulva or more proximal in the structures above the meatus.

❷ Vulvar or vaginal pathologies may result in the sensations of burning or pain when the tissues are bathed in urine during voiding. This discomfort may be sufficient to result in urinary retention, as in the case of herpetic vulvitis. Vulvar atrophy that results from the loss of estrogen may be sufficient to lose the normal protective cornified layers, resulting in a burning sensation when the tissue is exposed to the mild acids of urine.

❸ An effective, but optional, method of screening for urinary tract infection is the microscopic examination of urinary sediments. To perform this, approximately 10 ml of clean-catch midstream urine is centrifuged for 30 to 60 seconds in a table-top centrifuge, the fluid decanted, and the resulting button of sediment resuspended in the liquid that remains. This is then placed on a microscope slide, covered with a cover slip, and examined under high power. The presence of more than 10 white blood cells per high-power field suggests the presence of an infection. If a significant number of squamous cells are present, vaginal contamination is presumed and the evaluation is inconclusive.

❹ A formal urinalysis should be performed on any patient with the complaint of dysuria. The use of leukocyte esterase dipsticks is associated with a false-negative rate of up to 25% and may give false-positive tests if the sample is contaminated by vaginal white blood cells. Similarly, nitrate dipsticks fail to detect infections in 10% to 30% of patients. If the urinalysis is positive, a culture and sensitivity should be performed on the sample, though therapy should not be delayed pending the results.

❺ If a urinary tract infection is suspected based on the results of a microscopic examination, urinalysis or other means, a culture and sensitivity should be performed. Uncomplicated patients with frank urinary tract infections may not require this step for an initial infection, but those patients generally will present with a different symptom pattern than isolated dysuria. Empiric antibiotic therapy should be started while the results of the culture are awaited. Once these results are available, the correctness of the diagnosis should be evaluated along with the choice of antibiotics. A test of cure is generally not required unless there have been frequent recurrences, the patient is at high risk, or sensitivity has been demonstrated on culture was marginal.

❻ Patients who have "internal" symptoms and do not have an obvious urinary tract infections should undergo a careful examination of the urethra. Infection of the Skene's ducts, urinary diverticula, foreign bodies, and other potential causes of dysuria may be evident during this evaluation. Diffuse tenderness along and adjacent to the urethra is typical of urethritis or Reiter or Stevens–Johnson syndromes.

❼ A culture of the urethra, if not already obtained, should be performed. The most common urethral infections to present with symptoms of dysuria are *Chlamydia trachomatis* and *Neisseria gonorrhoeae*. When infection is documented, appropriate antibiotic therapy should be started. Patients with urethral atrophy due to uncorrected hypoestrogenism, those with acute or recurrent urethral trauma ("honeymoon cystitis"), or those who use or abuse some medications (such as amphetamines) may experience dysuria in the absence of specific findings. A careful history will suggest these in most cases.

REFERENCES

American College of Obstetricians and Gyneologists. Antimicrobial Therapy for Obstetric Patients. ACOG Technical Bulletin 117. Washington, DC: ACOG, 1988.

Bump RC. Urinary tract infection in women. Current role of single-dose therapy. J Repro Med 1990;35:785.

Greenberg RN, Reilly PM, Luppen KL, et al. Randomized study of single-dose, three-day, and seven-day treatment of cystitis in women. J Infect Dis 1986;153:277.

Kim JH, Schaeffer AJ. Female Urinary Tract Infection. In Sciarra JJ (ed): Gynecology and Obstetrics. Philadelphia: JB Lippincott, 1993;(1)80:1.

Pappas P. Laboratory in the diagnosis and management of urinary tract infections. Med Clin North Am 1991;75:313–325.

Powers R. New directions in the diagnosis and therapy of urinary tract infections. Am J Obstet Gynecol 1991;164:1387–1389.

Smith RP. Gynecology in Primary Care. Baltimore: Williams & Wilkins, 1997, pp 577–602.

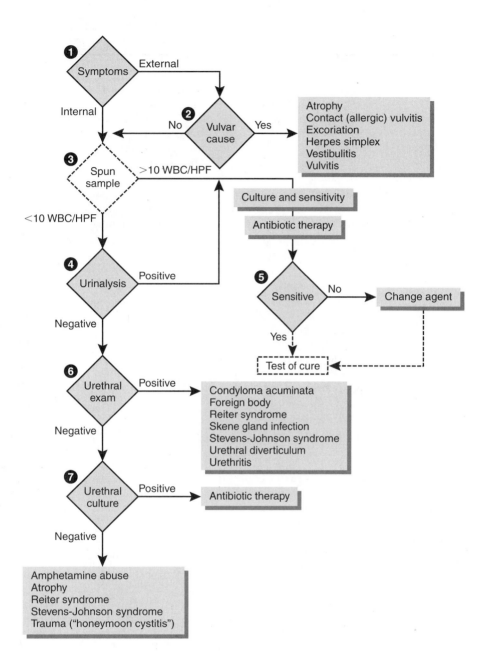

1 Symptoms
— External
— Internal

2 Vulvar cause
— No
— Yes → Atrophy / Contact (allergic) vulvitis / Excoriation / Herpes simplex / Vestibulitis / Vulvitis

3 Spun sample
— >10 WBC/HPF → Culture and sensitivity → Antibiotic therapy
— <10 WBC/HPF

4 Urinalysis
— Positive
— Negative

5 Sensitive
— No → Change agent
— Yes → Test of cure

6 Urethral exam
— Positive → Condyloma acuminata / Foreign body / Reiter syndrome / Skene gland infection / Stevens-Johnson syndrome / Urethral diverticulum / Urethritis
— Negative

7 Urethral culture
— Positive → Antibiotic therapy
— Negative → Amphetamine abuse / Atrophy / Reiter syndrome / Stevens-Johnson syndrome / Trauma ("honeymoon cystitis")

Ectopic Pregnancy

INTRODUCTION

Ectopic pregnancy is the leading cause of pregnancy-related death during the first trimester, and the second leading cause of maternal death overall. Tubal damage or altered motility may cause the fertilized egg to be improperly transported, resulting in implantation in an abnormal location. Between 10 and 30 of every 1000 pregnancies implant outside of the uterine cavity. This almost invariably dooms the pregnancy and can threaten the health and reproductive potential of the mother. The most common cause is acute salpingitis (50%). In the majority of remaining cases (40%) no risk factor is apparent. Abnormal embryonic development may play a role. Surgical intervention is generally required for symptomatic patients (salpingostomy, salpingectomy). Asymptomatic or mildly symptomatic patients may be considered for medical therapy.

1 The most important factor in the timely diagnosis of ectopic pregnancy is the recognition of its possibility, if not probability, in all reproductive-age patients with abdominal pain. Delayed or inaccurate diagnosis is present in roughly half of maternal deaths due to ectopic pregnancy. In one study one third of women with extrauterine pregnancies had been seen once and 11% seen twice before the diagnosis was established.

2 If a pregnancy test is negative, other sources of the patient's symptoms, such as torsion or bleeding in the adnexa or infection (appendicitis or pelvic inflammatory disease), must be sought. If the pregnancy test is positive, the possibility of an ectopic implantation must be presumed until proven otherwise.

3 Transabdominal ultrasonography will consistently show a gestational sac at 5 weeks, a fetal pole at 6 weeks, and cardiac activity at 7 weeks in the presence of a normal gestation. Reliable transabdominal ultrasonographic images of an intrauterine gestation should be possible when the beta-human chorionic gonadotropin (β-hCG) level reaches 5000 to 6000 mIU/ml. Transvaginal ultrasonography will generally provide identification of a gestational sac at 4 to 5 weeks, a yolk sac at 5 weeks, and fetal cardiac activity around 6 weeks. Transvaginal imaging of an intrauterine pregnancy should be routinely possible after the β-hCG level reaches 1500 mIU/ml. Because the diagnosis of ectopic pregnancy is made prior to 7 weeks in over one half of the cases, transvaginal ultrasonography the procedure of choice.

4 If an intrauterine gestation is confirmed by ultrasonography, the pregnancy may be observed and other sources for the patient's symptoms sought.

5 If the conceptional age is precisely known, the absence of a gestational sac on transvaginal ultrasonography by 24 days after conception (38 days from last period) is presumptive evidence of an ectopic implantation. When no gestational sac is seen and the adnexal structures are normal, dilatation and curettage can be helpful in the diagnosis of abnormal pregnancy. If villi cannot be identified, an ectopic implantation must be presumed and pursued by surgical or medical therapy. Sensitive serum assays of β-hCG and progesterone and the use of high-resolution ultrasonography have largely supplanted the use of dilatation and curettage. In many centers this option has been entirely abandoned in favor of management as outlined in step 9.

6 When products of conception (chorionic villi are found, ectopic pregnancy is essentially ruled out. In the case of a missed abortion or blighted ovum, β-hCG levels are usually stable or decreasing and chorionic villi will be found.

7 When chorionic villi are not found during dilatation and curettage, or when serum β-hCG levels plateau, an ectopic implantation should be presumed. Management by surgery or medical means is often a function of experience, the patient's condition, and physician or patient preference. Chemotherapeutic agents such as methotrexate and actinomycin D may be used to medically treat the pregnancy, resulting in involution and reabsorption. Methotrexate has been most commonly used and may be given orally, intramuscularly, or injected into the pregnancy, via a transvaginal route with ultrasonic guidance or via laparoscopy. The medical management of ectopic pregnancies is discussed separately.

8 Typical findings in ectopic pregnancy include a noncystic adnexal mass, cardiac activity in the adnexa (found in 20% to 25% of scans), and an empty uterine cavity. If a complex echogenic adnexal mass is identified by ultrasonography, the positive predictive value for ectopic pregnancy is 94%. Free intraperitoneal fluid may be helpful in the diagnosis of ectopic pregnancy, but is nonspecific.

9 The production of β-hCG is directly correlated with the proliferation of trophoblastic tissue, making serial determinations of β-hCG levels useful in assessing the health of a pregnancy. A single β-hCG value is of little value unless it is negative. The general rule of thumb given is that a doubling in value should occur in just over 48 hours, but the time may range from 1.4 to 3.5 days in normal pregnancies. Tubal pregnancies will generally plateau or have a decline in β-hCG levels, though this is not uniform.

10 Serum β-hCG levels that rise appropriately suggest, but do not guarantee, a normal gestation. Further follow-up to ensure that the pregnancy is progressing normally should be carried out based on the patient's history, physical findings, and symptoms.

REFERENCES

Ankum WM, Van der Veen F, Hamerlynck JVTH, Lammes FB. Suspected ectopic pregnancy: What to do when human chorionic gonadotropin levels are below the discrimination zone. J Reprod Med 1995;40:525–529.

American College of Obstetricians and Gynecologists. Medical Management of Tubal Pregnancy. ACOG Practice Bulletin 3. Washington, DC: ACOG, 1998.

Reich H, Freifeld ML, McGlynn F, et al. Laparoscopic treatment of tubal pregnancy. Obstet Gynecol 1987;69:275.

Russell JB. The etiology of ectopic pregnancy. Clin Obstet Gynecol 1987;30:181–190.

Shalev E, Yarom I, Bustan M, Weiner E, Ben-Shlomo I. Transvaginal sonography as the ultimate diagnostic tool for the management of ectopic pregnancy: Experience with 840 cases. Fertil Steril 1998;69:62.

Stovall TG, Ling FW, Buster JE. Outpatient chemotherapy of unruptured ectopic pregnancy. Fertil Steril 1989;51:435–438.

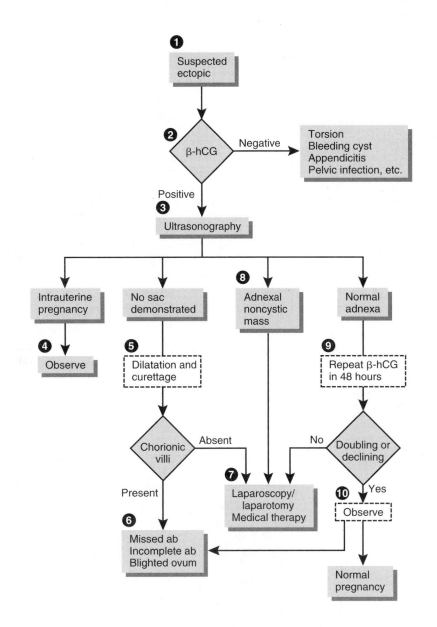

Ectopic Pregnancy

Medical Management

INTRODUCTION

Patients who are hemodynamically stable with an unruptured ectopic pregnancy 4 cm or less in diameter can be offered outpatient methotrexate treatment. Fertility outcomes in patients treated medically are similar to those treated with conservative surgery. Methotrexate antagonizes folic acid and inhibits dihydrofolate reductase, which is required for DNA synthesis and cell division. Patients who have contraindications to the use of methotrexate, are nursing, or have immunodeficiency, liver disease, active pulomonary or gastric disease, or blood dyscrasias should not be considered for this therapy.

❶ Only patients who are hemodynamically stable may be considered for medical therapy.

❷ If there are signs that the ectopic pregnancy has ruptured, surgical therapy by laparoscopy or laparotomy is indicated. Evidence of intraperitoneal leakage or the presence of a reactive increase in peritoneal fluid seen on ultrasonography are suggestive, but not diagnostic of tubal rupture. The use of culdocentesis has generally fallen out of favor as a diagnostic test for tubal rupture.

❸ If the adnexal structure presumed to be the ectopic pregnancy is less than 4 cm in diameter, the patient may be considered for medical therapy. At one time, the presence of fetal cardiac activity in an extrauterine gestation was thought to be a contraindication to medical management. Because of the inproved resolution of ultrasonography equipment (resulting in earlier detection) and experience with pregnancies with cardiac activity, this is now considered a relative contraindication only. These pregnancies are, however, at greater risk of failure or complication and require careful monitoring.

❹ To safely and effectively use medical management, it is imperative that the patient be compliant. Patients managed medically must return frequently for re-evaluation. The frequency of these visits de-

creases with time, but will often continue for 2 months or more.

❺ Before methotrexate can be safely administered, baseline assessments of serum beta-human chorionic gonadotropin (β-hCG) and aspartate transaminase (AST, to assess liver function), a complete blood count (CBC), and establishment of the patient's blood type and Rh factor must be carried out. If the patient is Rh negative, Rh immune globulin should be administered. Some centers set an arbitrary cut-off value above which the patient is not a candidate for medical therapy. This cut off has been reported to range from 6000 to 15,000 mIU/ml. Because of variations between assays and laboratories, as well as the existence of three international standards, thresholds for treatment (if any) must be set based on local experience.

❻ Methotrexate may be administered as a single dose of 50 mg/kg. Patients treated with methotrexate should be warned not to use alcohol or nonsteroidal anti-inflammatory drugs or to take vitamin preparations containing folic acid until completion of their therapy. Patients are generally asked to refrain from intercourse for the same period.

❼ Patients must return for measurement of serum β-hCG levels on days 4 and 7 of treatment. There is often a transient rise in β-hCG levels following therapy that reaches its peak around day 4 of therapy. Patients should be warned that there may be a increase in abdominal symptoms (such as pain, seen in up to two thirds of patients) between days 5 and 10. In some patients, these may be sufficient to require hospitalization for observation. The pain associated with therapy is generally milder and of limited duration compared with that associated with tubal rupture. Rarely do these patients require surgical intervention unless rupture and intra-abdominal bleeding is suspected. Mild vaginal bleeding may also occur, but heavy bleeding should prompt a reappraisal.

❽ When the results of the serum β-hCG assay drawn on day 7 are available, the value is compared to that obtained on day 4. When there has not been a decline of at least 15% between the two measurements, a repeat course of methotrexate or surgical evaluation and treatment are indicated. Up to 25% of patients managed successfully will require a second dose of methotrexate.

❾ The majority of patients will demonstrate a decline of more than 15% between the 4th and 7th days after the administration of methotrexate. These patients should be followed by weekly measurements of β-hCG titers until the value is undetectable (<5 mIU/ml). Single-dose therapy is associated with a median success rate of 84%, with reported values ranging from 67% to 100%. If β-hCG titers plateau or rise at any point, re-evaluation and re-treatment may be required. Fertility rates of 80% are reported, with recurrent ectopic implantations occurring in almost 30% of cases.

REFERENCES

Ankum WM, Van der Veen F, Hamerlynck JVTH, Lammes FB. Suspected ectopic pregnancy: What to do when human chorionic gonadotropin levels are below the discrimination zone. J Reprod Med 1995;40:525–529.

American College of Obstetricians and Gynecologists. Medical Management of Tubal Pregnancy. ACOG Practice Bulletin 3. Washington, DC: ACOG, 1998.

Carson S, Buster J. Current concepts: Ectopic pregnancy. N Engl J Med 1993;329:1174.

Glock J, Johnson J, Bunsted J. Efficacy and safety of single-dose systemic methotrexate in the treatment of ectopic pregnancy. Fertil Steril 1994;62:716.

Hajenius PJ, Engelsbel S, Mol BW, et al. Randomised trial of systemic methotrexate versus laparoscopic salpingostomy in tubal pregnancy. Lancet 1997;350:774.

Stovall TG, Ling FW, Buster JE. Outpatient chemotherapy of unruptured ectopic pregnancy. Fertil Steril 1989;51:435–438.

Stovall TG, Ling FW. Single-dose methotrexate: An expanded clinical trial. Am J Obstet Gynecol 1993;168:1759.

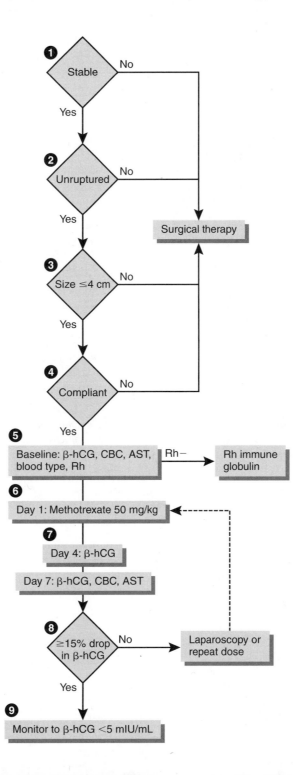

① Stable — No →

② Unruptured — No →

Surgical therapy

③ Size ≤4 cm — No →

④ Compliant — No →

⑤ Baseline: β-hCG, CBC, AST, blood type, Rh — Rh− → Rh immune globulin

⑥ Day 1: Methotrexate 50 mg/kg

⑦ Day 4: β-hCG

Day 7: β-hCG, CBC, AST

⑧ ≥15% drop in β-hCG — No → Laparoscopy or repeat dose

⑨ Monitor to β-hCG <5 mIU/mL

Endometrial Cancer Staging

INTRODUCTION

Malignant change of the endometrial tissues, generally of the adenocarcinoma, adenosquamous, clear cell, or papillary serous cell types, constitutes what is generally referred to as endometrial cancer. The grading of endometrial cancer is based on the percentage of nonsquamous and nonmorular solid growth patterns present: When these are less than 5% the grade is 1, when they represent 6% to 50% the grade is 2, and grade 3 lesions have greater than 50% of these elements present. The diagnosis is generally established by endometrial biopsy or curettage, while the staging of endometrial cancer is based on clinical examination, augmented by surgical findings and imaging studies of the pelvis and distant organs.

❶ Endometrial cancer confined to the endometrium itself is stage I. Five-year survival for patients with stage I disease is roughly 85%. Even when stage I disease is suspected, pelvic cytology and samples of lymph nodes must be obtained to adequately stage the patient's disease.

❷ Stage IA endometrial cancer is confined to the surface of the endometrium itself. This is occasionally an incidental finding at the time of histologic examination of specimens removed for other reasons.

❸ When invasion of the myometrium occurs, its depth, relative to the uterine wall thickness, must be measured. Invasion that does not extend beyond the inner half of the myometrium is classed as stage IB, while spread that extends beyond this toward the surface, but still confined to the uterus, is stage IC.

❹ Involvement of the cervix characterizes stage II disease. Roughly 60% of patients with stage II disease can be expected to survive 5 years or more.

❺ Involvement of the superficial endocervical tissues and glands is typical of stage IIA disease, while invasion into the stroma earns a stage IIB classification.

❻ Cancer that is limited to the uterus, vagina, or pelvic and para-aortic lymph nodes is stage III disease. Stage III disease is associated with only a 30% 5-year survival rate.

❼ When the tumor is confined to the uterus but involves the uterine serosa or the adnexa or there is positive peritoneal cytology, the patient is classified as having stage IIIA disease.

❽ Vaginal metastases signal the presence of stage IIIB disease, while metastases that involve the pelvic or para-aortic lymph nodes is classed as stage IIIC.

❾ Stage IV disease offers the poorest 5-year survival rate (10% or less) and is characterized by involvement of the bowel or bladder (stage IVA) or distant organs, including the abdominal or inguinal lymph nodes (stage IVB).

REFERENCES

American College of Obstetricians and Gynecologists. Classification and Staging of Gynecologic Malignancies. ACOG Technical Bulletin 155. Washington, DC: ACOG, 1991.

American College of Obstetricians and Gynecologists. Carcinoma of the Endometrium. ACOG Technical Bulletin 162. Washington, DC: ACOG, 1991.

Cushing KL, Weiss NS, Voigt LF, McKnight B, Beresford SAA. Risk of endometrial cancer in relation to use of low-dose, unopposed estrogens. Obstet Gynecol 1998;91:35.

Davies JL, Rosenshein NB, Antunes CMF, Stolley PD. A review of the risk factors for endometrial carcinoma. Obstet Gynecol Surv 1981;36:107.

Gallup DG, Stock RJ. Adenocarcinoma of the endometrium in women 40 years or younger. Obstet Gynecol 1984;64:417.

Reid PC, Brown VA, Fothergill DJ. Outpatient investigation of postmenopausal bleeding. Br J Obstet Gynaecol 1993;100:498.

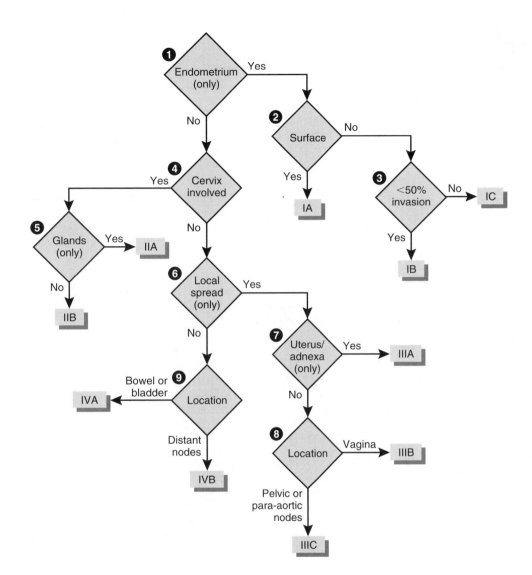

Endometrial Hyperplasia

INTRODUCTION

Overgrowth of the endometrium may occur in response to a number of conditions, but is most often associated with prolonged, unopposed estrogen stimulation. The risk of developing endometrial hyperplasia is increased in obese women (10-fold increase if more than 50 pounds above ideal), those with diabetes mellitus or delayed menopause, nulliparous patients, and those receiving tamoxifen therapy. Most often hyperplasia is suspected because of heavy or abnormal bleeding in an at-risk individual. It is becoming common that the diagnosis is suspected based on endometrial thickening found during ultrasound imaging of the uterus. The diagnosis must be established by histologic examination of tissue obtained by office biopsy, hysteroscopy, or dilatation and curettage.

❶ In determining the optimal therapy for endometrial hyperplasia, one of the most important aspects is the patient's fertility status. Those who are fertile and wish to keep the option of pregnancy are managed differently from those who are post-menopausal who use a sterilization method for contraception, or whose families are complete.

❷ Patients who desire fertility can generally be treated conservatively, but the treatment must be based on the presence and severity of atypia found in their endometrial sample. Irregular cell size, high nuclear/cytoplasmic ratios, nuclear pleomorphism, abnormal chromatin, mitoses, and prominent nucleoli characterize progressive atypia. The more severe the degree of atypia, the greater the malignant potential is thought to be, though up to half of these lesions may regress spontaneously.

❸ Moderate to severe hyperplasia is thought to be a premalignant condition and may be found to coexist with adenocarcinoma. Moderate to severe hyperplasia with a complex architecture is thought to have a greater malignant potential than simple hyperplasia with atypia of the same grade. The distinction between severe atypia and carcinoma in situ is not clear, though therapy is often similar. Patients wishing to preserve fertility may be treated with moderate- to high-dose continuous progestins for 3 to 6 months (e.g., megestrol acetate (Megace) 40 mg po qd).

❹ When atypia is more mild, progestin therapy may be either continuous or intermittent (cyclic, such as medroxyprogesterone acetate (Provera) 10 mg po qd for 10 to 14 days each month, or combination oral contraceptives). The presence or absence of bleeding or other symptoms often prompts the decision between these modes.

❺ Patients who receive progestin therapy for atypia, regardless of grade, should undergo endometrial sampling or other histologic evaluation after 6 months of therapy. When this follow-up sample is normal, the patient may be safely observed. If the follow-up evaluation reveals a continuing abnormality, hysterectomy must be seriously considered.

❻ The treatment of patients in whom fertility is not an issue is based on the presence or absence of atypia. Those with moderate to severe hyperplasia should be treated by surgical means. Those with mild atypia may be candidates for medical management, though many opt for hysterectomy because of the greater risk of malignancy in older patients. If progestin therapy is chosen, it may be given in either a continuous or an intermittent (cyclic) manner.

❼ Patients who receive progestin therapy should undergo endometrial sampling or other histologic evaluation after 6 months of therapy. When this follow-up demonstrates normal tissue, the patient may be safely observed. If the follow-up evaluation reveals a continuing abnormality, hysterectomy must be seriously considered.

❽ When no atypia is demonstrated on histologic examination, management decisions should be based on the character of the hyperplasia. Because the malignant potential of complex hyperplasia, even in the absence of atypia, is thought to be higher, these patients should undergo progestin therapy in either continuous or intermittent form.

❾ Following progestin therapy, endometrial sampling or other histologic evaluation should take place. When this follow-up demonstrates normal tissue, the patient may be safely observed. If the follow-up evaluation reveals a continuing abnormality, further management by either medical or surgical means must be offered.

❿ Patients with simple hyperplasia without atypia may be managed conservatively. Those with bleeding symptoms may be managed by intermittent progestin therapy, while asymptomatic patients need only observation. The risk of carcinoma in these patients is estimated to be about 2%.

REFERENCES

Copenhaver EH. Atypical endometrial hyperplasia. Obstet Gynecol 1959;13:264.

Eichner E, Abellera M. Endometrial hyperplasia treated by progestins. Obstet Gynecol 1971;38:739.

Gal D. Endometrial hyperplasia: Diagnosis and management. In Sciarra JJ (ed): Gynecology and Obstetrics. Philadelphia: JB Lippincott, 1991;(4)12:1.

Gusberg SB, Chen SY, Cohen CJ. Endometrial cancer: Factors influencing the choice of treatment. Gynecol Oncol 1974;2:308.

Kurman RJ, Kaminski PF, Norris HJ. The behavior of endometrial hyperplasia—a long-term study of "untreated" hyperplasia in 170 patients. Cancer 1985;56:403.

Pettersson B, Adami HO, Lindgren A, et al. Endometrial polyps and hyperplasia as risk factors for endometrial carcinoma. Acta Obstet Gynecol Scand 1985;64:653.

Wentz WB. Progestin therapy in endometrial hyperplasia. Gynecol Oncol 1974;2:362.

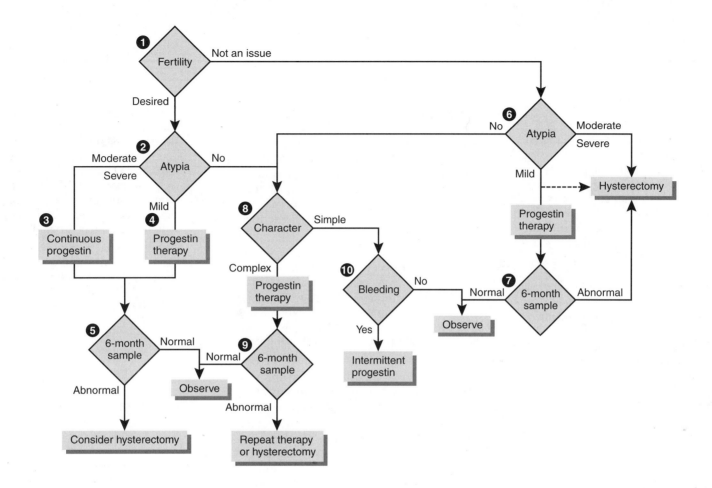

Endometriosis

INTRODUCTION

The prevalence of endometriosis is reported to range from 5% to 15% of patients due in part to selection bias and the observation that up to 30% of patients are asymptomatic. The clinical diagnosis is generally suggested by cyclic pelvic pain or dyspareunia (both worst 36 to 48 hours before menses), premenstrual and menstrual pain, dyschezia, and mid-cycle (ovulatory) pain. Between 30% and 50% of infertility patients are diagnosed as having endometriosis.

1 Even when the symptoms experienced by the patient are classic for endometriosis, the patient must still be carefully evaluated for symptoms and physical findings that may suggest other causes. Irritable bowel disease strongly mimics the timing and symptoms typical of endometriosis. The sequellae of pelvic inflammatory disease or urinary tract infection (including interstitial cystitis) should be considered. Infertility patients should have a complete evaluation, including semen analysis, assessments of ovulation and tubal patency, and other tests prior to pursuing the possibility of endometriosis.

2 Many authors suggest a trial of nonsteroidal anti-inflammatory agents before more invasive testing is considered. If the trial is successful, no further evaluation is warrented.

3 Some studies suggest that empiric treatment of presumed endometriosis may be cost effective. Based on the symptoms present, this may vary from low-dose monophasic oral contraceptives to gonadotropin-releasing hormone (GnRH) agonists. If these therapies are successful in resolving the patient's symptoms, further evaluation is not necessary. Empiric therapy is probably not appropriate where infertility is a major consideration.

4 The ultimate diagnosis of endometriosis rests on direct inspection of the involved area (laparoscopy), supported by histologic confirmation. Endometriosis may appear as brown "powder burns," red, blue, or white plaques, small petechial areas, or stellate areas of scarring. Care should be exercised to avoid rupturing endometriomas, if present. If no sign of endometriosis is evident, further evaluation and symptomatic therapies should be pursued.

5 An important aspect of determining optimal treatment is an assessment of the patient's plans for fertility. When fertility is not an issue there is greater flexibility in treatments possible. When the establishment or preservation of fertility is paramount, the thrust of therapy is necessarily different.

6 When fertility is not an issue and laparoscopy demonstrates mild endometriosis, expectant management or medical therapy are often sufficient.

7 Patients who do not wish future childbearing and who have moderate to severe disease are often best treated by hysterectomy with bilateral salpingo-oophorectomy. Ovarian conservation may be considered in younger patients, but recurrence and reoperation rates are high. If the ovaries are removed, estrogen replacement therapy can be started 6 weeks after surgery.

8 For patients pursuing fertility, observation or medical therapy may manage those who have minimal symptoms and mild endometriosis. Fifty to sixty percent of these patients will conceive without additional intervention. Pregnancy rates are not increased with surgery or medical therapy. Patients who fail to conceive may consider assisted reproductive technologies.

9 Moderate disease is best treated with medical therapy unless large (>5 cm) endometriomas are present. If this route is chosen, therapy must continue for 6 months or longer, and care must be given to side effects such as bone loss and menopausal symptoms. If severe pain or large endometriomas are present, laparoscopic resection of disease and reconstruction is recommended. Some authors suggest simultaneous ablation of the uterosacral ligaments for pain control, though no prospective studies document a benefit to this adjunctive procedure.

10 Severe disease generally requires open surgical therapy. Resection of implants, adhesions, and endometriomas, along with reconstruction as needed provides the best hope of preserving fertility. Pain and other symptoms may not be resolved by this conservative treatment, and assisted fertility may still be required for those who fail to conceive.

REFERENCES

Barbieri RL. Etiology and epidemiology of endometriosis. Am J Obstet Gynecol 1990;162:565.

Cook AS, Rock JA. The role of laparoscopy in the treatment of endometriosis. Fertil Steril 1991;55:663.

Friedman AJ, Hornstein MD. Gonadotropin-releasing hormone agonist plus estrogen–progestin "add-back" therapy for endometriosis-related pelvic pain. Fertil Steril 1993;60:236.

Hughes EG, Fedorkow DM, Collins JA. A quantitative overview of controlled trials in endometriosis-associated infertility. Fertil Steril 1993;59:963.

Hurst BS, Rock JA. Endometriosis: pathophysiology, diagnosis and treatment. Obstet Gynecol Surv 1989;44:297.

Olive DL, Schwartz LB. Endometriosis. N Engl J Med 1993;328:1759–1768.

Waller KG, Shaw RW. GnRH analogs in the treatment of endometriosis: long-term follow-up. Fertil Steril 1993;59:511.

Wright S, Valdes CT, Dunn RC, Franklin RR. Short-term Lupron or Danazol therapy for pelvic endometriosis. Fertil Steril 1995;63:504–507.

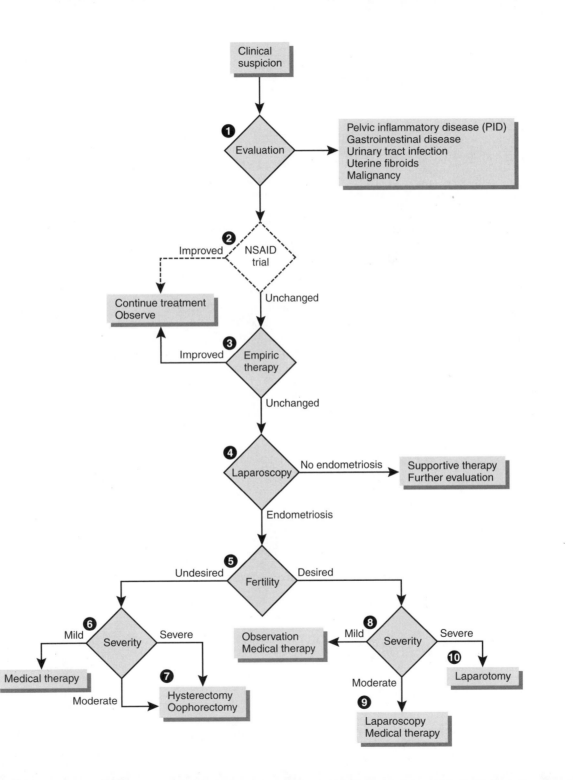

Galactorrhea

INTRODUCTION

Galactorrhea is most often caused by elevated levels of prolactin, though only about one third of patients with such elevations will have this symptom. (The absence of galactorrhea may be due to reduced levels of estrogen common in these patients.)

❶ While it should go without saying, the first issue to be addressed in the evaluation of galactorrhea is the establishment of the diagnosis. Unilateral nipple discharge, even if milky in character, should be evaluated as a nipple or breast problem and not galactorrhea. Similarly, the ability to express a small amount of discharge from the nipples is not the same as the spontaneous leakage that constitutes true galactorrhea.

❷ When serum levels of prolactin are elevated, the source of the elevation must be sought. (This evaluation is discussed separately.)

❸ Processes that involve the chest wall or spine may cause galactorrhea. Persistent nipple stimulation caused by such things as cutaneous lesions (herpes), suckling, or continuing manual stimulation caused by obsessive behavior or patterns of sexual expression may result in galactorrhea. The same neurologic arcs may be stimulated by thoracotomy scars or spinal lesions.

❹ While uncommon as causes of galactorrhea, stress, trauma (resulting in pituitary stalk damage), surgery or anesthetic agents, and unrecognized central nervous system disease may result in elevated levels of prolactin. Galactorrhea that follows pregnancy in the absence of nursing (Chiari–Frommel syndrome) may be physiologic, though it is prudent to remain vigilant for the possibility of unrecognized disease.

REFERENCES

American College of Obstetricians and Gynecologists. Amenorrhea. Technical Bulletin 128. Washington, DC: ACOG, 1989.

Chang RJ, Keye WR, Young JR, et al. Detection, evaluation, and treatment of pituitary microadnomas in patients with galactorrhea and amenorrhea. Am J Obstet Gynecol 1977;128: 356.

Schlechte J, Dolan K, Sherman B, et al. The natural history of untreated hyperprolactinemia: A prospective analysis. J Clin Endocrinol Metab 1989;68:412.

Smith RP. Gynecology in Primary Care. Baltimore: Williams & Wilkins, 1997, pp 405–426.

Speroff L, Glass RH, Kase NG. Clinical Gynecologic Endocrinology and Infertility, 5th ed. Baltimore: Williams & Wilkins, 1994, pp 404, 555–560.

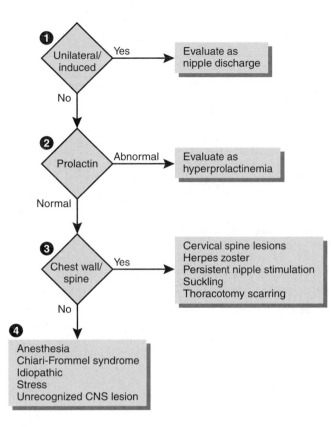

1 Unilateral/induced — Yes → Evaluate as nipple discharge

No ↓

2 Prolactin — Abnormal → Evaluate as hyperprolactinemia

Normal ↓

3 Chest wall/spine — Yes → Cervical spine lesions
Herpes zoster
Persistent nipple stimulation
Suckling
Thoracotomy scarring

No ↓

4 Anesthesia
Chiari-Frommel syndrome
Idiopathic
Stress
Unrecognized CNS lesion

Genital Herpes

Management in the Pregnant Patient

INTRODUCTION

Babies born to mothers with active herpes lesions have a 40% to 50% risk of acquiring the infection—an infection that carries an 80% mortality rate. Of those that survive, up to 50% will have neurologic, ophthalmic, and other sequellae. Approximately 80% of women with recently acquired infection will have recurrences during pregnancy (two to four symptomatic events). Despite efforts to identify those at risk, up to 70% of all neonates with herpes are born to asymptomatic mothers. In the absence of any reliable rapid tests for herpes infection, management continues to be problematic.

❶ Genital herpes infections that occur during the early stages of pregnancy may be treated symptomatically and do not usually affect the pregnancy itself. Some studies indicate a slightly increased risk of pregnancy loss when the infection occurs during the first few weeks after fertilization, though the risk is low. Suppressive therapy should not be used for pregnant patients, as these are class C drugs.

❷ The greatest risk of neonatal infection is during labor and the birth process, with preterm infants at greatest risk. Women with a history of herpes infections need not be routinely cultured during pregnancy, though careful inspection for lesions at the time of labor and questioning about the possibility of prodromal symptoms is important. Amniocentesis is not indicated to assess fetal infection.

❸ Patients with a history of herpes infections in the past who have neither prodrome nor lesions present require no special management during labor. The history should be noted and conveyed to the pediatrician as a matter of routine.

❹ Even though the results of culture will generally not be available to affect the direct management of the patient in labor, a culture to confirm the diagnosis should still be carried out. This will assist the pediatrician in the management of the infant and help in the counseling of the patient regarding future episodes, pregnancies, and other sexually transmitted diseases. Viral cultures of material are taken by swab from the lesions (95% sensitivity). Smears of vesicular material may also be stained with Wright's stain to visualize the giant multinucleated cells with characteristic eosinophilic intranuclear inclusions.

❺ Patients with active herpes infections should be considered for cesarean section delivery. When there has been prolonged (>4 to 6 hours) rupture of the amniotic membranes, infection may have already taken place, blunting the value of cesarean delivery. If the patient has a history of genital tract herpes during pregnancy, fetal scalp blood sampling and the use of fetal scalp electrodes should be avoided, if possible.

REFERENCES

American College of Obstetricians and Gynecologists. Gynecologic Herpes Simplex Virus Infections. ACOG Technical Bulletin 119. Washington, DC: ACOG, 1988.

Baker DA. Herpes and pregnancy: New management. Clin Obstet Gynecol 1990;33:253–257.

Binkin NJ, Koplan JP, Cates W Jr. Preventing neonatal herpes: The value of weekly viral cultures in pregnant women with recurrent genital herpes. JAMA 1984;251:2816.

Haddad J, Langer B, Astruc D, et al. Oral acyclovir and recurrent genital herpes during late pregnancy. Obstet Gynecol 1993;82:102–104.

Maccato ML, Kaufman RH. Herpes genitalis. Dermatol Clin 1992;10:415.

Randolph AG, Washington AE, Prober CG. Cesarean delivery for women presenting with genital herpes lesions. Efficacy, risks, and costs. JAMA 1993;270:77–82.

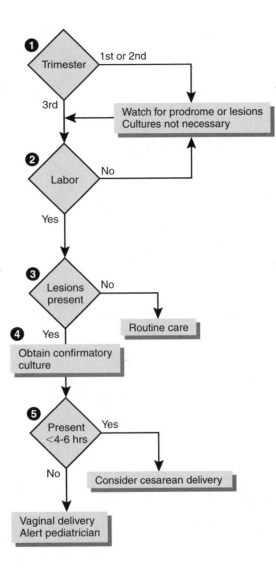

❶ Trimester — 1st or 2nd

3rd

Watch for prodrome or lesions
Cultures not necessary

❷ Labor — No

Yes

❸ Lesions present — No → Routine care

❹ Yes

Obtain confirmatory culture

❺ Present <4-6 hrs — Yes → Consider cesarean delivery

No

Vaginal delivery
Alert pediatrician

Genital Herpes

Management in the Nonpregnant Patient

INTRODUCTION

Infection by the herpes simplex virus results in recurrent symptoms that run from uncomfortable to disabling and carries special risk to the neonate when herpes complicates pregnancy. In the United States, there are an estimated 20 million recurrent cases, 300,000 to 500,000 new cases per year, and a prevalence 1 in 200 asymptomatic women. The infection is characterized by a prodromal phase: mild paresthesia and burning (beginning approximately 2 to 5 days after infection). This progresses to very painful vesicular and ulcerated lesions 3 to 7 days after exposure (may prompt hospitalization in up to 10% of cases). Dysuria due to vulvar lesions, urethral and bladder involvement, or autonomic dysfunction may lead to urinary retention. Malaise, low-grade fever, and inguinal adenopathy occur in 40% of patients. Systemic symptoms, including aseptic meningitis, fever, headache, and meningismus can be found in 70% of patients 5 to 7 days after the appearance of the genital lesions.

❶ The management of herpetic infections is stratified by acuity: primary, or initial, infections behave and are treated differently from the milder recurrent episodes.

❷ When the patient's symptoms and clinical findings strongly support the diagnosis, empiric treatment may be begun while confirmatory studies are underway. If the diagnosis is not certain, additional studies and considerations are warranted.

❸ Antiviral therapy has proven most efficacious if begun during the first 48 hours of the clinical signs of infection. Beyond this period, results do not justify the cost and a more symptomatic approach is appropriate.

❹ Symptomatic treatment of genital herpes lesions consists of topical cleansing, sitz baths, followed by drying with a heat lamp or hair dryer, and analgesics. Topical analgesics (lidocaine 2% jelly, or nonprescription throat spray with phenol) may be added. If secondary infections occur, therapy with a local antibacterial cream, such as Neosporin, is appropriate. Sexual continence during prodrome to full healing should be advised in an effort to reduce the risk of infecting the patient's partner. Healing of the lesions is generally complete. Inguinal adenopathy may persist for several weeks after the resolution of the vulvar lesions. Suppuration is uncommon. Complete resolution of all symptoms occurs in 2 to 4 weeks.

❺ When the classical vesicular lesions are absent or have healed, the diagnosis must be considered provisionary and other possibilities considered. If vesicles are present, but the diagnosis is uncertain because of an atypical course, location, or character, symptomatic therapy is appropriate while cultures or other diagnostic tests are undertaken.

❻ Viral cultures of material taken by swab from the lesions (95% sensitivity). Smears of vesicular material may also be stained with Wright's stain to visualize giant multinucleated cells with characteristic eosinophilic intranuclear inclusions. Scrapings from the base of vesicles may be stained using immunofluorescence techniques to detect the presence of viral particles. If these tests indicate a herpetic infection, antiviral therapy may be considered, though most patients will be beyond the point where this therapy will be useful. Establishing a correct diagnosis for future reference and counseling is valuable even if it does not affect current management.

❼ Recurrent infections may be successfully treated with antiviral agents if they are instituted during the prodromal phase or within the first 48 hours after the appearance of clinical lesions.

❽ Between 60% and 90% of patients will have a recurrence of herpetic lesions in the first 6 months after their initial infection. Though generally shorter and milder, these recurrent attacks are no less virulent. If the patient has experienced a limited number of recurrences, episodic care and observation is appropriate.

❾ Patients who experience periodic, but infrequent recurrences are best managed episodically. When recurrences occur frequently with a short interval, antiviral suppressive therapy is appropriate (acyclovir 200 mg po tid or 400 mg po bid, increased to 5 times/day with lesions, or famciclovir (Famvir) 125 mg po bid for 5 days). This has been shown to be effective in decreasing frequency and severity of flare-ups, but should be limited to less than 6 months of use.

REFERENCES

American College of Obstetricians and Gynecologists. Gynecologic Herpes Simplex Virus Infections. ACOG Technical Bulletin 119. Washington, DC: ACOG, 1988.

Bryson YJ, Dillon M, Bernsterin DI, et al. Risk of acquisition of genital herpes simplex virus type 2 in sex partners of persons with genital herpes: a prospective couple study. J Infect Dis 1993;167:942–946.

Centers for Disease Control and Prevention. 1998 Guidelines for treatment of sexually transmitted diseases. MMWR 1998;47(No. RR–1):21.

Cone RW, Swenson PD, Hobson AC, et al. Herpes simplex virus detection from genital lesions: a comparative study using antigen detection (HerpChek) and culture. J Clin Microbiol 1993;31:1774–1776.

deRuiter A, Thin RN. Genital herpes. A guide to pharmacological therapy. Drugs 1994;47:297–304.

Maccato ML, Kaufman RH. Herpes genitalis. Dermatol Clin 1992;10:415.

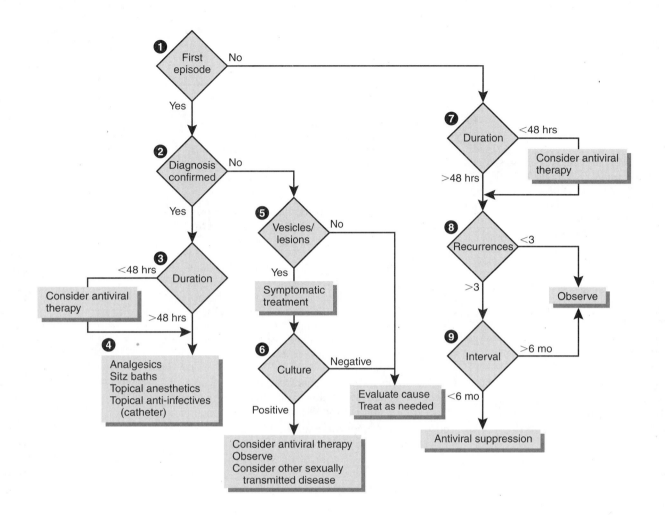

Hair Loss (Alopecia)

INTRODUCTION

Hair loss affects both men and women, but is uniquely distressing when it occurs to women. Hair growth and character is affected by diet, metabolism, hormonal fluctuations, and other factors, some of which are related to gynecologic or obstetric events. Hair follicles follow cycles of growth (anagen), followed by a resting phase (telogen) of 3 to 9 months, before resuming normal growth. Some conditions may synchronize the growth phase of the hair follicles, resulting in the reversible loss of large quantities of hair.

❶ When hair loss occurs over a long period, or begins later in life, it is most often familial and physiologic. Topical therapy (minoxidil) may be used if desired and has been shown to be effective in women (40% response rate in 1 year).

❷ Patchy hair loss suggests the possibility of scalp disease. This can generally be identified by simple observation, though occasionally consultation or biopsy may be required to establish a final diagnosis.

❸ If the base of a lost hair shaft is smooth, it came from natural (telogen) loss; if the base has the follicular bulb still attached (a white swelling at the end), the loss may be due to dermatologic or other disease conditions and consultation is suggested.

❹ Accelerated hair loss may come about any time there is an abrupt change in hormonal patterns, and is the result of a higher number of hair follicles entering into the resting, or telogen, phase of hair growth. If this is the situation, the lost hair will be regained in time. Stress and some medications (anticoagulants, retinoids, beta blockers, chemotherapeutic agents) may also cause similar hair loss. The relative androgen dominance found in postmenopausal women not on hormone replacement therapy may also cause male pattern hair loss (temporal balding, androgenic alopecia). The possibility of traction alopecia must be considered and results from hair styles that place the hair shafts under undue and prolonged traction.

❺ Endogenous sources for changes in estrogen such as pregnancy or masculinizing tumors may result in abrupt hair loss. These processes may result in synchrony of hair growth, which may not be apparent until approximately 3 months later, when the hair shaft is sloughed. This is the reason that pregnancy-related hair loss is most noticeable in the postpartum period.

❻ When exogenous hormones, such as contraceptive steroids, are identified as possible sources of the patient's hair loss, the need for these agents should be reassessed. Discontinuation of the agent will generally result in the regrowth of hair in 6 to 12 months.

REFERENCES

Burfke KE. Hair loss. What causes it and what can be done about it. Postgrad Med 1989;85:52.

Rook A, Dawber R. Diseases of the Hair and Scalp, 2nd ed. Boston: Blackwell Scientific Publications, 1992.

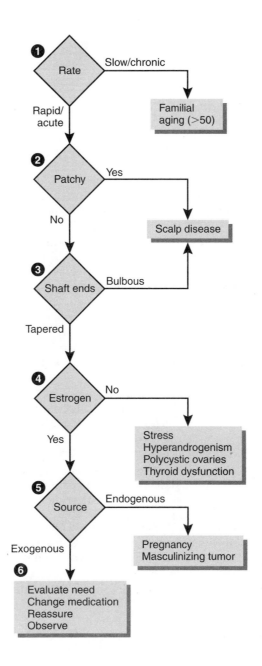

Headache

Acute, Severe

INTRODUCTION

Of all somatic complaints, headache is one of the most common and one that has a predilection for women, accounting for approximately 6 million visits by women yearly. Roughly, 80% of Americans experience some form of headache annually: half have severe headaches and 10% to 20% seek care with headache as a chief complaint. While the majority of headaches do not reflect serious underlying pathology, new-onset, acute, severe headaches may reflect serious pathology and do require careful evaluation.

❶ Most common headaches are recurrent, while a few are chronic. Because the risk of serious underlying pathology is significantly greater if the patient experiences a new-onset, acute, severe headache, this distinction should be made first in the evaluation. Headaches that are dramatically different from those experienced in the past, are consistently localized and prevent sleep, are associated with straining, have associated neurologic symptoms, vomiting or fever, or are progressive also suggest he need for an aggressive evaluation.

❷ Most patients with acute headaches do not have hypertension and most patients with hypertension do not have headaches because of their blood pressure. Regardless, measurement of the patient's blood pressure is fast, simple, and has often been carried out even before they are seen by the caregiver. Simple observation of the results will provide this diagnosis.

❸ A relatively brief but focused physical examination, based on the symptoms present, may suggest the presence of a neurologic abnormality. The presence of an abnormality should prompt an evaluation of the head by computed tomography or magnetic resonance imaging.

❹ Acute, severe headaches may result from a number of intracranial pathologies that may be detected by imaging studies. If the imaging studies are normal, an examination of cerebrospinal fluid should be made.

❺ Meningitis or encephalitis may be detected by an abnormal lumbar puncture. Acute-onset cluster or complex migraine headaches may produce abnormal findings on the neurologic examination and yet have normal imaging and cerebrospinal fluid studies.

❻ Not all cases of meningitis or encephalitis will present with abnormal neurologic findings. A lumbar puncture should be strongly considered for the patient with acute-onset, severe headaches.

❼ Following a negative cerebrospinal fluid evaluation, computed tomography should be considered for the unusual occurrences of bilateral subdural hematomas, dural sinus thrombosis, or sinusitis. Computed tomography is not required for all patients with headache, only those with severe, acute headaches that suggest the presence of underlying pathology as noted above.

❽ An erythrocyte sedimentation rate will be abnormal in patients with cranial arteritis, while patients with other causes will have normal or marginally elevated rates. While the list of remaining causes is long, history, associated factors or symptoms, and simple physical and laboratory evaluations will differentiate them.

REFERENCES

APGO Educational Series on Women's Health Issues: Strategies for the Management of Headache. Washington, DC: APGO, 1998.

Edelson RN. Menstrual migraine and other hormonal aspects of migraine. Headache 1985;25:376–379.

Granella F, Sances G, Zanferrari C, et al. Migraine without aura and preproductive life events. A clinical epidemiologic study in 1300 women. Headache 1993;33:385–389.

Headache Classification Committee of the International Headache Society. Classification and diagnostic criteria for headache disorders, cranial neuralgia, and facial pain. Cehpalagia 1988;8:1–96.

Kudrow L. The relationship of headache frequency to hormone use in migraine. Headache 1975;15:36.

Laube DW. Headache. In Ling FW, Laube DW, Nolan TE, et al (eds): Primary Care in Gynecology. Baltimore: Williams & Wilkins, 1996, pp 87–100.

Silberstein SD. The role of sex hormones in headache. Neurology 1992;42:37–42.

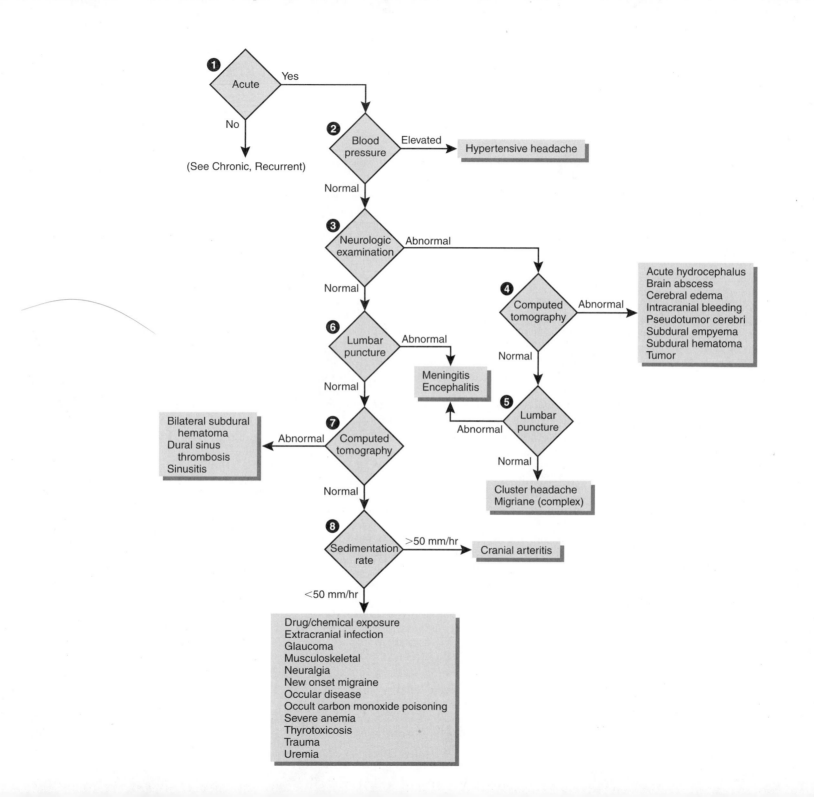

Headache

Chronic, Recurrent

INTRODUCTION

Of all somatic complaints, headache is one of the most common and one that has a predilection for women, accounting for approximately 6 million visits by women yearly. Roughly, 80% of Americans experience some form of headache annually: half have severe headaches and 10% to 20% seek care with headache as a chief complaint. The majority of recurrent headaches do not reflect serious underlying pathology, though they often lead to excessive, and often inappropriate tests and diagnostic procedures. Most recurring headaches are associated with muscle contraction or tension, disorders of neurotransmitter function and dural vasodilation (as in migraine and cluster headaches), or environmental or psychological disturbances (as with depression).

❶ Most common headaches are recurrent, while a few are chronic. Because the risk of serious underlying pathology is significantly greater if the patient experiences a new-onset, acute, severe headache, this distinction should be made first in the evaluation. Headaches that are dramatically different than those experienced in the past, are consistently localized and prevent sleep, are associated with straining, have associated neurologic symptoms, vomiting or fever, or are progressive also suggest the need for an aggressive evaluation.

❷ Fewer than 2% of patient over age 50 experience new-onset, severe headaches. A new-onset, unrelenting headache in these patients suggests the possibility of tumor, encephalitis or meningitis, or temporal arteritis, though the most common cause of chronic headache in these patients is depression. Associated or causal factors, location, physical examination and limited, focused laboratory studies will establish the diagnosis.

❸ The duration of the patient's symptoms may assist in establishing a possible cause. Studies in children

suggest that the majority of chronic headaches do not have organic disease.

❹ If a headache has been present for more than 4 weeks and there are no neurologic signs, a psychogenic origin is most probable. Patients with psychogenic or conversion-type headaches will describe their pain in vivid terms and with great affect but do not appear to be in great pain.

❺ Though the majority of patients with chronic (prolonged) headaches will have normal neurologic examinations, those with a documented abnormality must undergo further assessment with computed tomography or magnetic resonance imaging.

❻ Meningitis or encephalitis may be detected by an abnormal lumbar puncture. Cluster or complex migraine headaches may produce abnormal findings on the neurologic examination and yet have normal imaging and cerebrospinal fluid studies.

❼ Short-duration headaches of mild severity are the most commonly encountered type and are due to muscle contraction or tension. These headaches are 5 to 6 times more common than vascular types. Analgesics and reassurance is generally sufficient management for these patients. It is not uncommon for a patient to awaken with a muscle tension headache (such as with bruxism), but it is unusual for the patient to be awakened by one. If this occurs, additional evaluations are warranted.

❽ The presence of a prodrome suggests a vascular origin. Migraine headaches are 3 times more common in women; estimated to affect 15% to 20% of adult women. Menstrual migraine headaches occur on days 1 to 4 of the menstrual cycle and can be distinguished from other forms of migraine on this basis.

❾ Vascular headaches (migraines) that lateralize are most often of the classic type, while those that are bilateral are more typical of the common type. Because each may mimic the other, additional attri-

butes must be used to differentiate these two types of migraines.

❿ Moderate to severe headaches that are poorly localized are most typical of those caused by general conditions such as anemia, uremia, hypertension (uncommon), or thyrotoxicosis. Trauma, muscle tension, and arteriosclerosis may also present with this pattern.

⓫ Lateralized, well-localized headaches are typical of migraines but may also reflect pathologies of other structures in and around the head.

⓬ Lateralized, well-localized headaches are typical of migraines but may also reflect pathologies of other structures in and around the head.

⓭ While frontal headaches may arise from muscle tension or galial sources, sinusitis or dental diseases are more common causes.

REFERENCES

APGO Educational Series on Women's Health Issues: Strategies for the Management of Headache. Washington, DC: APGO, 1998.

Edelson RN. Menstrual migraine and other hormonal aspects of migraine. Headache 1985;25:376–379.

Granella F, Sances G, Zanferrari C, et al. Migraine without aura and preproductive life events. A clinical epidemiologic study in 1300 women. Headache 1993;33:385–389.

Headache Classification Committee of the International Headache Society. Classification and diagnostic criteria for headache disorders, cranial neuralgia, and facial pain. Cephalagia 1988;8:1–96.

Kudrow L. The relationship of headache frequency to hormone use in migraine. Headache 1975;15:36.

Laube DW. Headache. In: Ling FW, Laube DW, Nolan TE, et al (eds): Primary Care in Gynecology. Baltimore: Williams & Wilkins, 1996, pp 87–100.

Silberstein SD. The role of sex hormones in headache. Neurology 1992;42:37–42.

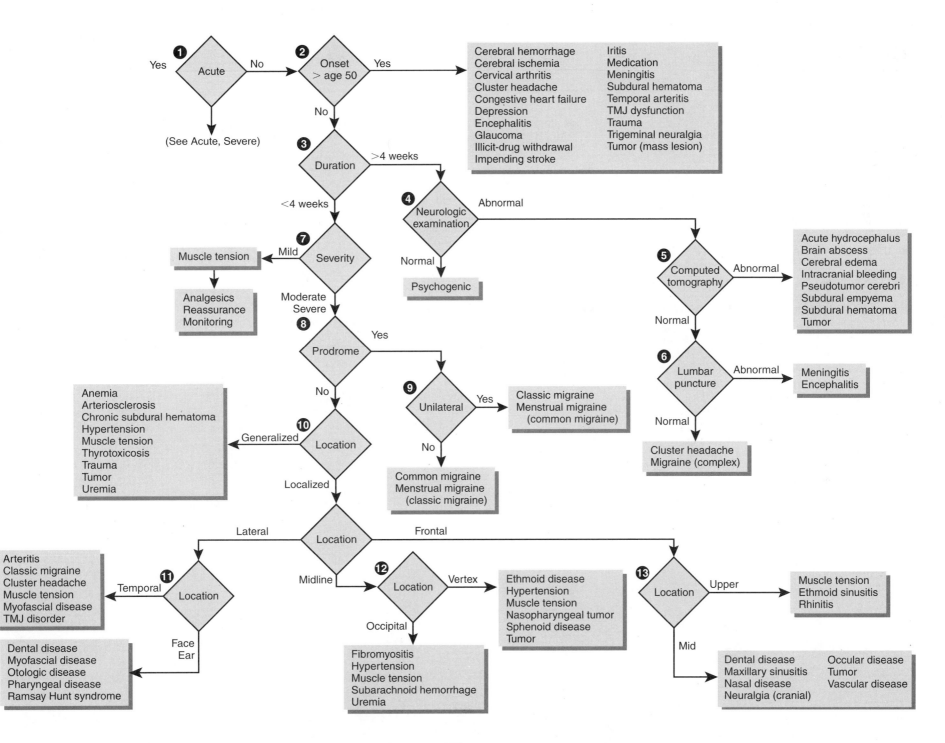

1 Acute — Yes → (See Acute, Severe)

No →

2 Onset > age 50 — Yes → Cerebral hemorrhage / Cerebral ischemia / Cervical arthritis / Cluster headache / Congestive heart failure / Depression / Encephalitis / Glaucoma / Illicit-drug withdrawal / Impending stroke / Iritis / Medication / Meningitis / Subdural hematoma / Temporal arteritis / TMJ dysfunction / Trauma / Trigeminal neuralgia / Tumor (mass lesion)

No →

3 Duration — >4 weeks → **4** Neurologic examination

<4 weeks → **7** Severity

4 Neurologic examination — Abnormal → **5** Computed tomography

Normal → Psychogenic

5 Computed tomography — Abnormal → Acute hydrocephalus / Brain abscess / Cerebral edema / Intracranial bleeding / Pseudotumor cerebri / Subdural empyema / Subdural hematoma / Tumor

Normal → **6** Lumbar puncture

6 Lumbar puncture — Abnormal → Meningitis / Encephalitis

Normal → Cluster headache / Migraine (complex)

7 Severity — Mild → Muscle tension → Analgesics / Reassurance / Monitoring

Moderate Severe → **8** Prodrome

8 Prodrome — Yes → **9** Unilateral

No → **10** Location

9 Unilateral — Yes → Classic migraine / Menstrual migraine (common migraine)

No → Common migraine / Menstrual migraine (classic migraine)

10 Location — Generalized → Anemia / Arteriosclerosis / Chronic subdural hematoma / Hypertension / Muscle tension / Thyrotoxicosis / Trauma / Tumor / Uremia

Localized → Location

Location — Lateral → **11** Location

Midline → **12** Location

Frontal → **13** Location

11 Location — Temporal → Arteritis / Classic migraine / Cluster headache / Muscle tension / Myofascial disease / TMJ disorder

Face Ear → Dental disease / Myofascial disease / Otologic disease / Pharyngeal disease / Ramsay Hunt syndrome

12 Location — Vertex → Ethmoid disease / Hypertension / Muscle tension / Nasopharyngeal tumor / Sphenoid disease / Tumor

Occipital → Fibromyositis / Hypertension / Muscle tension / Subarachnoid hemorrhage / Uremia

13 Location — Upper → Muscle tension / Ethmoid sinusitis / Rhinitis

Mid → Dental disease / Maxillary sinusitis / Nasal disease / Neuralgia (cranial) / Occular disease / Tumor / Vascular disease

Hematuria

INTRODUCTION

The symptom of blood in the urine may arise through misattribution, urinary tract infection, or causes that are more sinister. The first two, and most common, causes may be easily evaluated and treated. Patients with true hematuria not due to infection must be rapidly evaluated for the possibility of malignancy, which is presumed until another cause can be found or the possibility thoroughly eliminated.

❶ The first task when presented with the symptom of blood in the urine is to verify the source. Unlike in men, it is easy for blood from other sources to be admixed with urine, resulting in a misattribution as to source. A clean-catch urinalysis will usually resolve this issue. A catheterized specimen may be used, but is generally not necessary unless the patient is unable to comply or there is a suspicion of duplicity. Hematuria is generally defined as greater than 3 red blood cells per high-power field on routine urinalysis. Red cell casts suggest a renal source. Dipstick testing may give false-positive results in the presence of free hemoglobin.

❷ A urinary tract infection may cause hematuria without, or before, other symptoms become apparent. If the only symptom of infection was the presence of blood, a follow-up urinalysis should be performed at the conclusion of therapy to verify successful resolution.

❸ An abnormality of blood clotting, either natural or iatrogenic, may present with hematuria. Because up to 50% of patients with a coagulopathy have a coexisting cause, further evaluation by intravenous pyelography (IVP), cystoscopy, or other method should be strongly considered.

❹ The presence of significant proteinuria (>1 g/day) suggests significant renal parenchymal pathology and the need for a renal biopsy.

❺ The most common renal tumor (85%) is the renal cell carcinoma. More common sources of proteinuria and hematuria include acute and chronic glomerulonephritis, interstitial nephritis, and vasculitis. If the biopsy is negative, diagnoses such as benign familial hematuria and the hematuria associated with activity such as running should be considered.

❻ Intravenous pyelography may demonstrate the presence of renal tumors, polycystic kidneys, diverticula, or stones (renal or ureteral).

❼ Patients with hematuria but not proteinuria, who have normal pyelography, should be presumed to have a bladder or urethral source. Cystoscopy, with urethroscopy, is used to evaluate this possibility. Bladder and urethral tumors are more common in smokers.

❽ When no source for persistent hematuria is found, renal ateriography should be considered.

REFERENCES

Ahmed Z, Lee J. Asymptomatic urinary abnormalities. Hematuria and proteinuria. Med Clin North Am 1977;81(3):641.

Ahn JH, Morey AF, McAninch JW. Workup and management of traumatic hematuria. Emerg Med Clin North Am 1988;16:145.

Feld LG, Waz WR, Perez LM, Joseph DB. Hematuria. An integrated medical and surgical approach. Pediatr Clin North Am 1997;44:119.

Foresman WH, Messing EM. Bladder cancer: natural history, tumor markers, and early detection strategies. Semin Surg Oncol 1977;13:299.

Jayson M, Sanders H. Increased incidence of serendipitously discovered renal cell carcinoma. Urology 1998;51:203.

Mahan JD, Turman MA, Mentser MI. Evaluation of hematuria, proteinuria, and hypertension in adolescents. Pediatr Clin North Am 1997;44:1573.

McCarthy JJ. Outpatient evaluation of hematuria: locating the source of bleeding. Postgrad Med 1997;101:125.

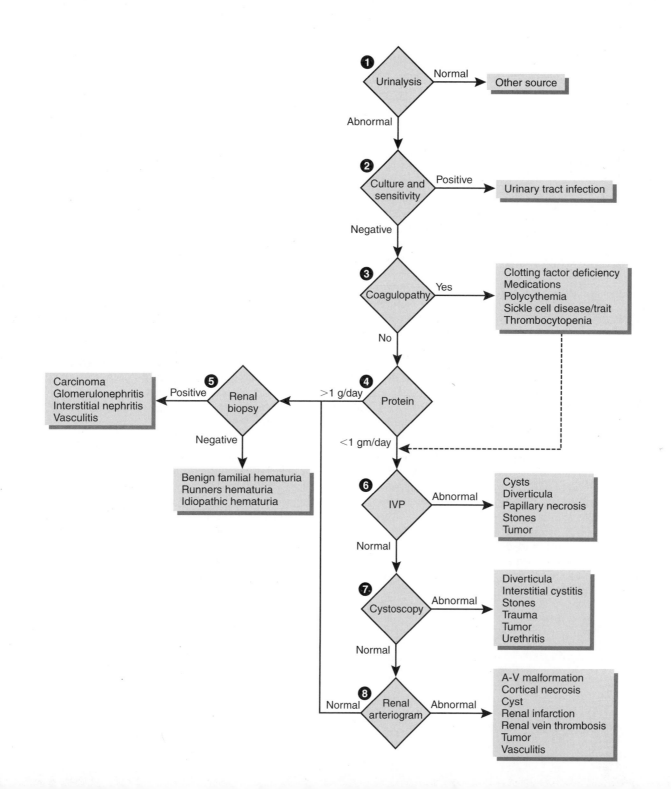

Hemorrhoids

INTRODUCTION

Symptomatic dilation of the hemorrhoidal venous plexus and the resulting perianal swelling, itching, pain, hematochezia, and fecal soiling are the hallmarks of what is traditionally referred to as "hemorrhoids." More common with increasing age, obesity, and heavy lifting, or in the presence of a chronic cough or bowel irregularity, for women they frequently become symptomatic during pregnancy and beyond. While a large percentage of patients will not seek help or will use over-the-counter or other remedies, the diagnosis and management of hemorrhoids in the office setting is straightforward. Symptoms may be acute, chronic, or relapsing.

❶ Small, external hemorrhoids are a common finding during the physical examination of parous women. If they are asymptomatic, observation and reinforcement of preventive measures such as perineal hygiene and bowel regularity are all that are required.

❷ When patients present with symptoms suggestive of hemorrhoids (rectal bleeding, itching, or fecal soiling) but no dilated vessels are found, a careful further evaluation is warranted. A number of other conditions (shown) can mimic the symptoms of hemorrhoids. Based on the patient's symptoms, flexible sigmoidoscopy or colonoscopy should be strongly considered. Some care must be used to differentiate large hemorrhoids from rectal prolapse, which requires surgical intervention.

❸ Thrombosis of a hemorrhoidal vessel is an indication for immediate surgical treatment. These are best treated by incision and drainage, which may be accomplished under local anesthesia in the office or emergency room setting.

❹ When symptoms are mild, simple treatments such as sitz baths and soothing witch hazel (methyl salicylate) pads are effective. Other therapies include stool softeners (docusate sodium (Colace, Dialose, Sof-Lax) 50 to 300 mg po qd (larger doses are generally divided over the day)); topical analgesic sprays or ointments such as benzocaine (Americaine, Hurricaine) 20% spray or gel and dibucaine (Nupercainal) 1% ointment; antipruritics and anti-inflammatory agents such as hydrocortisone (Anusol-HC, Analpram-HC, Cortenema, Cortifoam, Epifoam, Proctofoam-HC); and pramoxine 1% (Fleet rectal pads, Analpram-HC); and astringents (Preparation H). It should be remembered that docusate sodium may potentiate the hepatotoxicity of other drugs.

❺ Surgical therapy is appropriate for those patients with debilitating symptoms or failed medical therapy (15% to 20% of cases). The therapy chosen is based on the location of the hemorrhoids. Internal hemorrhoids are generally treated by rubber band ligation. Hemorrhoid banding may be performed in the office setting with a minimum of equipment. The hemorrhoid is gently grasped and brought into the band applier, two elastic bands are applied to the base and the hemorrhoid is left to necrose and slough. External hemorrhoids may be treated by a number of modalities, including cryosurgery, laser ablation, injection of sclerosing agents, and surgical excision.

❻ Following successful therapy of symptomatic hemorrhoids, it is important to stress perineal hygiene, adequate dietary fluids and fiber, and the reduction of modifiable risk factors if recurrent episodes are to be avoided.

REFERENCES

Bassford T. Treatment of common anorectal disorders (review). Am Fam Physician 1992;45:1787.

Bleday R, Pena JP, Rothenberger DA, et al. Symptomatic hemorrhoids: current incidence and complications of operative therapy. Dis Colon Rectum 1992;35:477–481.

Devine R, Ory S. Treatment of hemorrhoids in pregnancy. J Fam Pract 1992;17:65.

Guthri JF. The current management of hemorrhoid. Pract Gastroenterol 1987;11:56.

Mazier WP. Hemorrhoids, fissures, and pruritus ani (review). Surg Clin North Am 1994;74:1277.

Medich DS, Fazio VW. Hemorrhoids, anal fissure, and carcinoma of the colon, rectum, and anus during pregnancy. Surg Clin North Am 1995;75:77.

Schussman LC, Lutz LJ. Outpatient management of hemorrhoids. Prim Care 1986;13:527.

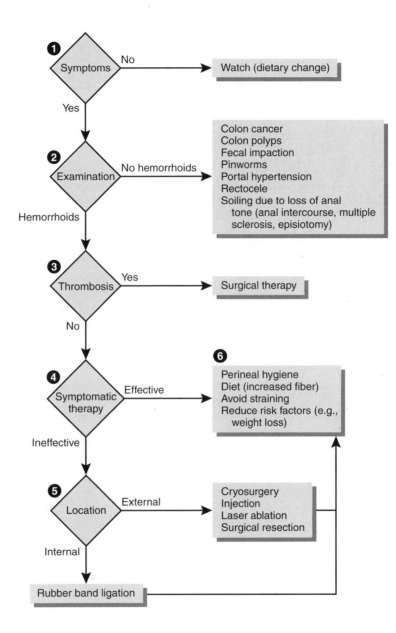

1 Symptoms — No → Watch (dietary change)

Yes ↓

2 Examination — No hemorrhoids → Colon cancer
Colon polyps
Fecal impaction
Pinworms
Portal hypertension
Rectocele
Soiling due to loss of anal
  tone (anal intercourse, multiple
  sclerosis, episiotomy)

Hemorrhoids ↓

3 Thrombosis — Yes → Surgical therapy

No ↓

4 Symptomatic therapy — Effective → **6** Perineal hygiene
Diet (increased fiber)
Avoid straining
Reduce risk factors (e.g.,
  weight loss)

Ineffective ↓

5 Location — External → Cryosurgery
Injection
Laser ablation
Surgical resection

Internal ↓

Rubber band ligation

Hidradenitis Suppurativa

INTRODUCTION

Hidradenitis suppurativa is a chronic, unrelenting, refractory infection of the skin and subcutaneous tissue, initiated by obstruction and subsequent inflammation of apocrine glands, with resultant sinus and abscess formation. This process may involve the axillae, vulva, and perineum. The infection is commonly a complex polymicrobial one that originates from organisms found on the surrounding skin, or vaginal and rectal flora. Vulvar abscess may rupture, dissect into surrounding tissues or form fistulae to adjacent areas.

❶ The clinical diagnosis of hidradenitis suppurativa may be difficult and often requires the use of biopsy. Biopsy of the lesions will reveal inflammation of the apocrine glands with occlusion of ducts, cystic dilation, and inspissation of keratin material. Multiple draining sinuses and abscesses are common.

❷ Because of the progesterone-mediated changes in apocrine function, some women will experience cyclic symptoms early in the course of the disease. This may be modified by the use of oral contraceptives.

❸ If oral contraceptive therapy is chosen, a monophasic agent with one of the newer progestins may give the best results. If satisfactory results are not obtained, the patient should be managed in the same manner as those cases without a cyclic character.

❹ Antibiotic therapy directed toward anaerobes and facultative anaerobes may provide some transient relief, though a complete cure is seldom obtained. Antibiotics such as tetracycline (2 gm po qd) or clindamycin (topical qd) have been suggested. Some authors advocate the addition of a topical steroid to help reduce inflammation.

❺ Isotretinoin (Accutane) has been shown to provide relief in roughly half of patients treated. This agent must be used with care because of its teratogenic effects. For this reason, it is often combined with oral contraceptive therapy.

❻ Surgical therapy must consist of wide local excision. Unroofing of abscesses or less than complete removal of the apocrine tissues will result in recurrences. Simple incision and drainage are not effective. The wound may be closed primarily or allowed to heal by secondary intention. Because of the amount of tissue that may be involved, skin grafts or flaps may be required in some cases.

REFERENCES

Basta A, Madej JG Jr. Hidradenoma of the vulva. Incidence and clinical observations. Eur J Gynecol Oncol 1990;11:185.

Sherman AL, Reid R. CO₂ laser for supperative hidradenitis of the vulva. J Reprod Med 1991;36:113.

Thomas R, Barnhill D, Bibro M, et al. Hidradenitis suppurativa: a case presentation and review of the literature. Obstet Gynecol 1985;66:592.

Wilkinson EJ, Stone IK. Atlas of Vulvar Disease. Baltimore: Williams & Wilkins, 1995, p 148.

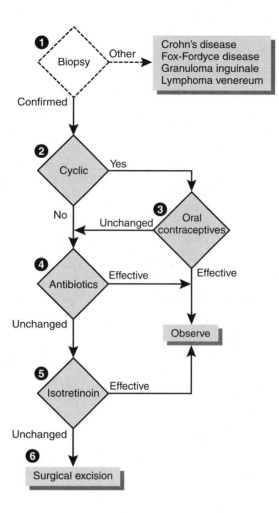

Hirsutism

INTRODUCTION

Hirsutism is generally defined as the presence of hair in locations where it is not normally found in a woman, such as the midline of the body, upper lip, chin, back, and intermammary region. Hirsutism depends on the genetically determined hair density, degree of androgen-mediated induction of terminal hairs, the ratio of growing to resting hairs, and the pigmentation of individual hairs. The degree of hirsutism is often quantitated using the Ferriman–Gallwey score, which assesses hair growth in 11 areas of the body.

❶ The first step in the evaluation of hirsutism is to determine if the diagnosis is correct. Patients with increased hair number, density, or coarseness that is predominantly peripheral and who lack midline hair are more correctly classed as having hypertrichosis. While this may be cosmetically distressing, it is most often familial or idiopathic in origin, stable, and best treated (if at all) by electrolysis or other hair removal methods.

❷ The next step in the evaluation of hirsutism is to inquire about other members of the family. Many ethnic groups and individual families have a greater or lesser density of hair follicles. As a result, some women may express an exaggerated response to normal levels of androgens, while others, such as Japanese women, have little response even in the face of excessive levels. When the family history indicates sporadic occurrences of others with similar hair distributions, the possibility of mosaicism should be considered.

❸ The patient should be carefully questioned about the use of medications, diet supplements, and over-the-counter heath or nutrition supplements. Many medications have androgenic side effects or can alter sex-binding globulin levels sufficiently to result in hirsutism or virilization. Examples include phenytoin, diazoxide, minoxidil, cyclosporine, glucocorticoids, penicillamine, and psoralens. Hirsutism has been reported by patients using danazol, metyrapone, some 19-nortestosterone derivatives used in oral contraceptives and androgens (for vulvar conditions). Performance-enhancing agents (anabolic steroids) used by athletes can have the same effect.

❹ A number of medical conditions, such as anorexia nervosa, Cushing's disease, hyperprolactinemia, hypothyroidism, obesity, porphyria, and some neurologic conditions may be associated with hypertrichosis. The patient's skin should be inspected for signs of acanthosis nigricans (verrucous, velvety, hyperpigmented skin changes) on the neck, axillae, and groin. This is a marker for insulin resistance. Acromegaly and chronic skin irritation can also result in increased hair growth.

❺ A careful search must be made for signs of virilization. Signs such as the loss of female sexual characteristics (body contour, breast volume) and the acquisition of masculine qualities such as increased muscle mass, temporal balding, deepening of the voice, and clitoromegaly suggest virilization. Virilization suggests the possibility of a serious medical condition that requires prompt and aggressive evaluation (discussed separately).

❻ Ultrasonography (abdominal or transvaginal) may suggest the presence of polycystic ovaries, stromal thickening, or a tumor. The clinical history will generally be sufficient to suggest polycystic ovary syndrome, but it may be confirmed by measuring the serum luteinizing hormore level. Selective catheterization of the ovarian veins or surgical exploration may be required when there is a strong suspicion of an ovarian tumor that is not found by imaging techniques.

❼ Elevations of 3α-androstanediol glucuronide (3α-AG) suggest an abnormality of the peripheral conversion of precursors into 5α-dihydrotestosterone (DHT) by the enzyme 5α-reductase. This abnormal conversion rate is typical in cases of idiopathic hirsutism. Elevations of dehydroepiandrosterone sulfate (DHEA-s) suggest an adrenal source, while ovarian causes generally result in elevated serum testosterone levels.

❽ Patients with familial or idiopathic hirsutism may be treated with antiandrogens such as cyproterone acetate, flutamine, or spironolactone. Cyproterone acetate competes for binding with androgen receptors and reduces the activity of 5α-reductase in the skin, though finasteride is a more potent blocker of this enzyme. Flutamine has been shown to be an effective antiandrogen, but a moderate rate of side effects has generally limited it use. Spironolactone has a long history of use and effectiveness. No treatment will reverse the growth of hair follicles that have already undergone induction. As a result, most treatment should be combined with mechanical means of hair removal as well.

❾ Suppression of nontumor adrenal sources of androgen is usually accomplished with corticosteroid therapy based on the specific pathology present. The antifungal, ketoconazole, has also been found to be effective through its alteration of the cytochrome P-450 enzyme system.

❿ When the source of excess androgens is from the ovary, oral contraceptives or gonadotropin-releasing hormone (GnRH) agonists may be effective. Tumors will require surgical evaluation and treatment.

REFERENCES

American College of Obstetricians and Gynecologists. Evaluation and Treatment of Hirsute Women. ACOG Technical Bulletin 203. Washington, DC: ACOG, 1995.

Carr BR, Breslau NA, Givens C, et al. Oral contraceptive pills, gonadotropin-releasing hormone agonists for use in combinations for treatment of hirsutism: A clinical research center study. J Clin Endocrinol Metab 1995;80:1169–1178.

Ferriman D, Gallwey JD. Clinical assessment of body hair growth in women. J Clin Endocrinol Metab 1961;21:1440.

Fruzzetti F, De Lorenzo D, Parrini D, Ricci C. Effects of finasteride, a 5α-reductase inhibitor, on circulating androgens and gonadotropin secretion in hirsute women. J Clin Endocrinol Metab 1994;79:831–835.

Kuttenn F, Couillin P, Girard F, et al. Late-onset adrenal hyperplasia in hirsutism. N Engl J Med 1985;313:224.

Rittmaster RS, Loriaux DL. Hirsuitism. Ann Intern Med 1987;106:95–107.

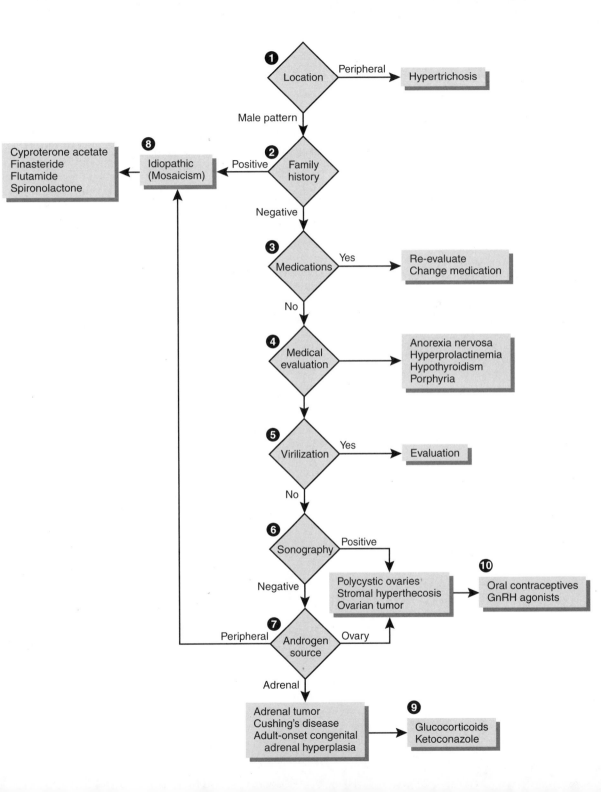

Hymeneal Stenosis

INTRODUCTION

Hymeneal stenosis is a thickening or narrowing of the hymeneal opening that causes difficulty with tampon use or intercourse. This may result from congenital narrowing of the hymen or scarring following trauma or surgery (e.g., previous excision).

❶ The most common symptoms of hymeneal stenosis are difficulty with the insertion of tampons and difficulty with intercourse. Care should be taken to distinguish a normal hymeneal remnant from symptoms caused by vestibulitis or vaginismus. Younger girls may develop recurrent vaginitis or vaginal odors due to trapping of urine behind a thickened or stenotic hymeneal rim.

❷ The character of the stenotic band can suggest the route of therapy: stiff tissues may require excision, while softer tissues may be treated more conservatively.

❸ If the stenotic band is soft in character, gentle stretching using the patient's fingers or progressively sized dilators may be sufficient to provide relief. Based on the patient's age, the addition of topical estrogen therapy may be helpful. If this is unsuccessful despite an adequate trial, surgical excision may be required.

❹ Care must be take to establish a correct diagnosis before surgical intervention is attempted. Vaginismus or phobic conditions often worsen after surgical therapy, and secondary scarring may result in as much disability as the original condition. When a stenotic hymen is incised surgically, incisions should be limited to the 4 to 5 and 7 to 8 o'clock positions and should extend only to base of the hymen, avoiding the base of the labia minora. Excision of the posterior hymeneal band is not required if it is soft and mobile. Tight bands or severe narrowing may require the use of a Z-plasty.

REFERENCES

Bachmann GA. Superficial dyspareunia and vestibulitis. In Sciarra JJ (ed): Gynecology and Obstetrics. Philadelphia: JB Lippincott, 1998;(1)77:1.

Smith RP. Gynecology in Primary Care. Baltimore: Williams & Wilkins, 1997, p 517.

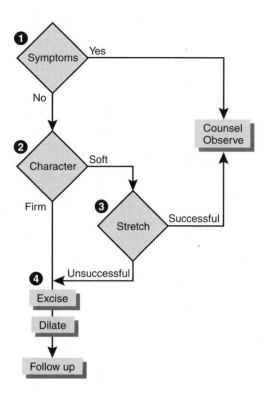

Hyperprolactinemia

INTRODUCTION

Elevated levels of prolactin may result in galactorrhea, though only about one third of patients with such elevations will have this symptom. (The absence of galactorrhea may be due to reduced levels of estrogen common in these patients.) Hyperprolactinemia may result in menstrual irregularities or amenorrhea. Roughly, one third of patients with secondary amenorrhea not due to pregnancy will have an elevated prolactin level.

❶ When serum levels of prolactin are greater than 100 ng/ml, the evaluation should proceed directly to imaging of the pituitary and surrounding structures. This should also be the first step if visual changes develop or there is a sudden appearance of, or change in, headaches.

❷ Hypothalamic lesions, stalk lesions, compression or transection, or pituitary tumors maybe visible using coned-down roentgenography, computed tomography, or magnetic resonance imaging. Most patients with prolactin levels in this range (>100 ng/ml) will have demonstrable lesions. The inability of these modalities to demonstrate an abnormality does not rule out the possibility of a small lesion. The evaluation of these patients should continue in the same manner as in those with lower prolactin levels.

❸ A large number of medications can cause increased levels of prolactin. These include amphetamines, α-methyldopa, butyrophenones, diazepam, estrogens, isoniazid, metoclopramide, opioids, oral contraceptives (high-dose), phenothiazines, reserpine, tricyclic antidepressants, and verapamil. If any of these agents are used by the patient, the need for them should be re-evaluated, and the medication either changed or withdrawn. If the medication is at fault, serum levels and symptoms should resolve over the subsequent 6 months. Endogenous sources of elevated estrogen should also be considered.

❹ A large number of medical diseases or conditions can result in elevated levels of prolactin by unregulated production (e.g., bronchogenic carcinoma) or altered metabolism (e.g., renal failure). While it is uncommon for these diseases to present through symptoms of galactorrhea, they must be considered.

❺ Persistent nipple stimulation caused by such things as cutaneous lesions (herpes), suckling, or continuing manual stimulation caused by obsessive behavior or patterns of sexual expression may result in elevated prolactin levels. The same neurologic arcs may be stimulated by thoracotomy scars or spinal lesions.

❻ While uncommon as causes of hyperprolactinemia, stress, trauma (resulting in pituitary stalk damage), surgery or anesthetic agents, and unrecognized central nervous system disease may result in elevated levels of prolactin. Galactorrhea that follows pregnancy in the absence of nursing (Chiari–Frommel syndrome) may be physiologic, though it is prudent to remain vigilant for the possibility of unrecognized disease.

REFERENCES

American College of Obstetricians and Gynecologists. Amenorrhea. Technical Bulletin 128, Washington, DC:ACOG, 1989.

Chang RJ, Keye WR, Young JR, et al. Detection, evaluation, and treatment of pituitary microadnomas in patients with galactorrhea and amenorrhea. Am J Obstet Gynecol 1977;128:356.

Schlechte J, Dolan K, Sherman B, et al. The natural history of untreated hyperprolactinemia: A prospective analysis. J Clin Endocrinol Metab 1989;68:412.

Smith RP. Gynecology in Primary Care. Baltimore: Williams & Wilkins, 1997, pp 405–426.

Speroff L, Glass RH, Kase NG. Clinical Gynecologic Endocrinology and Infertility, 5th ed. Baltimore: Williams & Wilkins, 1994, pp 404, 555–560.

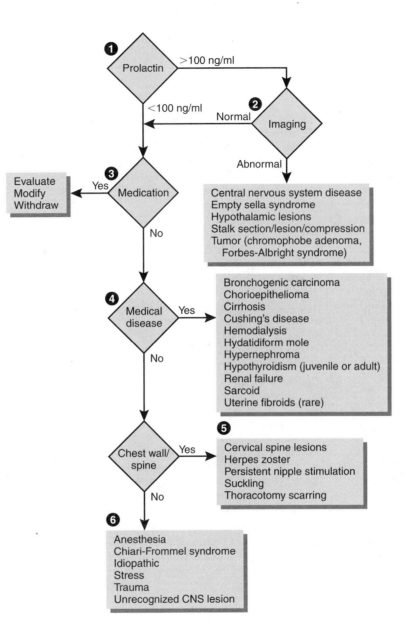

1 Prolactin

>100 ng/ml

<100 ng/ml

2 Imaging

Normal

Abnormal

3 Medication

Yes → Evaluate
Modify
Withdraw

No

Central nervous system disease
Empty sella syndrome
Hypothalamic lesions
Stalk section/lesion/compression
Tumor (chromophobe adenoma,
    Forbes-Albright syndrome)

4 Medical disease

Yes →

Bronchogenic carcinoma
Chorioepithelioma
Cirrhosis
Cushing's disease
Hemodialysis
Hydatidiform mole
Hypernephroma
Hypothyroidism (juvenile or adult)
Renal failure
Sarcoid
Uterine fibroids (rare)

No

Chest wall/ spine

Yes →

5
Cervical spine lesions
Herpes zoster
Persistent nipple stimulation
Suckling
Thoracotomy scarring

No

6
Anesthesia
Chiari-Frommel syndrome
Idiopathic
Stress
Trauma
Unrecognized CNS lesion

Immunizations During Pregnancy

INTRODUCTION

Ideally, all immunizations should be carried out prior to pregnancy. On occasion, immunization may need to be considered during pregnancy, or an immunization may be inadvertently given during an undiagnosed pregnancy. Active vaccination as prophylaxis should generally be deferred until after the pregnancy has ended. More common is the use of immune globulin to provide passive immunity after acute exposure. Examples of this include hepatitis A and B, rabies, tetanus, varicella, *Haemophilus influenzae* type B, *Neisseria meningitidis, Streptococcus pneumoniae*, and measles. (Erythroblastosis fetalis prevention represents an example of passive immunization using an immune globulin that does not involve an infective organism.)

❶ If immunization, either active or passive, is being considered for women of reproductive age, the possibility of an ongoing pregnancy must be considered. Live virus vaccines are generally not given electively during pregnancy and patients are generally advised to delay pregnancy for 3 months after their use. Passive immunization or immunization using other vaccines is possible, but other factors should be considered.

❷ Criteria for defining immunity vary by disease, requiring careful attention to the history of prior illness, previous immunization, and the results of serologic testing. In many cases (such as rubella) the history of disease is not sufficiently reliable to establish probable immunity. It is estimated that roughly 6% to 11% of reproductive-age women are not immune to rubella. These patients, and others, who lack immunity to other infections, potentially face the dilemma of immunization during pregnancy if they become exposed. (Persons born before 1957 are presumed to be immune to measles and mumps.)

❸ The risk of exposure to disease must be considered. While the patient may lack immunity to a given disease, if the prevalence or virulence of the disease is low, immunization by not be necessary. Risk factors such as occupation, social habits (drug use, multiple sexual partners), past medical history (splenectomy), and other factors should be considered in determining the likelihood of exposure or infection. Efforts should be made to reduce risk where possible (such as avoiding travel to areas of endemic disease and reducing risky behaviors).

❹ The risk to the mother or fetus posed by the disease must be considered. Infections such as influenza are not materially altered during pregnancy and do not pose extraordinary risk to the fetus, making immunization of otherwise healthy pregnant women unnecessary. Infections such as polio, tetanus, and hepatitis B pose special risks to the mother, fetus, or both, making prevention a priority when exposure has occurred, or is likely to occur.

❺ The final aspect that should be considered is the risk of the immunobiologic agent involved. Live viral or bacterial vaccine agents that pose a theoretical risk are generally avoided during pregnancy. The level of this risk is thought to be low: Roughly 275 patients who were given live virus rubella vaccine (RA27/3) have been followed to term without showing signs of ill effect, giving an estimated risk of 0% to 1.7%. Inactivated vaccines, immune globulins, and antitoxins appear to be safe for use in pregnancy, though in many cases the use of immune globulin to that the place of active immunization have not been shown to alter the risk of fetal infection or maternal disease.

REFERENCES

American College of Obstetricians and Gynecologists. Immunization During Pregnancy. ACOG Technical Bulletin 160. Washington, DC: ACOG, 1991.

Centers for Disease Control and Prevention. Prevention and control of influenza recommendations of the Advisory Committee on Immunization Practices (ACIP). MMWR 1995;44(RR-3):1–22.

Hayward RS, Steinberg EP, Ford DE, et al. Preventive care guidelines: 1991. Ann Intern Med 1991;114:758–783.

Task Force on Adult Immunization. Adult immunizations 1994. Ann Intern Med 1994;121:540.

Task Force on Primary and Preventive Health Care of the American College of Obstetricians and Gynecologists. The Obstetrician–Gynecologist and Primary–Preventive Health Care. Washington, DC: ACOG, 1993.

Update on adult immunization: Recommendations of the Immunization Practices Advisory Committee. MMWR 1991;40(No. RR–12):Table 7.

U.S. Preventive Services Task Force. Guide to Clinical Preventive Services, 2nd ed. Baltimore: Williams and Wilkins, 1995.

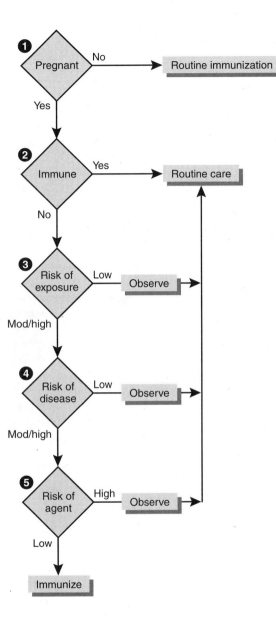

Imperforate Hymen

INTRODUCTION

An imperforate hymen is the most commonly encountered anomaly due to abnormalities in the development or canalization of the müllerian ducts. This abnormality results from a failure of the endoderm of the urogenital sinus and the epithelium of the vaginal vestibule to fuse and perforate during embryonic development. Although most commonly diagnosed during adolescence, an imperforate hymen may be diagnosed during infancy, though the redundancy of the labial folds caused by maternal estrogen generally obscures the condition at birth.

❶ A bulging mass at the introitus in young girls, or primary amenorrhea in the presence of well-established secondary sex characteristics, should suggest the possibility of an imperforate hymen. Up to a liter of mucus or blood can be contained in the vagina behind the obstructing membrane. Compression by this mass may result in compromise of urinary or intestinal function. Because endometriosis is common with long-standing cryptomenorrhea and retrograde flow, adnexal masses are also common. Rarely, the inability to use a tampon or have intercourse will be the presenting complaint.

❷ The first step in management is to establish the diagnosis. If the physical examination establishes the presence of a normal vaginal opening, the source of the symptoms the patient is experiencing must be sought elsewhere. A cribriform or stenotic hymen may produce some of the same symptoms, but is treated more conservatively (see Hymeneal Stenosis).

❸ When no apparent opening is present, the patient should be asked to strain. (Younger patients may be examined while crying to produce the same effect.) Patients with a true imperforate hymen will demonstrate a bulging of the introitus, while patients with labial fusion will not.

❹ Before treatment for a presumed imperforate hymen, some form of evaluation of the upper genital tract must be made. Gentle rectal examination, pelvic ultrasonography, or other imaging technique must be used to determine the presence or absence of a cervix and uterus. Patients with complete vaginal or uterine agenesis must be evaluated and treated in a very specialized manner.

❺ Surgical treatment of an imperforate hymen consists of complete excision of the membrane, not simple incision. Carbon dioxide laser is preferred by many because it allows superior hemostasis while producing less tissue damage and fewer postoperative complications. If an hydrometrocolpos or hematometra is present, it must be drained and antibiotic coverage provided. Postoperative topical estrogen treatment may reduce the risk of scarring even in women of reproductive age.

REFERENCES

Baramki TA. The treatment of congenital anomalies in girls and women. J Reprod Med 1984;29:376.

Greiss FC, Mauzy CH. Congenital anomalies in women: an evaluation of diagnosis, incidence, and obstetric performance. Am J Obstet Gynecol 1961;82:330.

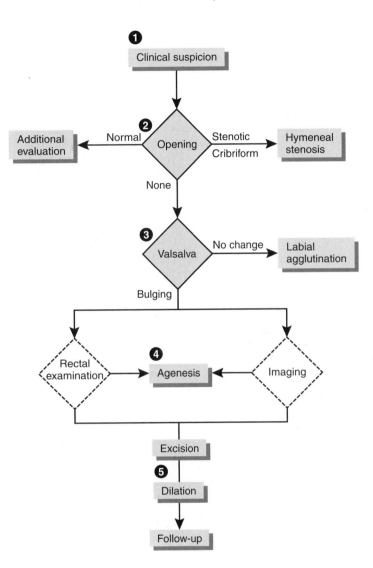

In Utero Diethylstilbestrol Exposure

INTRODUCTION

In utero exposure to diethylstilbestrol (DES) is associated with an increased risk of several reproductive sequellae: vaginal adenosis, cervical ectropion, structural abnormalities of the cervix and upper vagina (including transverse ridges, cervical collars, hoods, cockscombs, cervical hypoplasia, and pseudopolyps), and alterations in the shape of the uterine cavity. The association of in utero DES exposure and clear cell adenocarcinoma (risk approxiamately 1:4,000) has prompted recommendations that these women undergo more vigorous cancer surveillance.

❶ Most women recall medications taken during pregnancy and may pass this information to their daughters or be available to answer questions. The actual use of DES during pregnancy should be confirmed through the medical records of the pregnancy when ever possible.

❷ Women exposed to DES in utero should begin periodic examinations by age 14 (or menarche, which ever is earlier). The evaluation begins with careful inspection and palpation, before the collection of cytologic specimens from the cervix and vaginal fornicies. Lubricants should not be used because they interfere with the interpretation of the specimens. The pelvic examination should involve a speculum examination that includes inspection of the entire vaginal wall and standard cervical cytology (Pap smear). Any abnormality found should prompt a colposcopic evaluation. Normal patients may be reassured, but should continue annual examinations for life.

❸ The colposcopic examination of DES-exposed women should involve careful inspection of the vaginal walls as well as the cervix itself. Cytologic specimens should be obtained and labeled separately to identify the location of any abnormality found. Vaginal adenosis generally has a grapelike appearance, while squamous metaplasia may have a punctate or mosaic pattern similar to that of intraepithelial neoplasia in unexposed women. Any area of abnormality should be biopsied to obtain a final diagnosis.

❹ If biopsies are normal, the suspicious area should be documented in the chart and the patient re-evaluated every 6 months.

❺ Normal colposcopic evaluations should be supplemented by the application of half-strength Lugol's solution. This will help to identify areas of metaplasia, adenosis, or ectropion. If abnormalities are identified, the location should be documented in the medical record and the patient followed at intervals of 6 months until the examinations are again normal. If no abnormalities are identified, annual examinations will suffice.

REFERENCES

Herbst AL, Ulfelder H, Poskanzer DC. Adenocarcinoma of the vagina: Association of maternal stilbestrol therapy with tumor appearance in young women. N Engl J Med 1971;284:878.

Hillard PA. Benign diseases of the female reproductive tract: Symptoms and signs. In Berek JS, Adashi EY, Hillard PA (eds). Novak's Gynecology, 12th ed. Baltimore: Williams & Wilkins, 1996, p 390.

Melnick D, Cole P, Anderson D, Horbst A. Rates and risks of diethylstilbestrol-related clear cell adenocarcinoma of the vagina and cervix. N Engl J Med 1987;316:514.

Mishell DR, Stenchever MA, Droegemueller W, Herbst AL. Comprehensive Gynecology, 3rd ed. St Louis: CV Mosby, 1997, p 389.

Sedlacek TV, Riva JM, Magen AB, et al. Vaginal and vulvar adenosis: an unsuspected side effect of CO_2 laser vaporization. J Reprod Med 1990;35:995.

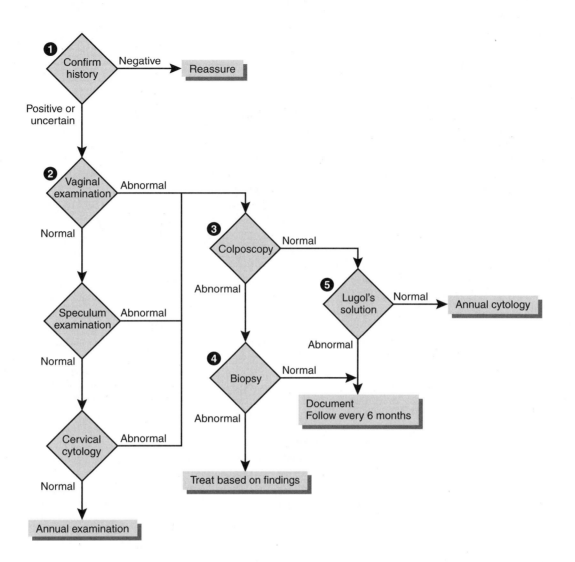

Infertility

INTRODUCTION

Infertility affects approximately 15% of all couples who attempt to conceive. The evaluation of infertility is independent of whether there has been a previous conception or not. Roughly 10% to 20% of couples have no identifiable cause for their infertility (idiopathic).

❶ As with many conditions, the evaluation of infertility begins with a complete history and physical examination. This should focus on factors associated with reduced fertility in either partner (pelvic infections, surgery, mumps) and physical findings that suggest an impediment to conception (vericocele, genital tract anomaly).

❷ Because up to 40% of infertility is of male origin, the first step in the evaluation of an infertile couple is a semen analysis. This test is quick to perform and will assesses a major source of infertility. This test should be performed even when the male partner has fathered children in the past. The evaluation of male-factor infertility is discussed separately.

❸ The next step is to assess ovulatory function in the female. Between 10% and 15% of infertility is caused by an ovulatory disorder. The presence of ovulation may be inferred on the basis of a basal body temperature chart recorded over a period of two or three cycles. This chart can also record the frequency and timing of intercourse relative to ovulation. Other methods of ovulation detection (urinary luteinizing hormone, salivary progesterone) may be substituted if desired.

❹ Because basal body temperature evaluations may not completely reflect ovulation, patients who have a flat or equivocal study should have an endometrial biopsy performed. This is a more sensitive test of ovulation and can allow assessment of the endometrial response to hormonal stimulation at the same time.

❺ If anovulation is confirmed, hysterosalpingography should be performed to assess tubal patency. Tubal factors are present in 20% to 30% of infertile couples. For this reason, tubal patency must be established prior to ovulation induction.

❻ An assessment of the function and suitability of cervical mucus may be appropriate for patients who are ovulatory. The Huhner–Sims (postcoital) test has generally fallen out of favor, but may be useful to confirm sperm deposition and to look for evidence of antisperm antibodies, though more direct tests are now available.

❼ Laparoscopy may be required to asses tubal status and to look for other factors such as pelvic adhesive disease or endometriosis. Surgical therapy at the time of laparoscopy or at a later date may be instituted based on the pathology present. When this examination is normal, assisted reproductive technologies may be indicated.

REFERENCES

American College of Obstetricians and Gynecologists. Infertility. ACOG Technical Bulletin 125. Washington, DC: ACOG, 1989.

American College of Obstetricians and Gynecologists. Male Infertility. ACOG Technical Bulletin 142. Washington, DC: ACOG, 1990.

American College of Obstetricians and Gynecologists. Managing the Anovulatory State: Medical Induction of Ovulation. ACOG Technical Bulletin 142. Washington, DC: ACOG, 1997.

Office of Technology Assessment. Infertility: Medical and Social Choices. Washington, DC: Congress of the United States, 1988:25.

Mosher WD, Pratt WF. Fecundity and infertility in the United States, 1965–1988. Advance Data 1990;192:1–6.

Smith RP. Gynecology in Primary Care. Baltimore: Williams & Wilkins, 1997, pp 339–358.

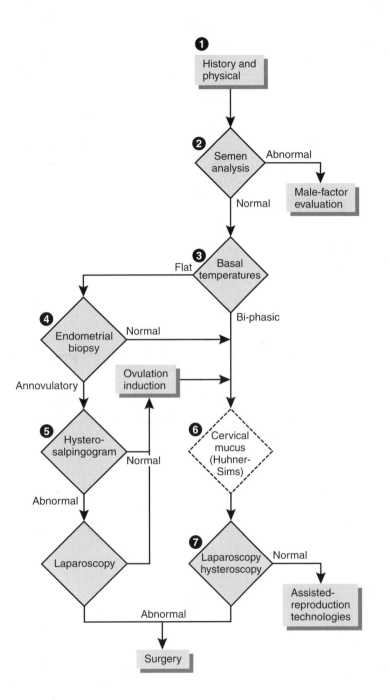

Infertility

Male Factor

INTRODUCTION

While many providers of gynecologic care will prefer to refer patients with male-factor infertility, an acquaintance with the testing procedures is still valuable in counseling the infertile couple.

❶ As with many conditions, the evaluation of infertility begins with a complete history and physical examination. This should focus on factors associated with reduced fertility in either partner (pelvic infections, surgery, mumps) and physical findings that suggest an impediment to conception (varicocele, genital tract anomaly). When the semen analysis is normal, the evaluation should proceed as outlined separately. Consideration should be given to a sperm penetration assay in those few couples in whom evaluation of the female partner is fruitless.

❷ Classification of the male is based on two or three semen analyses. Semen analysis is carried out after a minimum of 48 hours of abstinence. When a semen analysis is abnormal, it should be repeated, with careful attention given to appropriate abstinence and sample collection. If the repeat analysis is normal, evaluation of the female partner can proceed.

❸ Equivocal semen analysis tests may be followed by a sperm penetration test. The sperm penetration assay is best used to evaluate men with inconsistent or inconclusive semen analysis and those undergoing treatment for infertility, prior to expensive or invasive tests or therapies, and couples with prolonged unexplained infertility. This test indicates the functionality of the sperm present. If abnormalities are found, a referral is indicated.

❹ If the semen analysis is persistently abnormal, possible causes should be sought and consideration should be given to referral. Some conditions, such as varicocele, may be corrected, resulting in a return of fertility.

REFERENCES

American College of Obstetricians and Gynecologists. Infertility. ACOG Technical Bulletin 125. Washington, DC: ACOG, 1989.

American College of Obstetricians and Gynecologists. New Reproductive Technologies. ACOG Technical Bulletin 140. Washington, DC: ACOG, 1990.

American College of Obstetricians and Gynecologists. Male Infertility. ACOG Technical Bulletin 142. Washington, DC: ACOG, 1990.

Office of Technology Assessment. Infertility: Medical and social choices. Washington, DC: Congress of the United States, 1988:25.

Rogers BJ. The sperm penetration assay: Its usefulness reevaluated. Fertil Steril 1985;43:821.

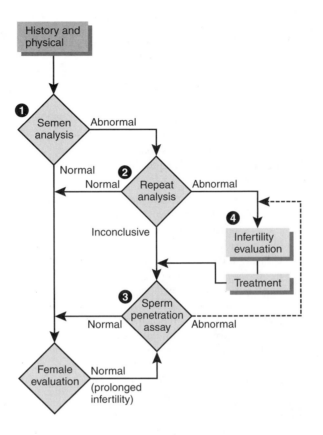

Intermenstrual Bleeding (Dysfunctional Uterine Bleeding)

Diagnosis

INTRODUCTION

The evaluation of irregular or intermenstrual bleeding with no clinically identifiable underlying cause can be broken down by the most common causes encountered over the patient's lifetime. Therapy for the most commonly encountered form (anovulatory bleeding) is discussed separately.

❶ Soon after birth, some female infants will have vaginal spotting due to the loss of stimulation from maternal estrogens. Tumors, vaginal irritation, or lacerations must be ruled out.

❷ In prepubescent girls, the possibility of foreign bodies or infection should be considered. This may take the form of mechanical or chemical irritation from toilet or bathing products, toilet paper, or laundry products. Less common causes include tumors (ovarian or sarcoma botryoides). The prospect of trauma must also be considered.

❸ Irregular periods are common during the early stages of a woman's menstrual function and are caused by immaturity of the pituitary–hypothalamic–ovarian axis, which results in anovulation. This may also be induced by psychosocial stress, including that associated with eating disorders. Blood dyscrasias that may have gone undetected may manifest with intermenstrual bleeding or menorrhagia.

❹ Dysfunctional bleeding is most commonly encountered during the reproductive years. The possibility of pregnancy must always be considered first in these patients. Uterine, cervical, and vaginal causes, including cancer, must be sought and treated when encountered. Sometimes, our own interventions may result in dysfunctional bleeding or other menstrual disturbances through side effects or direct actions of medications, surgery, or other therapy. Systemic illnesses such as hypothyroidism may cause intermenstrual bleeding and should be considered before the diagnosis of anovulation is rendered. (The evaluation of anovulation is discussed under Secondary Amenorrhea.)

❺ Climacteric patients (those around the age of menopause) may experience dysfunctional bleeding as ovulation become less certain and serum levels of hormones fluctuate. The possibility of endometrial cancer or cervical lesions must always be evaluated.

❻ While the possibility of sinister sources of bleeding such as uterine or ovarian cancer must be considered, vaginal atrophy and bleeding induced by hormone therapy are more common causes of dysfunctional bleeding in postmenopausal women.

REFERENCES

Aksel S, Jones GS. Etiology and treatment of dysfunctional uterine bleeding. Obstet Gynecol 1974;44:1.

American College of Obstetricians and Gynecologists. Dysfunctional Uterine Bleeding. ACOG Technical Bulletin 134. Washington, DC: ACOG, 1989.

Bayer RL, DeCherney AH. Clinical manifestations and treatment of dysfunctional uterine bleeding. JAMA 1993;269:1823.

Cowan BD, Morrison JC. Management of abnormal genital bleeding in girls and women. N Engl J Med 1991;324:1710.

Field CS. Dysfunctional uterine bleeding. Prim Care 1988;15:561.

Neese RE. Managing abnormal vaginal bleeding. Postgrad Med 1991;89:205.

Smith RP. Gynecology in Primary Care. Baltimore: Williams & Wilkins, 1997, pp 25–48.

Smith RP. Gynecology in Primary Care. Baltimore: Williams & Wilkins, 1997, pp 375–388.

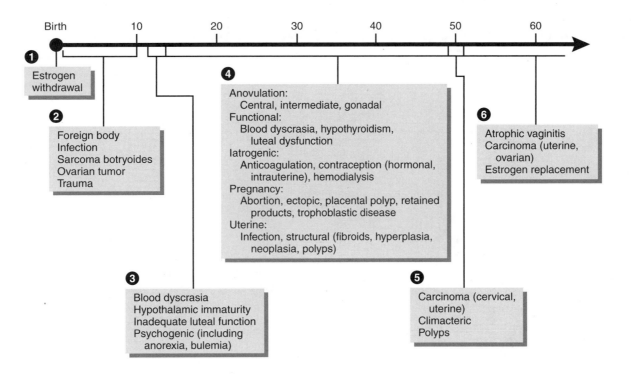

Birth   10   20   30   40   50   60

❶
Estrogen
withdrawal

❷
Foreign body
Infection
Sarcoma botryoides
Ovarian tumor
Trauma

❸
Blood dyscrasia
Hypothalamic immaturity
Inadequate luteal function
Psychogenic (including
    anorexia, bulemia)

❹
Anovulation:
    Central, intermediate, gonadal
Functional:
    Blood dyscrasia, hypothyroidism,
    luteal dysfunction
Iatrogenic:
    Anticoagulation, contraception (hormonal,
    intrauterine), hemodialysis
Pregnancy:
    Abortion, ectopic, placental polyp, retained
    products, trophoblastic disease
Uterine:
    Infection, structural (fibroids, hyperplasia,
    neoplasia, polyps)

❺
Carcinoma (cervical,
    uterine)
Climacteric
Polyps

❻
Atrophic vaginitis
Carcinoma (uterine,
    ovarian)
Estrogen replacement

Intermenstrual Bleeding (Dysfunctional Uterine Bleeding)

Therapy

INTRODUCTION

For menstrual-age women with dysfunctional uterine bleeding (intermenstrual bleeding with no clinically apparent cause), effective therapy can be instituted after a minimal evaluation. If a prompt relief of symptoms is not obtained, further evaluation is required.

❶ Based on the age of the patient, certain minimum evaluations should be performed prior to instituting therapy. (A full discussion of possible causes of dysfunctional uterine bleeding is carried out separately.) All patients must be assessed for the possibility of pregnancy-related bleeding.

❷ Patients below the age of 15 should undergo a pelvic and rectal examination and have their bleeding time evaluated prior to therapy.

❸ Patients between the ages of 15 and 20 should have a pelvic examination to rule out causes other than anovulation.

❹ Patients above the age of 20 should have a routine pelvic examination (including cervical cytology) and should be considered for endometrial biopsy based on the character of the bleeding and the presence or absence of risk factors. Transvaginal ultrasonography to evaluate the endometrial thickness may be used to augment other evaluations. Its reliability remains to be fully established and is dependent on the skill and technique of the person performing the test.

❺ When bleeding is determined to be anovulatory (or without clinically identifiable cause) and is heavy, moderate- to high-dose combined estrogen and progestin therapy for 7 days will generally result in control. When estrogen levels are thought to be normal, medroxyprogesterone acetate may be substituted. (In roughly 85% of patients who have been ovulatory in the past, a single cycle provides adequate response.)

❻ Once initial cycle control is obtained, consideration should be given to cyclic estrogen and progestin (oral contraceptive) therapy for period of 3 months. (Medroxyprogesterone acetate may be substituted at a rate of 5 to 10 mg for 1 to 14 days each month.)

❼ Long-term therapy (if any) should be determined by the contraceptive needs of the patient and any history of previous occurrences of similar bleeding episodes. Cyclic progestin therapy can be very effective in these patients but does not provide contraceptive protection. For those patients who need contraception, continued oral contraceptive therapy is more appropriate.

REFERENCES

American College of Obstetricians and Gynecologists. Dysfunctional Uterine Bleeding. ACOG Technical Bulletin 134. Washington, DC: ACOG, 1989.

Bayer RL, DeCherney AH. Clinical manifestations and treatment of dysfunctional uterine bleeding. JAMA 1993;269:1823.

Cowan BD, Morrison JC. Management of abnormal genital bleeding in girls and women. N Engl J Med 1991;324:1710.

Field CS. Dysfunctional uterine bleeding. Prim Care 1988;15:561.

Neese RE. Managing abnormal vaginal bleeding. Postgrad Med 1991;89:205.

Smith RP. Gynecology in Primary Care. Baltimore: Williams & Wilkins, 1997, pp 375–388.

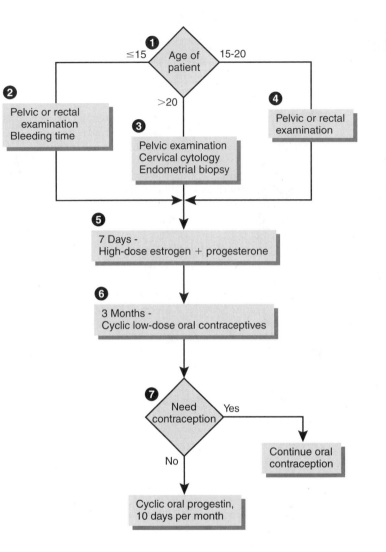

❶ Age of patient

≤15   15-20

>20

❷
Pelvic or rectal
examination
Bleeding time

❸
Pelvic examination
Cervical cytology
Endometrial biopsy

❹
Pelvic or rectal
examination

❺
7 Days -
High-dose estrogen + progesterone

❻
3 Months -
Cyclic low-dose oral contraceptives

❼ Need contraception

Yes

No

Continue oral
contraception

Cyclic oral progestin,
10 days per month

Labial Agglutination (Fusion)

INTRODUCTION

Labial agglutination is the most common form of vaginal obstruction found in young girls. While most often asymptomatic, retention of urine in the vestibule or vagina can result in irritation, discharge, and odor. Generally, fusion of the labia majora occurs in the midline and extends from just below the clitoris to the posterior fourchette. It is rare in neonates and in reproductive-age women because of their higher estrogen levels. Fusion arises when friction, infection, or injury results in epithelial damage. Subsequent healing results in midline scarring.

❶ If urinary retention is present, it constitutes a surgical emergency. Immediate suprapubic drainage of the bladder should be established, with subsequent sharp dissection of the obstructing fusion.

❷ The presence of a mass suggests complete obstruction. The origin of the mass must be determined before therapeutic options are considered.

❸ The most expeditious way of determining the source of the mass is to perform ultrasonography. If the mass is a distended bladder, immediate drainage must be established. If the mass is an obstructed vagina, sharp dissection of the fusion should be performed. If surgical incision is performed, appropriate antibiosis should be considered and topical estrogen treatment should be instituted.

❹ While examining the patient thought to have labial fusion, the presence of a thin lucent midline line should be noted. If this is absent, the obstruction is most probably an imperforate hymen and not labial fusion. Patients with an imperforate hymen require a different course of management and treatment (discussed separately).

❺ Patients with labial fusion should be treated with topical estrogen cream. The labia should never be separated manually because doing so results in acute pain, dysuria, and a loss of cooperation in young patients that will impede further evaluation or treatment. Manual separation also results in denuded epithelial edges, which will either produce scarring or recurrence of fusion. Topical estrogen therapy will generally cause spontaneous separation within 4 to 8 weeks. Transient side effects, such as breast tenderness or vulvar hyperpigmentation, may occur, but regress after treatment stops.

REFERENCES

Slupik R. Pediatric gynecology. In Sciarra JJ (ed): Obstetrics and Gynecology. Philadelphia: JB Lippincott, 1991;1–19:14.

Smith RP. Gynecology in Primary Care. Baltimore: Williams & Wilkins, 1997, p 177.

Stovall TG, Murman D. Urinary retention secondary to labial adhesions. Adolesc Pediatr Gynecol 1988;1:203.

Wells EC. Simple operation of the vulva. In Sciarra JJ (ed): Obstetrics and Gynecology. Philadelphia: JB Lippincott, 1998;(1)11:10.

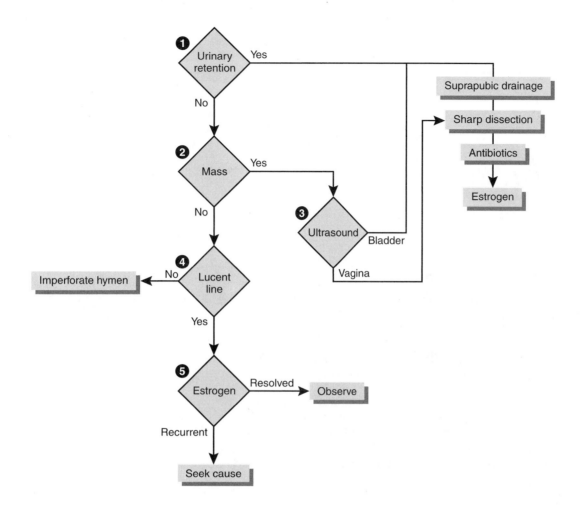

Menopause

Management Strategies

INTRODUCTION

The physiology of menopause has not changed, but our view of it has. Menopause is now viewed as an endocrinopathy: the loss of an endocrine function with adverse health consequences. This may occur as a result of the loss of normal ovarian steroidogenesis due to age, chemotherapy, radiation, or surgical therapy. Estrogen replacement therapy has evolved from an option to treat persistent symptoms to a prophylactic option to promote long-term health. The diagnosis is most often clinical, but when the diagnosis of ovarian failure must be confirmed, measurement of serum follicle-stimulating hormone (FSH) is sufficient. Levels of greater than 100 mlU/ml are diagnostic, though lower levels (40 to 50 mlU/ml) may be sufficient to establish a diagnosis when symptoms are also present. Serum estradiol levels may be determined (generally less than 15 pg/ml) but are less reliable as a marker of ovarian failure. A pregnancy test is always indicated in sexually active climacteric women who are not using contraception.

❶ Ninety-five percent of American women will go through natural menopause between the ages of 45 and 55 years. When spontaneous menopause occurs prior to age 45, the possibility of a polyendocrinopathy must be considered. Deletions of a portion of the X chromosome are associated with shortened stature and premature menopause. When this is suspected, a karyotype should be performed.

❷ The loss of ovarian steroids, whether by natural, surgical, or other causes, is often associated with symptoms. Hot flashes, flushes, and disturbances of sleep most often accompany abrupt loss. Gradual loss often results in dysfunctional uterine bleeding. Both can result in atrophic changes in the bladder and genital tract, and increased risks for cardiovascular disease, osteoporosis, and other sequellae.

❸ The loss of ovarian function represents a major change in body and personal image for many women. These changes often prompt a new receptivity to health issues. As a result, an important aspect of care for these women must be the encouragement of a healthy life-style, good diet, and exercise programs. Systemic estrogen replacement is an important part of dealing with the symptoms of estrogen loss. (Less than 1% of women will not benefit from therapy. Only 17% of women use estrogen, 55% never start, and 28% try but discontinue therapy.)

❹ Systemic estrogen therapy is associated with a roughly eight-fold increase in the risk of endometrial cancer. If a progestin is added to the hormone replacement (in adequate amounts and for an adequate duration) the risk of uterine cancer is reduced to below the untreated rate.

❺ If symptoms respond to therapy, periodic health maintenance, including annual mammography, cervical cytology (if indicated), and periodic sigmoidoscopy, thyroid function, and serum cholesterol, are indicated.

❻ If symptoms do not resolve, increasing the dose of estrogen, or moving to a more potent preparation (such as β-estradiol) will generally provide relief. Symptoms of breast tenderness, bloating, or depression often resolve in the first few months of treatment or respond to a reduction in the dose or potency of the progestin.

❼ Asymptomatic patient (roughly 15% of menopausal women) should be evaluated for special risk factors that suggest a need for the prophylactic effects of estrogen treatment. Patients with a family history of cardiovascular disease or osteoporosis derive significant protective effects from estrogen therapy. Reductions in the risk of ovarian, uterine, and colon cancer, Alzheimer's disease, and other conditions is less well defined.

❽ As with symptomatic women, those who are receiving prophylactic hormone replacement therapy and still retain their uterus must receive progestin therapy at the same time. This may be supplied as a continuous low-dose supplement, or as periodic progestin therapy.

❾ Often the start of hormone replacement therapy is associated with transient symptoms. If symptoms do not resolve, altering the dose of estrogen, or moving to a different route or more potent preparation (such as β-estradiol), will generally provide relief. Symptoms of breast tenderness, bloating, or depression often resolve in the first few months of treatment or respond to a reduction in the dose or potency of the progestin.

❿ Not all women will have apparent risk factors that recommend hormone replacement therapy. These patients should still be counseled about healthy choices in lifestyle, diet, and exercise.

⓫ Studies suggest that even in the absence of risk factors, hormone replacement therapy may still provide a protective effect for cardiovascular disease, osteoporosis, urogenital function, and other hormone-based effects. These effects should be discussed in an open manner, allowing the patient free choice in the use of replacement.

⓬ The patient who chooses not to, or cannot, use hormone replacement therapy should still be accorded the benefit of annual mammography, cervical cytology (if indicated), and periodic sigmoidoscopy, thyroid function checks, and measurements of serum cholesterol. The patient should also be periodically re-evaluated for the emergence of symptoms or risk factors that would prompt a reconsideration of replacement therapy.

REFERENCES

American College of Obstetricians and Gynecologists. Hormone Replacement Therapy. ACOG Technical Bulletin 247. Washington, DC: ACOG, 1998.

American College of Obstetricians and Gynecologists. Health Maintenance for Perimenopausal Women. ACOG Technical Bulletin 210. Washington, DC: ACOG, 1995.

Grodstein F, Stampfer MJ, Colditz GA. Postmenopausal hormone therapy and mortality. N Engl J Med 1997;336:1769.

Lobo RA. Benefits and risks of estrogen replacement therapy. Am J Obstet Gynecol 1995;173:982.

Sherwin BB. Hormones, mood and cognitive functioning in postmenopausal women. Obstet Gynecol 1996;87:20S.

Udoff L, Langenberg P, Adashi EY. Combined continuous hormone replacement therapy: a critical review. Obstet Gynecol 1995;86:306.

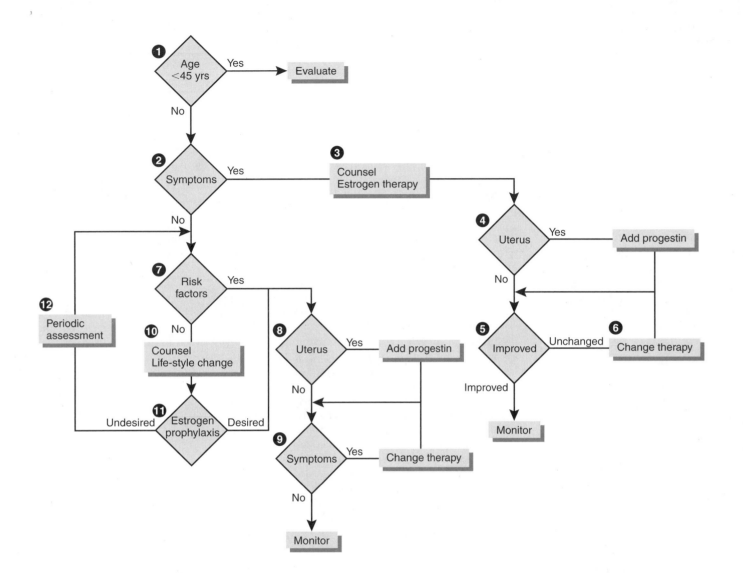

147

Menorrhagia

INTRODUCTION

Heavy vaginal bleeding may arise from many causes and represent a continuing inconvenience or an acute threat to life. By its nature, even the diagnosis of heavy vaginal bleeding is difficult to establish in all but the extreme cases. Even when quantitation is not possible, the complaint of excessive bleeding deserves at least cursory evaluation.

❶ Acute vaginal bleeding has both a different significance and a different set of causes from that which is chronic or intermittent (true menorrhagia). Because the volume of blood lost can be significant, acute bleeding requires an aggressive evaluation and treatment strategy.

❷ Acute vaginal bleeding in a reproductive-age woman must always be presumed to be due to an accident of pregnancy until proven otherwise. Spontaneous pregnancy loss, ectopic implantation, or retained products of conception following the end of a pregnancy may all cause acute, heavy vaginal bleeding. The treatment is directed by the cause, but often requires curettage of the endometrial cavity.

❸ Patients who are not pregnant but experience acute loss should be stabilized with fluids or blood products in the rare instances when hemodynamic instability results from vaginal losses.

❹ Women who are postmenopausal and experience acute vaginal bleeding should be aggressively evaluated for the possibility (if not the probability) of a tumor. Premenopausal women may be stabilized with high-dose hormonal therapy or curettage. Advocated treatments include conjugated estrogen (20 to 25 mg IV), intramuscular progestins, oral estrogen (conjugated estrogen 2.5 mg, micronized estradiol 3 to 6 mg q2h until bleeding improves, then for 20 to 25 additional days, a progestin added last 10 days), or combination oral contraceptives with estradiol and norgestrel (Ovral, 4 tablets a day

for 3 to 5 days or until bleeding stops, then 1 qd for the duration of the pack or 4 tablets the first day, then 3 for 1 day, 2 the next day, and then 1qd until finished).

❺ When recurrent heavy menstrual flow is the problem (true menorrhagia), the age of the patient affects the evaluation. Periods that are heavy from menarche may be symptomatic of a systemic problem; those acquired later in life are more likely the result of local factors.

❻ Adolescent patients who experience heavy menstrual flow at the menarche or soon after should be evaluated for the possibility of a blood dyscrasia or other abnormality of clotting. While uncommon, this is often the first indication of a partially compensated abnormality. Hypothyroidism and leukemia may rarely present in this manner as well.

❼ Women who develop heavy periods later in the course of their menstruation should be examined for the possibility of cervical or uterine causes (secondary menorrhagia). Uterine leiomyoma (one third of patients will have menorrhagia), endometrial or cervical polyps, or adenomyosis (40% to 50% have menorrhagia) may all be associated with increased blood loss during menstruation.

❽ If a pathologic source for the excessive menstrual flow is found, the management will be determined, in part, by the patient's wishes for fertility. Those who wish to preserve the possibility of future children have a more limited range of options than those whose families are complete.

❾ Women without an obvious cause of their menorrhagia, and those with secondary menorrhagia but who want to preserve fertility, must be treated through the modification of the periods themselves. Those who wish, or will accept, short-term contraception may be managed using oral contraceptives to produce an atrophic endometrium and hence a lighter flow. Long-acting progestin contraception often results in lighter or even absent menses, but the possibility of irregular bleeding early in therapy and the ease of reversal limit acceptance

for some patients. Progestin-containing intrauterine contraceptive devices (IUCDs) may reduce menstrual blood loss, while copper-bearing devices may even contribute to heavier flow.

❿ Patients who are ovulatory, do not have a clinically identifiable cause for their heavy flow (primary menorrhagia), and do not want contraception may be treated effectively using nonsteroidal anti-inflammatory agents. This efficacy is based on the ability of these agents to reduce endometrial levels of prostaglandin E_2, which is found in elevated levels in these patients. When taken for this indication, these medications must be taken continuously for the duration of flow. Anovulatory patients may be successfully managed with cyclic progestins or oral contraceptives until they are ready to conceive. In intractable cases, or in patients being prepared for extirpative surgery or endometrial ablation, therapy with gonadotropin-releasing hormone agonists may be considered.

REFERENCES

Anderson ABM, Haynes PJ, Cuillebaud J, et al. Reduction of menstrual blood loss by prostaglandin synthetase inhibitors. Lancet 1976;1:774.

Cohen BJB, Gibor J. Anemia and menstrual blood loss. Obstet Gynecol Survey 1980;35:597.

Duncan KM, Hart LL. Nonsteroidal antiinflammatory drugs in menorrhagia. Ann Pharmacother 1993;27:1353.

Fraser IS. Hysteroscopy and laparoscopy in women with menorrhagia. Am J Obstet Gynecol 1990;165:1264.

Higham JM. The medical management of menorrhagia. Br J Hosp Med 1991;45:19.

Liddell H. Menorrhagia. N Z Med J 1993;106:255.

Long CA, Gast MJ. Menorrhagia. Obstet Gynecol Clin North Am 1990;17:343.

Shaw RW. Treating the patient with menorrhagia. Br J Obstet Gynaecol 1994;101 (Suppl 11):1.

Wood C. Treatment of menorrhagia. Aust Fam Phys 1995;24(5):825.

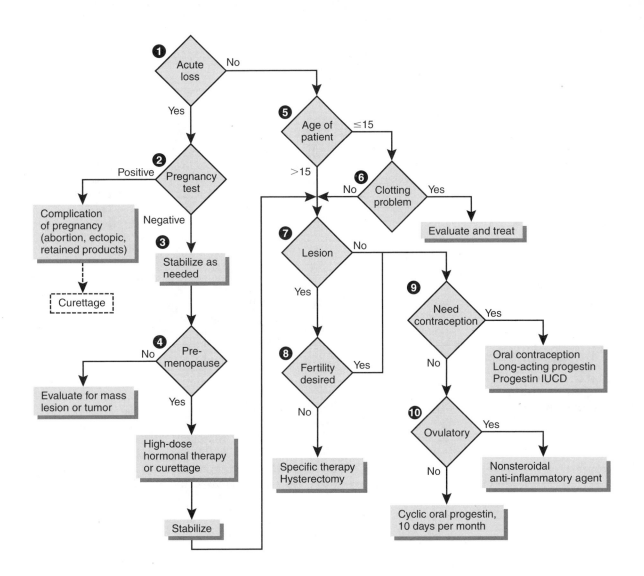

Myofascial Syndromes

INTRODUCTION

Musculoskeletal pain frequently radiates to, or is referred to, areas quite distant from the source of the nociceptive signal. Myofascial syndromes can mimic many gynecologic conditions and are an often-overlooked source of chronic pelvic pain. On occasion, a "trigger point" may be identified that induces, or reproduces, the patient's symptoms. Variously called trigger points, spots, zones, or areas, these hypersensitive areas overlying muscles induce spasm and pain. Myofascial pain syndromes and fibromyalgia frequently demonstrate trigger-point involvement.

❶ Myofascial syndromes often present as pain that is worse in the morning, with stress or weather change, and after nonrestorative sleep. The symptoms are frequently better with activity, stress reduction, or rest. Because symptoms may become entrained with the menstrual cycle, it is easy for these symptoms to be mistaken as evidence for reproductive pathology. The first step in establishing the diagnosis, therefore, is to consider the possibility.

❷ Trigger points may be found throughout the body, but are most common in the abdominal wall, back, and pelvic floor when pelvic pain is the symptom. Abnormal spasm of a small portion of a muscle results in an extremely taut, tender band of muscle (trigger point). Compression of this site will elicit local tenderness, and often reproduce the referred pain. Most trigger points are located at or near areas of moving or sliding muscle surfaces, though they are not limited to these locations. While the absence of these findings does not completely rule out a myofascial syndrome, other diagnoses must be considered.

❸ The initial treatments for pain of myofascial origin are analgesics, heat (hot packs, ultrasound therapy), and general conditioning exercises. For many, these will be sufficient to provide relief.

❹ Patients who do not respond to simple measures should be considered for more specific therapy options such as transcutaneous electrical nerve stimulation (TENS) or trigger-point injections. Trigger-point injections may be easily accomplished using a 22-gauge needle and a small amount (0.5 to 2 ml) of anesthetic agent infiltrated into the area. No more than 10 ml of any anesthetic agent should be used. Superficial trigger points may also be treated will a "spray-and-stretch" technique. The area overlying the trigger point is sprayed with a coolant or freezing spray (e.g., ethyl chloride) for several seconds and the muscle forcibly stretched by passive extension. If these fail, hypnosis, antidepressants, sleep aids, and muscle relaxants may also be used.

REFERENCES

Campbell SM. Regional myofascial pain syndromes. Rheumatic Dis Clin North Am 1989;15:31.

Garvey TA, Marks MR, Wiesel SW. A prospective, randomized, double-blind evaluation of trigger-point injection therapy for low-back pain. Spine 1989;14:962.

Ling FW, Slocumb JC. Use of trigger point injections in chronic pelvic pain. Obstet Gynecol Clin North Am 1993;20:809.

McClaflin RR. Myofascial pain syndrome. Primary care strategies for early intervention. Postgrad Med 1994;96:56.

Rothschild B. Diagnosing and treating fibrositis and fibromyalgia. Geriatr Consult 1990;9:26.

Slocumb JC. Neurologic factors in chronic pelvic pain: Trigger points and the abdominal pelvic pain syndrome. Am J Obstet Gynecol 1984;149:536.

Wolfe F, Smythe HA, Yunus MB, et al. The American College of Rheumatology criteria for the classification of fibromyalgia. Arthritis Rheum 1990;33:160.

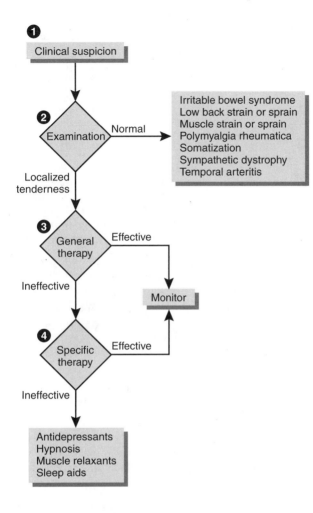

❶ Clinical suspicion

❷ Examination — Normal →
- Irritable bowel syndrome
- Low back strain or sprain
- Muscle strain or sprain
- Polymyalgia rheumatica
- Somatization
- Sympathetic dystrophy
- Temporal arteritis

Localized tenderness

❸ General therapy — Effective → Monitor

Ineffective

❹ Specific therapy — Effective → Monitor

Ineffective

- Antidepressants
- Hypnosis
- Muscle relaxants
- Sleep aids

Ovarian Cancer Staging

INTRODUCTION

Ovarian cancer represents the second most common malignancy of the genital tract (after endometrial cancer), but is the most common fatal gynecologic cancer. Ovarian cancer accounts for 26,700 cases annually in the United States, resulting in 14,800 deaths. Overall, there is a 1/70 lifetime risk of ovarian cancer. Over 90% of ovarian cancer is of the epithelial cell type, thought to arise from pluripotential mesothelial cells of the visceral peritoneum of the ovarian capsule. Lymphatic spread occurs in roughly 20% of tumors that appear grossly confined to the ovary.

1 Ovarian cancer that is confined to the ovary is stage I disease. Stage I disease is further subdivided into stages A, B, and C.

2 If malignant cells are found in peritoneal washings, there is tumor on the exterior surface of the ovary, or the capsule of the ovary is ruptured during the process of the surgical removal, the disease is automatically staged as IC.

3 Stage IA disease must be confined to one ovary, with no malignant cells in the peritoneal fluid, no external tumor, and no disruption of the capsule.

If both ovaries are involved, the staging is increased to stage IB.

4 Tumors that are not confined to the ovary but are limited to the pelvis are stage II.

5 As in stage I disease, if malignant cells are found in peritoneal washings, there is tumor on the exterior surface of the ovary, or the capsule of the ovary is ruptured during the process of the surgical removal, the disease is automatically staged as IIC.

6 Tumor that has spread only to the uterus or fallopian tubes is stage IIA, while extension to other pelvic tissues results in a IIB staging.

7 Tumor that is confined to the abdominal cavity is stage III disease. This includes peritoneal implants outside the pelvis, positive lymph nodes, superficial liver metastasis, or extension to small bowel or omentum.

8 When tumor is grossly limited to the pelvis but malignant nodes or microscopic seeding is found, the sub classification is stage IIIA.

9 Patients with peritoneal implants that are less than 2 cm in size with spread to lymph nodes have stage IIIB disease, but if the implants are larger than

2 cm or there are retroperitoneal or inguinal nodes, the disease is stage IIIC.

10 Patients with distant metastases or a malignant pleural effusion are classified as having stage IV disease. The presence of parenchymal liver disease results in a special classification (IVA).

REFERENCES

American College of Obstetricians and Gynecologists. Cancer of the Ovary. ACOG Technical Bulletin 141. Washington, DC: ACOG, 1990.

American College of Obstetricians and Gynecologists. Classification and Staging of Gynecologic Malignancies. ACOG Technical Bulletin 155. Washington, DC: ACOG, 1991.

Averette HE, Nguyen HN. The role of prophylactic oophorectomy in cancer prevention. Gynecol Oncol 1994;55:S38–S41.

Bell R, Petticrew M, Sheldon T. The performance of screening tests for ovarian cancer: Results of a systematic review. Br J Obstet Gynaecol 1998;105:1136–1147.

Boente MP, Godwin AK, Hogan WM. Screening, imaging and early diagnosis of ovarian cancer. Clin Obstet Gynecol 1994;37:377–391.

Lynch HT, Watson P, Conway T, Lynch J. Hereditary ovarian cancer: natural history, surveillance, management, and genetic counseling. Hematol Oncol Ann 1994;2:107–117.

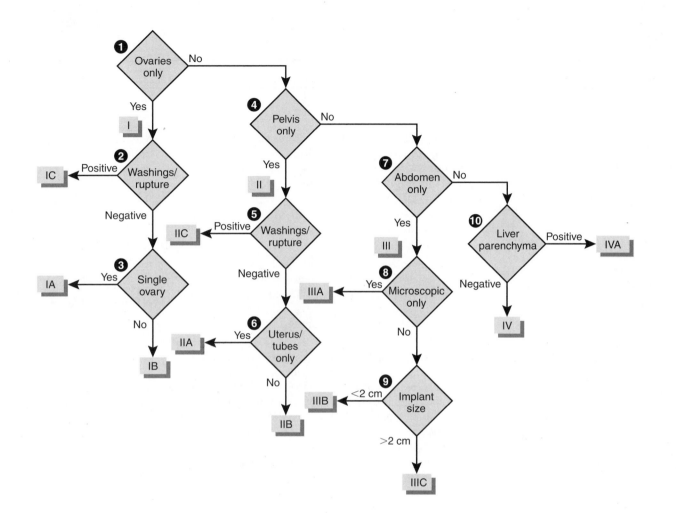

Ovarian Cysts

Postmenopausal

INTRODUCTION

The character of the cyst encountered may suggest a benign or malignant process, but a final diagnosis can only be established by histology. The most important objective of the management of an ovarian cyst is the timely diagnosis of its type and origin. Subsequent therapy and assessment of risk is based on the correctness of the diagnosis. In cases of acutely symptomatic cysts, rapid evaluation and intervention may be necessary. Because of the metabolic inactivity of the ovaries following menopause, any adnexal mass must be view with suspicion in these women.

1 Symptomatic adnexal masses in postmenopausal women engender the greatest concern. Symptoms of pain arise when the mass grows rapidly, the patient experiences internal bleeding, or the mass undergoes torsion. These processes are uncommon in the normally quiescent menopausal ovary. Therefore, aggressive assessment through imaging is required. The most appropriate modalities are computed tomography or magnetic resonance imaging because of their ability to evaluate the entire abdominal cavity and the retroperitoneal nodes. Some surgeons recommend the measurement of tumor markers (as a baseline, not for diagnosis) prior to surgical intervention.

2 Asymptomatic adnexal masses are often managed based on their size: Masses under 4 to 6 cm may be managed in a more conservative manner than those of larger size.

3 While simple masses are most likely to be benign in character, surgical exploration is generally recommended for larger masses. The extent of preoperative evaluations indicated should be based on any additional findings suggested by the physical examination, history, or review of symptoms.

4 While the majority of adnexal masses encountered in postmenopausal women will be benign, only surgical exploration and histologic evaluation can confirm this. The choice between open laparotomy and laparoscopy will depend on the presence and character of symptoms (if any), the risk of malignancy, and operator experience.

5 Complex masses have a greater likelihood of malignancy than do simple cystic structures. For this reason, imaging studies, including an assessment of the retroperitoneal lymph nodes and other pelvic organs, must be carried out before the correct surgical approach can be determined. If tumor markers are drawn, they should only be used as a baseline for further management, not for the purposes of diagnosis.

6 Smaller, asymptomatic masses may be safely followed if the patient is willing to return for periodic reassessment and an adequate evaluation of the mass through pelvic examination (or imaging) is possible. Stable masses, or those that regress, are managed conservatively unless other factors (such as family history or patient preference) supervene.

REFERENCES

Fenoglio CM, Richart RM. Common epithelial ovarian tumors. In Sciarra JJ (ed): Gynecology and Obstetrics. Philadelphia: JB Lippincott, 1989;(4)30:1.

Fleischer AC. Transabdominal and transvaginal sonography of ovarian masses. Clin Obstet Gynecol 1991;34:433.

Petersen WF, Prevost EC, Edmunds FT, et al. Benign cystic teratomas of the ovary. Am J Obstet Gynecol 1955;70:368–382.

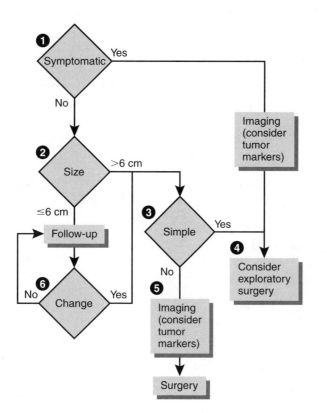

Ovarian Cysts

Premenopausal

INTRODUCTION

Around 90% of ovarian tumors encountered in younger women are benign and metabolically inactive. Over 75% of the benign adnexal masses are functional, arising from the normal processes of ovulation and hormone production. About 25% of ovarian enlargements in reproductive-age women represent true neoplasia, with only about 10% being malignant. The largest group of benign ovarian tumors are those that arise from the epithelium of the ovary and its capsule. Despite the diversity of tumors with epithelial beginnings, the most common ovarian tumor in young reproductive-age women is the cystic teratoma, or dermoid, which is germ cell in origin. The character of the cyst encountered may suggest a benign or malignant process, but a final diagnosis can only be established by histology. The most important objective of the management of an ovarian cyst is the timely diagnosis of its type and origin. Subsequent therapy and assessment of risk is based on the correctness of the diagnosis. In cases of acutely symptomatic cysts, rapid evaluation and intervention may be necessary.

❶ Benign ovarian tumors are most frequently diagnosed at the time of routine examination and are asymptomatic. When symptoms do occur, they will generally be either catastrophic (as when bleeding, rupture, or torsion occur), or indolent and nonspecific (such as a vague sense of pressure or fullness). Catastrophically symptomatic patients must be stabilized and considered for immediate surgical evaluation and treatment. Those with milder or no symptoms may be evaluated in a more orderly manner. There are no laboratory tests that are of specific help in the global diagnosis of ovarian cysts. Laboratory investigations may support specific diagnoses.

❷ Mildly symptomatic masses that have a complex character require surgical evaluation and management because they are less likely to be functional in origin or transient in nature.

❸ Large simple masses are most often managed surgically, though suppression with hormones (oral contraceptives or long-acting progestins) or gonadotropin-releasing hormone (GnRH) agonists may be considered. Smaller cysts are often transient and may resolve with time or suppression.

❹ Regression rates of 65% to 75% are often cited for hormonal suppression, but this strategy is in great measure a matter of personal choice, since definitive studies are lacking. Physiologic ovarian enlargements, including follicular or corpus luteum cysts, should not be present in oral contraceptive users. For this reason, patients who are already using oral contraceptives and develop adnexal masses are more likely to have pathology that will not regress, increasing the possibility that eventual surgical exploration may be required.

❺ Simple adnexal cysts are most likely to be benign, while complex masses carry a greater risk of malignancy, although the majority are still benign in character.

❻ When there is a significant concern about the possibility of malignancy, preoperative imaging and other studies must be undertaken to determine the proper management. Characteristics that should suggest malignancy include a significant solid component, a thickened (>3 mm) or papillary wall, or suggestions of fixation to the lateral pelvic wall or adjacent structures.

❼ When a cyst is simple with only a single cavity with no additional cysts, it can be managed based on size alone. When the cyst is multiple, or there are bilateral cysts, additional considerations must be made.

❽ Bilateral simple cysts are most likely to be functional and may represent either physiologic processes or polycystic ovary syndrome. When there are multiple cysts found in the same adnexa, surgical evaluation is indicated.

❾ The diagnosis of polycystic ovary syndrome may be made by measurements of serum luteinizing hormone (LH). LH levels may be abnormal even without other stigmata of the disease.

❿ Though most large simple cysts are benign, most physicians and patients feel safest managing them though surgical evaluation and extirpation. Smaller cysts may be managed though observation or suppression with oral contraceptives, long-acting progestins, or GnRH agonists, though the latter are not commonly used because of their expense and side effects.

REFERENCES

Fenoglio CM, Richart RM. Common epithelial ovarian tumors. In Sciarra JJ (ed): Gynecology and Obstetrics. Philadelphia: JB Lippincott, 1989;(4)30:1.

Fleischer AC. Transabdominal and transvaginal sonography of ovarian masses. Clin Obstet Gynecol 1991;34:433.

Petersen WF, Prevost EC, Edmunds FT, Hundley JM, Morriss FK. Benign cystic teratomas of the ovary. Am J Obstet Gynecol 1955;70:368–382.

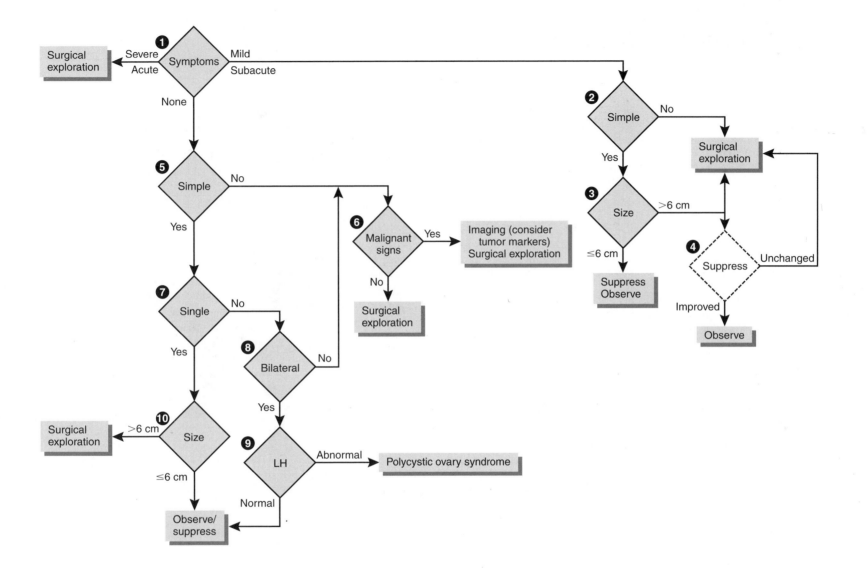

Ovarian Remnant Syndrome

INTRODUCTION

Ovarian remnant syndrome is characterized by chronic pelvic pain secondary to an area of functioning ovarian tissue remaining after bilateral oophorectomy. This functionally active tissue becomes entrapped within postoperative scar tissue.

❶ Ovarian remnant syndrome should be suspected when chronic pelvic or abdominal pain (cyclic or constant), dyspareunia, or dyskesia occurs following bilateral oophorectomy. These symptoms are often exacerbated by intercourse. This is most common in women who undergo hysterectomy for endometriosis or chronic pelvic inflammatory disease and have extensive adhesions found at the time of surgery.

❷ Pelvic examination may demonstrate a small (average 3 cm) tender mass located in the retroperitoneal space near the lateral pelvic wall. The presence of such a lesion, in conjunction with a pattern of clinical symptoms consistent with this syndrome, supports the presumptive diagnosis.

❸ Imaging with ultrasonography or magnetic resonance imaging may demonstrate functional ovarian tissue. While loculated peritoneal fluid, loops of bowel, or matted omental tissue may be mistaken for retained ovarian tissue, the presence of a suggestive finding on imaging may be sufficient to justify surgical exploration in symptomatic patients.

❹ Measurement of serum levels of follicle-stimulating hormone (FSH) may be helpful in establishing the diagnosis. If enough functional tissue remains, FSH levels may be normal. Elevated serum levels of FSH are not sufficient to rule out the diagnosis.

❺ When necessary, suppression of presumed ovarian function with oral contraceptives or gonadotropin-releasing hormone agonists should establish the diagnosis. If significant improvements in symptoms are not achieved with these therapies, other causes should be sought.

❻ Long-term therapy with oral contraceptives or long-acting progestins may be acceptable for some patients. When this not an option, surgical exploration is indicated.

❼ The most effective treatment of ovarian remnant syndrome is surgical extirpation of the retained tissue. The tissue must be removed by wide excision with care to protect the ureter that is invariably near the site of scarring.

REFERENCES

Minke T, DePond W, Winkelmann T, Blythe J. Ovarian remnant syndrome: study in laboratory rats. Am J Obstet Gynecol 1994;171:1440.

Price FV, Edwards R, Buchsbaum HJ. Ovarian remnant syndrome: difficulties in diagnosis and management. Obstet Gynecol Surv 1990;45:151.

Siddall-Allum J, Rae T, Rogers V, et al. Chronic pelvic pain caused by residual ovaries and ovarian remnants. Br J Obstet Gynaecol 1994;101:979.

Steege JF. Ovarian remnant syndrome. Obstet Gynecol 1987;70:64.

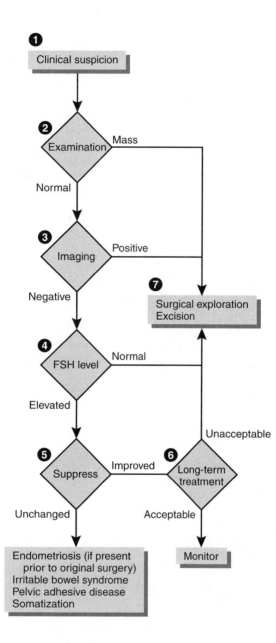

1 Clinical suspicion

2 Examination — Mass

Normal

3 Imaging — Positive

Negative

7 Surgical exploration
Excision

4 FSH level — Normal

Elevated

Unacceptable

5 Suppress — Improved — **6** Long-term treatment

Unchanged   Acceptable

Endometriosis (if present
  prior to original surgery)
Irritable bowel syndrome
Pelvic adhesive disease
Somatization

Monitor

Pelvic Inflammatory Disease

INTRODUCTION

Pelvic inflammatory disease (PID) is a serious, diffuse, frequently multiorganism infection of the pelvic organs that results in significant morbidity. Pelvic infections affect more than three quarters of a million women in the United States annually, resulting in an estimated health care cost of $3.5 billion. This infection is most often the result of sexually transmitted organisms (85%) but may also arise after medical manipulations, including intrauterine contraceptive device placement, endometrial sampling, or sonohysterography. Patients at increased risk include sexually active teens, women with multiple sexual partners, and those with a history of previous infections. Patients who use oral or barrier contraceptives have a reduced risk.

❶ The diagnosis and management of PID begins with a clinical suspicion. Because tubal obstruction occurs in more than 10% of women after a single episode, patients suspected of having PID should be aggressively treated even when the diagnosis is uncertain. The most common presenting findings are pain (99%), pelvic tenderness (95%), and a vaginal discharge (80%). A pelvic mass may be present in almost half of these patients. Fever (>38°C) is an unreliable sign, being present in only about a third of patients. Laparoscopy confirms the diagnosis in only two thirds of cases diagnosed by clinical criteria.

❷ While the laboratory assessment of PID is often supportive of the diagnosis, it cannot be the deciding factor. Less than 50% of patients with the clinical diagnosis of PID have a white blood cell count above 10,000 (WBC/ml) and only 25% to 30% of patients will have a positive cervical culture for chlamydia or gonorrhea (respectively). (Despite the poor prognostic significance of culture and the inherent delay in obtaining results, cultures should always be obtained along with screening tests for other sexually transmitted diseases, including human immunodeficiency virus.)

❸ Ultrasonography may be of assistance in when the pelvic examination is difficult or impossible (obe-

sity, uncooperative patient). Imaging may demonstrate free fluid (though the character of the fluid cannot be known), the presence of tubo-ovarian abscesses, or mimicking noninfectious causes for the patient's symptoms. If an abscess is identified, inpatient antibiotic therapy should be strongly considered.

❹ When complications such as pregnancy, gastrointestinal symptoms, or an intrauterine contraceptive devise are present, serious consideration should be given to inpatient treatment. Many authors suggest that young patients and those who are nulliparous should also be hospitalized for their treatment. Any time the diagnosis is uncertain, inpatient therapy is appropriate.

❺ Antibiotic therapy should be tailored to the needs of the individual patient, but common treatments include: cefoxitin 2 g im with probenecid 1 g po, ceftriaxone 250 mg im and doxycycline 100 mg po bid for 10 to 14 days, or tetracycline 500 mg po qid for 10 to 14 days. Erythromycin (500 mg po qid for 10 to 14 days) may be substituted for tetracycline.

❻ Patients who are treated as outpatients must be carefully monitored at 48 hours after the start of therapy. If the response has been suboptimal, or there has been any adverse change in the patient's condition, hospitalization and further evaluation are indicate.

❼ Inpatients who do not have high-risk factors such as an abscess should be treated with an intravenous cephalosporin with good coverage for gonococcal and other facultative gram-negative organisms and doxycycline 100 mg q12h by either intravenous or oral routes. High-risk patients should be treated with double- or triple-antibiotic regimens such as clindamycin plus gentamicin.

❽ Inpatients must be monitored carefully for signs of improvement, which should be apparent by 48 hours of treatment.

❾ When treatment does not result in signs of improvement, the original diagnosis as well as the

treatment chosen should be re-evaluated. The evaluation should include all possible diagnoses and may require invasive measures such as laparoscopy to obtain cultures and establish a diagnosis.

❿ Once the patient has remained afebrile for 24 to 48 hours and her symptoms have improved, a transition to oral therapy can be made and discharge planning begun.

⓫ Whether treated as an inpatient or outpatient, patients should be seen in follow-up after 1 week. Progress since treatment and the results of other screening tests may be reviewed at this visit.

⓬ The 1-week post discharge visit should include an assessment of the adnexa. When this examination is normal, the patient is encouraged to complete her course of treatment and resume routine care. This is also an opportunity to discuss contraception, sexually transmitted disease, possible infertility, and sexual risk taking.

⓭ When pelvic examination documents a persistent mass, careful follow-up is indicated and the possibility of diagnostic or therapeutic surgical intervention considered.

REFERENCES

Dodson MG. Antibiotic regimens for treating acute pelvic inflammatory disease: An evaluation. J Reprod Med 1994;39:285–296.

Hager WE, Eschenbach DA, Spence MR, Sweet RL. Criteria for diagnosis and grading of salpintitis. Obstet Gynecol 1983;61:113.

Jacobson LJ. Differntial diagnosis of acute pelvic inflammatory disease. Am J Obstet Gynecol 1980;138:1006–1011.

Ledger WJ. Laparoscopy in the diagnosis and management of patients with suspected salpingo-oophoritis. Am J Obstet Gynecol 1980;138:1012.

Washington AE, Cates W, Zaidi AA. Hospitalization for pelvic inflammatory disease. JAMA 1984;25:2529.

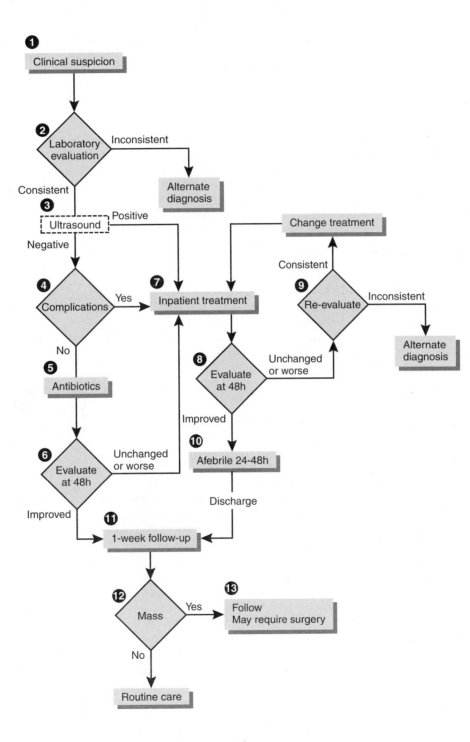

Pelvic Mass

INTRODUCTION

Almost any structure in or abutting the pelvis may be the source of enlargement, distention, or neoplasia, resulting in the formation of a mass. The most common pelvic masses found in women during their reproductive years are related to the uterus: pregnancy and leiomyomata (fibroids). The possibility of a pregnancy, intrauterine or otherwise, must always be considered when a pelvic mass is found. Adnexal masses constitute the fourth most common reason for hospital admission for women in the United States. Ovarian tumors may be either solid or cystic and arise from any of the histologic elements of the ovary. Most common of these are the benign serous and mucinous cystadenomas of epithelial origin. Ectopic pregnancies, tubo-ovarian abscess, and hydrosalpinx are the most commonly encountered nonovarian causes of an adnexal mass.

❶ The character of the mass is generally apparent from the pelvic examination. Only when the patient is uncooperative or obese, or the character of the mass is not apparent, is ultrasonography initially required. Ultrasonographic imaging provides limited information beyond the these situations and should not be used when the character is clinically evident.

❷ Ultrasonography is best used to characterize masses that cannot be adequately evaluated by clinical means. Cystic masses with solid components or those with multiple loculations should be evaluated in the same manner as completely solid masses. Patients with grossly malignant disease should be evaluated in preparation for definitive surgical staging and treatment.

❸ Solid masses of gynecologic origin should be considered suspicious for malignancy and evaluated with computed tomography (CT) and prepared for surgical exploration and diagnosis. The possibility that the mass has arisen from other pelvic or nonpelvic organs must always be considered.

❹ Cystic masses can arise from structures other than the ovary itself. The most common of these is a hydrosalpinx. These masses are usually oblong or tubular in shape. When viewed by ultrasonography, these will be asymmetric in their dimensions and separate from the ovary. Most symptomatic nonovarian cystic masses will require surgical evaluation and treatment.

❺ As noted in No. 2, simple ovarian cysts are managed differently from those with multiple internal components.

❻ Patients with solid pelvic masses, those with multiple cysts, and those with frankly malignant disease require several additional evaluations before undergoing surgical exploration and treatment. Preoperative imaging to evaluate the overall abdominal cavity and retroperitoneal lymph nodes can help to determine the optimal therapeutic approach. Serum tumor markers should be drawn in these patients, but this is obtained to assist with follow-up, not to establish a diagnosis.

❼ Large, simple ovarian cysts (>6 cm) are best treated by surgical excision. Masses below this size may be managed more conservatively if they are asymptomatic.

❽ Small, unilocular masses may be followed or suppressed. Spontaneous regression of small cysts occur frequently enough that watchful waiting for 2 to 8 weeks may be appropriate if symptoms are minimal or absent. Masses that grow should undergo surgical extirpation, while those that remain unchanged may respond to hormonal suppression (such as oral contraceptives). If the mass spontaneously resolves, follow-up is dictated by the level of comfort of the patient and provider because the risk of recurrence is low.

REFERENCES

Barbieri RL. Etiology and epidemiology of endometriosis. Am J Obstet Gynecol 1990;162:565.

Cramer SF, Patel D. The frequency of uterine leiomyomas. Am J Clin Pathol 1990;94:435.

Fleischer AC. Transabdominal and transvaginal sonography of ovarian masses. Clin Obstet Gynecol 1991;34:433.

Goldstein SR. Conservative management of small postmenopausal cystic masses. Clin Obstet Gynecol 1993;36:395.

Herman JR, Locher GW, Goldhirsch A. Sonographic patterns of ovarian tumors: prediction of malignancy. Obstet Gynecol 1987;69:777.

Kroon E, Andolf E. Diagnosis and follow-up of simple ovarian cysts detected by ultrasound in postmenopausal women. Obstet Gynecol 1995;85:211–214.

Vollenhoven BJ, Lawrence AS, Healy DL. Uterine fibroids: A clinical review. Br J Obstet Gynaecol 1990;97:285–298.

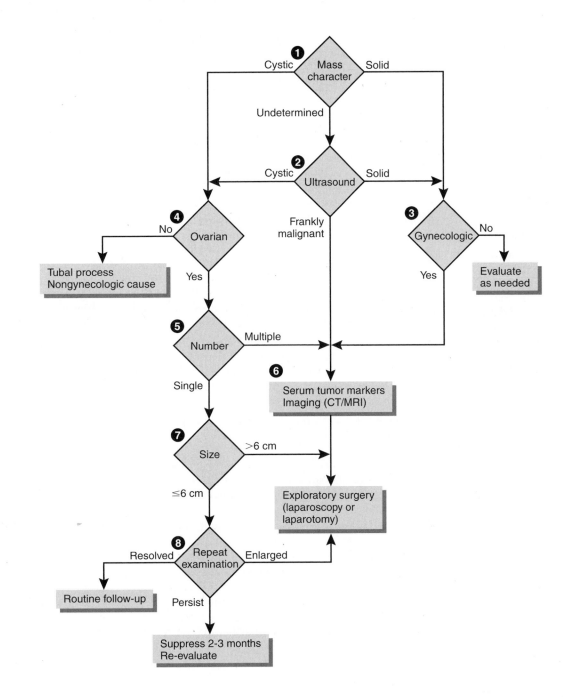

Pelvic Pain

Acute

INTRODUCTION

Acute abdominal and pelvic pain accounts for an extremely large number of emergency room and short-notice office visits. While most acute abdominal pain is of nongynecologic origin, pelvic organs are not infrequently involved. Acute pelvic pain is almost always associated with morbidity of at least some degree. This can vary from an inconvenient interruption to catastrophic collapse. Acute pelvic and abdominal pain frequently is a harbinger of significant physiologic disturbances that can carry life-threatening significance. For example, ectopic pregnancies still account for approximately 5% of deaths associated with reproduction.

❶ The first step in the evaluation of any patient with acute pain is to ascertain her hemodynamic stability. Acute pain may be the only sign of abrupt, life-threatening intra-abdominal blood loss, perforation of a hollow viscus, abrupt ischemia of a structure or organ, or disection of an aortic aneurysm. A cursory examination, supplemented by measurements such as blood pressure and pulse rate should establish the immediate threat to the patient. Indications of instability require that resuscitative efforts precede any effort at specific diagnosis.

❷ The presence of peritonitis should prompt an aggressive evaluation plan, including the possibility of surgical evaluation. Subacute pain with peritonitis is common for patients with pelvic infections or appendicitis. If the diagnosis is apparent, non-surgical management may be appropriate even with peritonitis present.

❸ Acute abdominal pain that carries a component that is outside the pelvis should suggest the probable involvement of organ systems other than the reproductive tract.

❹ Pelvic pain that is bilateral in character is typical of diffuse inflammatory conditions or the involvement of midline structures such as the bladder. In bilateral pelvic pain, the midline is often paradoxically spared. Pain well localized to the pelvic midline usually results from pathology involving midline structures, though they may not be confined to those within the abdominal cavity.

❺ Careful history and pelvic examination will generally the reproductive tract as the source of pain. The possibility, if not the probability, that the pelvic pain arises from sources other than the reproductive tract must always be considered.

❻ If the reproductive tract is suspected as the source of the patient's pain, the timing of the last menstrual period (LMP) should be established. When the time of the last period is unknown or more than 4 weeks prior to presentation, adnexal accidents or complications of pregnancy (ectopic implantation) must be strongly considered.

❼ When the last menstrual period was normal and approximately 2 weeks prior to the onset of pain, ovulation or complications thereof must be considered if the patient is not using hormonal contraception. Adnexal torsion may occur at any point in the menstrual cycle but is most common near the time of menses or when menses are delayed. The possibility of an ectopic implantation is not ruled out by a menstrual period in the preceding few weeks, especially if the period was abnormal and no contraception has been used. Endometriosis and bleeding into a corpus luteum cyst are most common around the time of the anticipated menses.

REFERENCES

American College of Obstetricians and Gynecologists. Medical Management of Tubal Pregnancy. ACOG Practice Bulletin 3. Washington, DC: ACOG, 1998.

Fiddian-Green RG, Acute right lower quadrant pain. In Norton LW, Steele G, Jr, Eisemen B (eds): Surgical Decision Making, 3rd ed. Philadelphia: WB Saunders, 1993, p 154.

Healey PM, Jacobson EJ. Common Medical Diagnoses: An Algorithmic Approach, 2nd ed. Philadelphia: WB Saunders, 1993, p 58.

Nichols DH, Julian PJ. Torsion of the adnexa. Clin Obstet Gynecol 1985;28:375.

Oelsner G, Bider D, Goldenberg M, et al. Long-term follow-up of the twisted ischemic adnexa managed by detorsion. Fertil Steril 1993;60:976.

Reich H, Freifeld ML, McGlynn F, et al. Laparoscopic treatment of tubal pregnancy. Obstet Gynecol 1987;69:275.

Shalev E, Yarom I, Bustan M, et al. Transvaginal sonography as the ultimate diagnostic tool for the management of ectopic pregnancy: Experience with 840 cases. Fertil Steril 1998;69:62.

Smith RP. Gynecology in Primary Care. Baltimore: Williams & Wilkins, 1997, p 471.

Zweizig S, Perron J, Grubb D, Mishell DR Jr. Conservative management of adnexal torsion. Am J Obstet Gynecol 1993;168:1791.

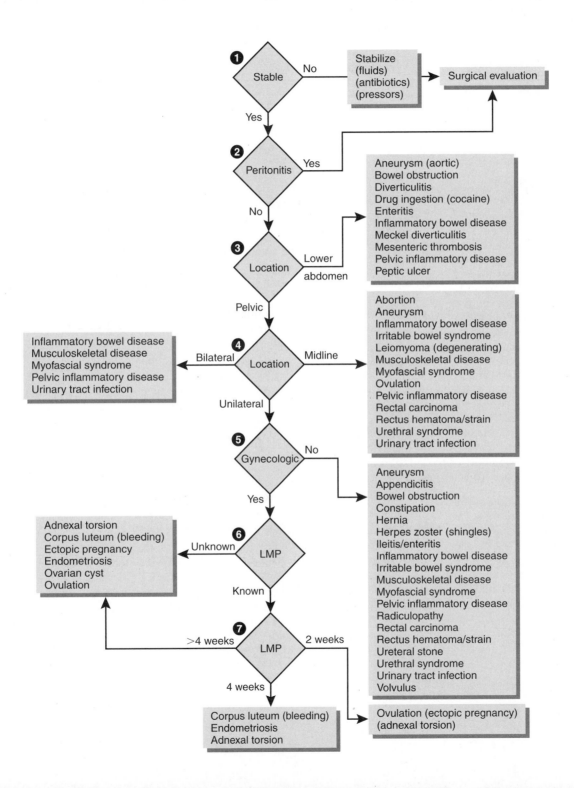

❶ Stable

No → Stabilize (fluids) (antibiotics) (pressors) → Surgical evaluation

Yes ↓

❷ Peritonitis

Yes →
- Aneurysm (aortic)
- Bowel obstruction
- Diverticulitis
- Drug ingestion (cocaine)
- Enteritis
- Inflammatory bowel disease
- Meckel diverticulitis
- Mesenteric thrombosis
- Pelvic inflammatory disease
- Peptic ulcer

No ↓

❸ Location

Lower abdomen → (to surgical evaluation)

Pelvic ↓

❹ Location

Bilateral ←
- Inflammatory bowel disease
- Musculoskeletal disease
- Myofascial syndrome
- Pelvic inflammatory disease
- Urinary tract infection

Midline →
- Abortion
- Aneurysm
- Inflammatory bowel disease
- Irritable bowel syndrome
- Leiomyoma (degenerating)
- Musculoskeletal disease
- Myofascial syndrome
- Ovulation
- Pelvic inflammatory disease
- Rectal carcinoma
- Rectus hematoma/strain
- Urethral syndrome
- Urinary tract infection

Unilateral ↓

❺ Gynecologic

No →
- Aneurysm
- Appendicitis
- Bowel obstruction
- Constipation
- Hernia
- Herpes zoster (shingles)
- Ileitis/enteritis
- Inflammatory bowel disease
- Irritable bowel syndrome
- Musculoskeletal disease
- Myofascial syndrome
- Pelvic inflammatory disease
- Radiculopathy
- Rectal carcinoma
- Rectus hematoma/strain
- Ureteral stone
- Urethral syndrome
- Urinary tract infection
- Volvulus

Yes ↓

❻ LMP

Unknown ←
- Adnexal torsion
- Corpus luteum (bleeding)
- Ectopic pregnancy
- Endometriosis
- Ovarian cyst
- Ovulation

Known ↓

❼ LMP

>4 weeks → (to Adnexal torsion box)

2 weeks → Ovulation (ectopic pregnancy) (adnexal torsion)

4 weeks ↓
- Corpus luteum (bleeding)
- Endometriosis
- Adnexal torsion

Pelvic Pain

Chronic

INTRODUCTION

Pelvic pain is by far the most common type of chronic pain suffered by women, accounting for up to 10% of all outpatient gynecology visits. The investigation, diagnosis, and treatment of chronic pelvic pain accounts for one third of laparoscopic procedures and 15% of hysterectomies performed.

The events that evoke pain signals are few: thermal (heat or cold), mechanical (stretch, distention, or muscular contraction), and chemical irritation (liberation of acetylcholine, acids, bradykinin, histamines, potassium ions, prostaglandins, proteolytic enzymes, and serotonin). The processes that create chronic or recurrent pain may be lumped into those that are structural (ongoing processes such as arthritis or metastatic cancer), psycho-physiologic (such as continuing muscle spasm creating pain after the original insult has passed), and somatizational (as found in those who internalize stress and express it in the form of pain). Chronic pelvic pain may be produced by gynecologic, urologic, gastrointestinal, musculoskeletal, or other processes, most of which have parallels with the causes of acute pain.

❶ The most important part of the evaluation of any patient with chronic pelvic pain is the history. The character, location and radiation, onset, duration, and evolution of the pain over time must be elicited. The distinction between diffuse and well-localized pain provides a rational separation of possible causes and represents the first decision point in the evaluation.

❷ Vague, diffuse symptoms more often arise from somatizational sources than specific organic pathology. Therefore, office screening for the presence of depression, somatization, or sleep disorders is appropriate. The Beck Depression Inventory is a quick and simple instrument to both take and score as an indication of subclinical depression.

❸ Sleep disorders may be uncovered through simple history.

❹ When chronic pain is well localized, an attempt should be made to determine the cyclicity of the pain. Simple history will often suffice though a menstrual calendar may be required in cases with a more obscure relationship.

❺ Patients with chronic pain that has a tie to the menstrual flow should receive hormonal suppression. Oral contraceptives, long-acting progestins, or gonadotropin-releasing hormone agonists can effectively suppress the symptoms of a number of gynecologic conditions. The absence of symptom relief with this therapy suggests a nongynecologic cause.

❻ A careful pelvic examination may suggest a cause in patients with well-localized pain that has a cyclic, but nonsuppressible character.

❼ Attention should be paid to factors that make the patient's symptoms change, not just improve or worsen. The impact of factors such as diet, activity, bowel movements, voiding, bladder filling, and sexual activity must all be explored.

❽ Diagnostic laparoscopy may be of help in the evaluation and treatment of patients experiencing chronic pelvic pain with no clinically evident cause. Even though laparoscopy will not identify pathology in up to a third of chronic pain patients, this lack of findings may be reassuring, though the absence of findings does not exclude the possibility of somatic disease. Laparoscopy is of greatest help when the pelvic examination is abnormal, initial therapy fails, or negative findings are significant (as in patients with morbid fears of cancer).

❾ The presence of associated symptoms may suggest other organ systems to be evaluated.

REFERENCES

American College of Obstetricians and Gynecologists. Chronic Pelvic Pain. ACOG Technical Bulletin 223. Washington, DC: ACOG, 1996.

Bass C, Benjamin S. The management of chronic somatisation. Br J Psychiatry 1993;162:472–480.

Beck A. Depression Inventory. Philadelphia: Center for Cognitive Therapy, 1991.

Drife JO. The pelvic pain syndrome. Br J Obstet Gynaecol 1993;100(6):508–510.

International Association for the Study of Pain. Classification of chronic pain, descriptions of chronic pain syndromes and definitions of pain terms. Pain 1986;3(Suppl):S1–S225.

Ling FW (ed). Contemporary management of chronic pelvic pain. Obstet Gynecol Clin North Am 1993;20(4):627–853.

Steege JF, Stout AL, Somkuti SG. Chronic pelvic pain in women: Toward an integrative model. Obstet Gynecol Surv 1991;12:95–110.

Smith RP, Metheny WP, Nolan TE: A tool for the assessment of chronic pelvic pain. J Psych Obstet Gynecol 1992; 13(4): 281–286.

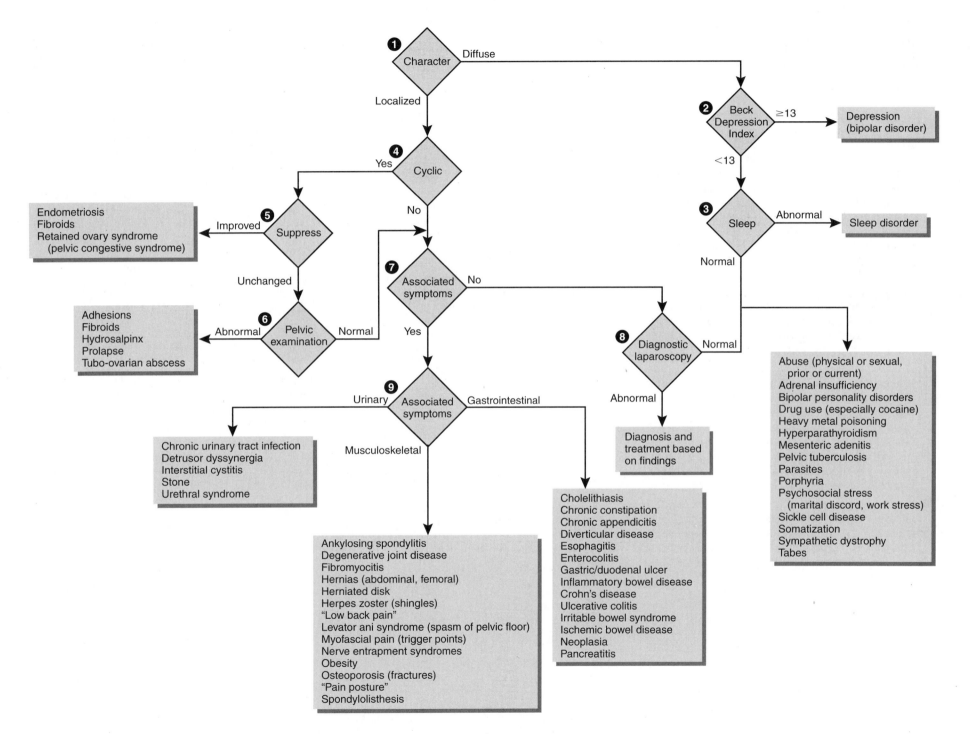

1. Character
   - Diffuse
   - Localized

2. Beck Depression Index
   - ≥13 → Depression (bipolar disorder)
   - <13

3. Sleep
   - Abnormal → Sleep disorder
   - Normal

4. Cyclic
   - Yes
   - No

5. Suppress
   - Improved → Endometriosis / Fibroids / Retained ovary syndrome (pelvic congestive syndrome)
   - Unchanged

6. Pelvic examination
   - Abnormal → Adhesions / Fibroids / Hydrosalpinx / Prolapse / Tubo-ovarian abscess
   - Normal

7. Associated symptoms
   - No
   - Yes

8. Diagnostic laparoscopy
   - Normal
   - Abnormal → Diagnosis and treatment based on findings

9. Associated symptoms
   - Urinary → Chronic urinary tract infection / Detrusor dyssynergia / Interstitial cystitis / Stone / Urethral syndrome
   - Musculoskeletal → Ankylosing spondylitis / Degenerative joint disease / Fibromyocitis / Hernias (abdominal, femoral) / Herniated disk / Herpes zoster (shingles) / "Low back pain" / Levator ani syndrome (spasm of pelvic floor) / Myofascial pain (trigger points) / Nerve entrapment syndromes / Obesity / Osteoporosis (fractures) / "Pain posture" / Spondylolisthesis
   - Gastrointestinal → Cholelithiasis / Chronic constipation / Chronic appendicitis / Diverticular disease / Esophagitis / Enterocolitis / Gastric/duodenal ulcer / Inflammatory bowel disease / Crohn's disease / Ulcerative colitis / Irritable bowel syndrome / Ischemic bowel disease / Neoplasia / Pancreatitis

Abuse (physical or sexual, prior or current)
Adrenal insufficiency
Bipolar personality disorders
Drug use (especially cocaine)
Heavy metal poisoning
Hyperparathyroidism
Mesenteric adenitis
Pelvic tuberculosis
Parasites
Porphyria
Psychosocial stress (marital discord, work stress)
Sickle cell disease
Somatization
Sympathetic dystrophy
Tabes

167

Pessary Therapy

INTRODUCTION

Available in a variety of types and sizes, pessaries are worn in the vagina to replace the missing structural support and to diffuse the forces of descent over a wide area. To varying degrees, the pessary occludes the vagina and holds the pelvic organs in a relatively normal position. Pessaries offer an excellent alternative to surgical repair, but the use of a pessary requires the cooperation and involvement of the patient.

❶ Patients who are unable, or unwilling, to manage the periodic insertion and removal of the device are poor candidates for their use. This may include those with severe limitations of movement or dexterity, such as arthritics, and those with memory impairment.

❷ Because all pessaries provide some degree of pressure on the vaginal wall, the vaginal tissues should be inspected for their general condition before a trial of pessary therapy. Pessaries will not be well tolerated or provide optimal support in the poorly estrogenized patient. Vaginal atrophy should be treated with topical or systemic estrogens for a sufficient period to provide a supple, thickened, and well-moistened epithelium.

❸ Prior to fitting a pessary, careful assessment of the anatomic defects present must be made along with a determination of the complaints to be addressed. The presence or absence or normal pelvic support will help to determine the type of pessary best suited for the patient at hand. The choice of pessary type is based on the indication for which the therapy is indicated. While some pessaries may be used for more than one indication, better results may often be obtained through the use of a device with more specific applications.

❹ Pessaries are fitted and placed in the vagina in much the same way as a contraceptive diaphragm: The depth of the vagina and the integrity of the supporting structures are gauged as a part of the pelvic examination. The size of pessary to be fitted is based on the findings of the pelvic examination. The pessary is lubricated with a water-soluble lubricant, folded or compressed, and inserted into the vagina. The pessary is next adjusted so that it is in the proper position based on the type. All pessaries must allow the easy passage of an examining finger between the pessary and the vaginal wall in all areas. The only situation in which a pessary is allowed to exert any significant pressure beneath the urethra is in cases of urinary incontinence.

❺ Patients who are to use a pessary should be instructed on both proper insertion and removal techniques. Patients fitted with a pessary need careful initial monitoring. Examination 5 to 7 days after initial fitting is required to confirm proper placement, hygiene, and the absence of pressure-related problems (vaginal trauma or necrosis). Earlier evaluation (in 24 to 48 hours) may be advisable for patients who are debilitated or require additional assistance.

❻ At the initial evaluation, the fit, function, and suitability of the pessary should be assessed. At this point, changes in the size or type of pessary used are not uncommonly required and the patient should be reassured that this does not alter the long-term suitability or satisfaction expected with pessary therapy. If the pessary is well tolerated and providing relief of the patient's symptoms, the patient should return to vaginal checks on a monthly basis. Under selected circumstances this interval may be lenghtened, but close follow-up is a lifetime requirement of therapy.

REFERENCES

American College of Obstetricians and Gynecologists. Pelvic Organ Prolapse. ACOG Technical Bulletin 214. Washington, DC: ACOG, 1995.

Deger RB, Menzin AW, Mikuta JJ. The vaginal pessary: Past and present. Postgrad Obstet Gynecol 1993;13:1.

Greenhill JP. The nonsurgical management of vaginal relaxation. Clin Obstet Gynecol 1972;15:1083.

Miller DS. Contemporary use of the pessary. In Sciarra JJ (ed): Obstetrics and Gynecology. Philadelphia: JB Lippincott, 1998;(1)39:1–12.

Sulak PJ, Kuehl TJ, Shull BL. Vaginal pessaries and their use in pelvic relaxation. J Reprod Med 1993;38:919–923.

Smith RP, Ling FW. Procedures in Women's Health Care. Baltimore: Williams & Wilkins, 1997, pp 127–136.

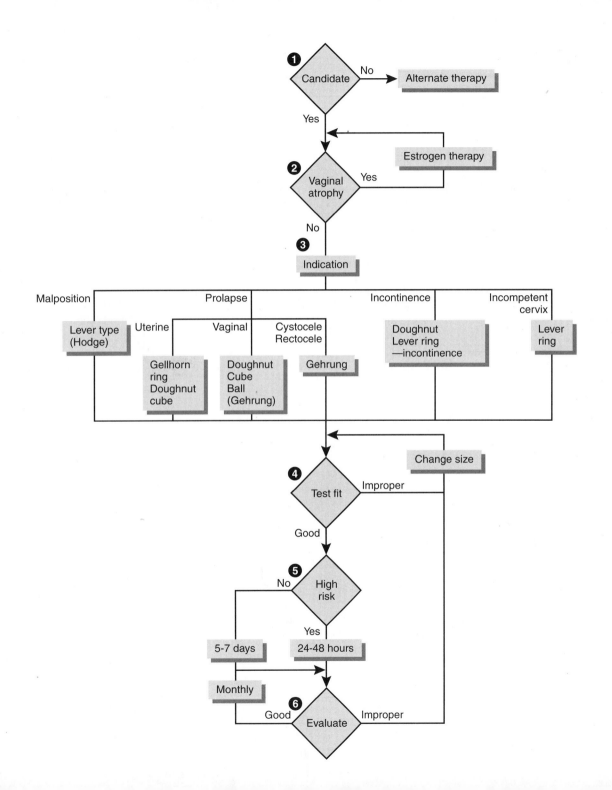

Postcoital Bleeding

INTRODUCTION

Vaginal bleeding following intercourse is at best distressing and at worse a harbinger of serious pathology. The timely evaluation of this symptom can allay fear and provided for opportune therapy.

❶ The acute bleeding after intercourse is often of different cause than that which has occurred episodically. Simple questioning provides this distinction. If a patient experiences an abrupt, dramatic change in the character of bleeding experienced in the past, the evaluation should proceed as for acute, first-time bleeding.

❷ The volume of blood loss experienced may be assessed by questioning or by direct inspection. Small-volume blood loss may be associated with minor coital trauma, atrophy, cervical lesions, or coincidental uterine bleeding related only by chance. Vaginal and pelvic examination, combined with other elements of the patient's history, will suggest the appropriate evaluations to pursue.

❸ On rare occasions, the volume of blood lost can be life threatening. Patients who are hemodynamically unstable should be stabilized with fluids, blood, and other measures as needed to protect their lives. These patients will generally require surgical evaluation and treatment to assess the cause and to provide control of the bleeding.

❹ Stabile patients who experience large-volume blood loss should be carefully examined for lacerations, tumors, and accidents of pregnancy. Here too, surgical evaluation and repair are often required.

❺ Small-volume, episodic vaginal bleeding after intercourse may arise from many sources. Vaginal inspection and careful pelvic examination will often suggest a cause. Many causes, such as inappropriate attribution, hormonal contraceptive use, and endometrial changes, will not be apparent on physical examination. History, imaging, and other studies will generally provide clues to the cause.

REFERENCES

American College of Obstetricians and Gynecologists. Dysfunctional Uterine Bleeding. ACOG Technical Bulletin 134. Washington, DC: ACOG, 1989.

Cowan BD, Morrison JC. Management of abnormal genital bleeding in girls and women. N Engl J Med 1991;324:1710.

Field CS. Dysfunctional uterine bleeding. Prim Care 1988;15:561.

Neese RE. Managing abnormal vaginal bleeding. Postgrad Med 1991;89:205.

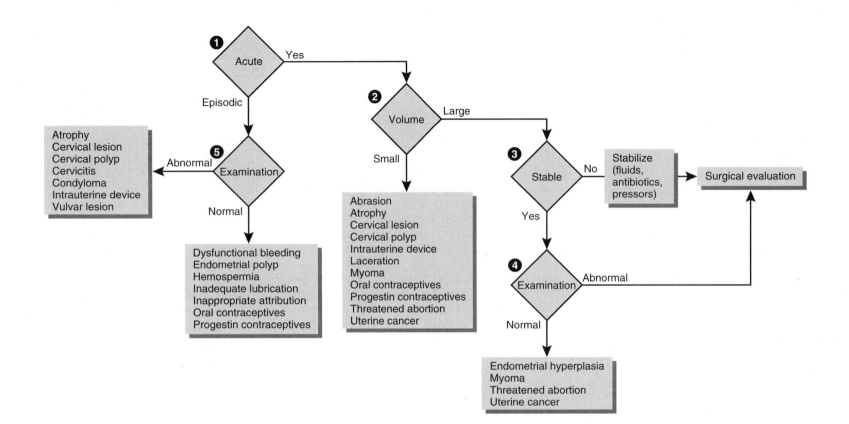

Atrophy
Cervical lesion
Cervical polyp
Cervicitis
Condyloma
Intrauterine device
Vulvar lesion

Dysfunctional bleeding
Endometrial polyp
Hemospermia
Inadequate lubrication
Inappropriate attribution
Oral contraceptives
Progestin contraceptives

Abrasion
Atrophy
Cervical lesion
Cervical polyp
Intrauterine device
Laceration
Myoma
Oral contraceptives
Progestin contraceptives
Threatened abortion
Uterine cancer

Endometrial hyperplasia
Myoma
Threatened abortion
Uterine cancer

❶ Acute
Yes
Episodic
❷ Volume
Large
Small
❺ Examination
Abnormal
Normal
❸ Stable
No
Stabilize (fluids, antibiotics, pressors)
Yes
Surgical evaluation
❹ Examination
Abnormal
Normal

Postmenopausal Vaginal Bleeding

INTRODUCTION

As a symptom only, postmenopausal bleeding requires evaluation to rule out processes that may threaten the long-term health of the patient.

❶ Acute postmenopausal bleeding often reflects a different set of possible causes than those responsible for recurrent or episodic bleeding. While the evaluation of these patients is often similar, the assessment can be expedited to some extent based on this distinction.

❷ Postmenopausal women are at increased risk for coital trauma as a consequence of genital atrophy, potentially resulting in abrasions, splits, or frank lacerations. Cervical polyps or cancers of the cervix or uterus may also present as postcoital bleeding.

❸ Acute episodes of vaginal bleeding in women who are not receiving hormonal replacement therapy may be due to cancers of the cervix or body of the uterus. This possibility must be evaluated by cervical cytology and endometrial biopsy or other technique of endometrial sampling.

❹ Recurrent episodes of vaginal bleeding in women who are not receiving hormonal replacement ther-apy may also be due to cancers of the cervix or body of the uterus. These women, too, must be evaluated by cervical cytology and endometrial biopsy or other technique of endometrial sampling.

❺ If the vaginal bleeding that the patient experiences is temporally related to hormone withdrawal it may be presumed to be pharmacologic. Recurrent episodes of this type of bleeding should suggest a need to re-evaluate the dosage and balance of hormones used. When the bleeding is not related to a withdrawal of hormones, the possibility of uterine cancer must be evaluated even though most episodes will be proven to be related to endometrial atrophy ("breakthrough bleeding").

❻ The advent of simple office endometrial sampling systems makes endometrial biopsy quick, easy, inexpensive, and safer compared to the traditional dilatation and curettage. A number of sampling devices (e.g., Accurette, Explora, Gynocheck, Pipelle, Z-Sampler) have been shown to provide reliable tissue diagnosis in 90% to 100% of cases. This office diagnostic technique is a valuable method of evaluating patients suspected of having endometrial cancer based on irregular perimenopausal or postmenopausal bleeding. Because it is associated with some discomfort and a small but not insignificant risk of perforation or infections, and carries not only the cost of the procedure but also the cost of histologic diagnosis, this procedure is best suited for diagnosis, not screening.

REFERENCES

Feldman S, Berkowitz RS, Tosteson ANA. Cost-effectiveness of strategies to evaluate postmenopausal bleeding. Obstet Gynecol 1993, 81:968–975.

Ferry J, Farnsworth A, Webster M, Wren B. The efficacy of the pipelle endometrial biopsy in detecting endometrial carcinoma. Aust NZ J Obstet Gynaecol 1993, 33:76–78.

Goldchmit R, Katz Z, Blickstein I, et al. The accuracy of endometrial pipell sampling with and without sonographic measurement of endometrial thickness. Obstet Gynecol 1993, 82:727–730.

Goldstein SR. Use of ultrasono-hysterography for triage of perimenoapusal patients with unexplained uterine bleeding. Am J Obstet Gynecol 1994, 170:565–570.

Reid PC, Brown VA, Fothergill DJ. Outpatient investigation of postmenopausal bleeding. Br J Obstet Gynaecol 1993, 100:498.

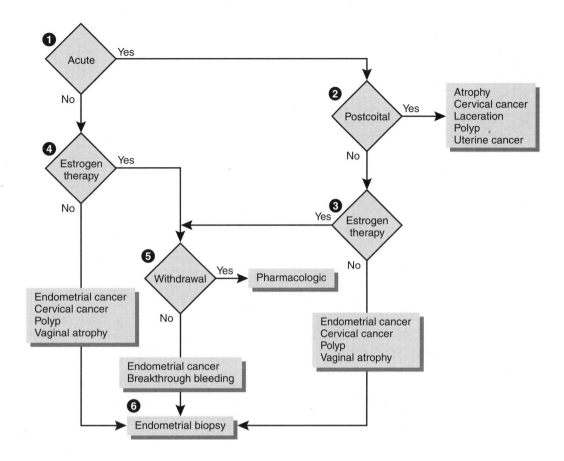

Premenstrual Syndrome

INTRODUCTION

Premenstrual syndrome (PMS) is a syndrome of physical and emotional symptoms characterized by its relationship to menses: symptoms are confined to a period or not more than 14 days prior to the onset of menstrual flow and resolve completely at, or soon after, the end of menstrual flow. It is estimated to effect 25% to 85% of reproductive-age women, though only 2% to 5% meet strict diagnostic criteria. The physiologic basis of PMS, premenstrual dysphoric disorder (PMDD), and premenstrual magnification (PMM) have yet to be established. The most promising research into a cause of PMS has been in the areas of β-endorphins and serotonin.

❶ Because patients with many diverse problems and pathologies will present for care with the self-applied label of "PMS," one of the first tasks it to consider the possibility of somatic diseases or psychological disturbances masquerading as PMS.

❷ To establish the diagnosis of PMS, a prospective menstrual calendar or other diary for a 3-month period must be obtained. Physical or emotional symptoms are confined to a period or not more than 14 days before the onset of menstrual flow and resolve completely at, or soon after, the end of menstrual flow. (The character of the symptoms is not important, only the timing of their appearance. Symptoms that are present at all times but worsen prior to menses or those that appear at irregular intervals do not meet the criteria for PMS.)

❸ A number of therapies for PMS have been proposed, including lifestyle changes (aerobic exercise (20 to 45 minutes, 3 times weekly), smoking cessation, stress reduction) and dietary changes or supplementation. When specific symptoms predominate, therapies directed toward reducing the severity of these symptoms may be implemented. Antidepressants, third-generation oral contraceptives, danazol and even gonadotropin-releasing hormone agonists have been studied and advocated.

❹ Whatever course is chosen, the patient should be followed up after 2 to 3 cycles (with a symptom calendar) to assess the effects of therapy.

❺ If there is a good response to therapy, plans should be made to taper and stop therapy after approximately 6 months. This duration should provide long-term relief of symptoms. If symptoms recur, the diagnosis should once again be carefully established.

❻ Patients who fail to obtain at least partial relief with therapy or who experience a recurrence of symptoms after withdrawal of treatment should have their diagnosis carefully re-evaluated. If the diagnosis is again established, therapy may be reintroduced or an alternate therapy may be chosen.

REFERENCES

American College of Obstetricians and Gynecologists. Premenstrual syndrome. ACOG Committee Opinion 155. Washington, DC: ACOG, 1995.

American Psychiatric Association. Diagnostic and Statistical Manual of Mental Disorders, 4th ed. Washington, DC: American Psychiatric Association, 1994.

Freeman E, Rickels K, Sondheimer S, Scharlop B. Diagnostic classifications from daily symptom ratings of women who seek treatment for premenstrual symptoms. Am J Gynecol Health 1987;1:17.

Garris PD, Sokol MS, Kelly K, et al. Leuprolide acetate treatment of catamenial pneumothorax. Fertil Steril 1994;61:173–174.

Moline ML. Pharmacologic strategies for managing premenstrual syndrome. Clin Pharm 1993;12:181–196.

Plouffe L Jr, Trott EA. Premenstrual syndrome: New concepts and recent therapeutic breakthroughs. Postgrad Obstet Gynecol 1995;15:1–7.

Rubinow DR. The premenstrual syndrome: new views. JAMA 1992;268:1998.

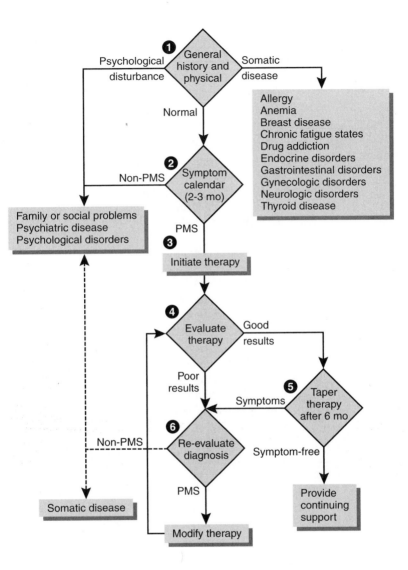

Pruritus Ani

INTRODUCTION

Perianal itching is often intense, distracting, and chronic. Pruritus ani is a symptom, not a diagnosis. Patients may present with complaints of vulvar itching or of a vaginal infection that has not responded to therapy. Successful treatment is predicated on establishing the diagnosis from a long list of possibilities.

❶ The evaluation of perianal itching begins with an examination of the vulva and perianal area.

❷ A number of skin and vulvar conditions can produce symptoms of itching. Many of these conditions are manifest by broken skin. Conditions that lack breaks in the integrity of the perineal epithelium may still be apparent. Punch biopsy should be considered to rule out malignancy or to clarify a difficult diagnosis. Treatment will be directed to the pathology encountered.

❸ If the pelvic examination is normal, anoscopy should be performed to evaluate the possibility of rectal pathology and to evaluate sphincter tone.

❹ Systemic diseases such as diabetes and chronic hepatic disease are frequently associated with perianal itching. If these are present, management of the systemic disease may improve the patient's symptoms. Gentle cleansing with nonabrasive materials (such as cotton balls), or the application of soothing solutions such as Burow's solution, along with thorough drying may provide soothing. Patients should be advised to wear loose-fitting clothing and keep the area dry and well ventilated.

❺ Studies to diagnose the presence of parasites or worms can establish these as a cause in the absence of physical signs.

❻ Some patients are extremely sensitive to contact allergens such as emollients, scented or colored toilet paper, and feminine hygiene products. These should be eliminated and the perineum cleansed with only clear water or unscented baby wipes.

Because of the possibility of food allergies, alcohol, caffeine, milk products, and chocolate should be eliminated for a period of 2 months. If symptoms abate, they may be added back individually until the offending agent is found. Drying agents, such as talc, may be of help. Antihistamines, especially at night when itching is often intense, and sedation may be desirable. Crotamiton (Eurax) may be applied topically, twice daily, to suppress itching. Occasionally, the use of a topical anesthetic, such as 2% lidocaine jelly, may be required.

REFERENCES

Alexander S. Dermatological aspects of anorectal disease. Clin Gastroenterol 1975;4:651.

Beart RW. Common anorectal problems. In Sciarra JJ (ed): Gynecology and Obstetrics. Philadelphia: JB Lippincott, 1992;(1)97:1.

Schrock TR. Diseases of the rectum and anus. In Wyngaarden JB, Smith LH, Jr, Bennett JC (eds): Cecil Textbook of Medicine, 19th ed. Philadelphia: WB Saunders, 1992, p 735.

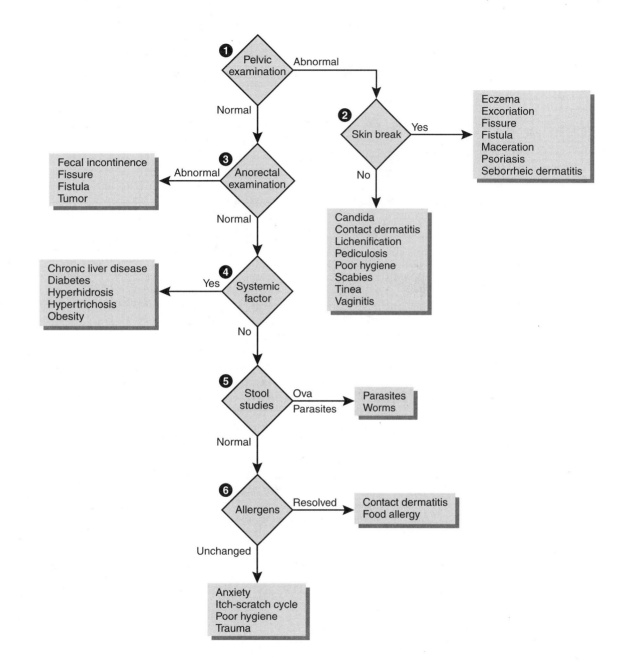

Pruritus Vulvae

INTRODUCTION

Intense itching and irritation of the vulva frequently leads to a self-perpetuation cycle of itching, scratching, dermal damage, healing with itching, and so forth.

❶ A careful history will frequently reveal one or more possible causes of vulvar itching. Gentle pelvic examination follows. Inspection of the vulva may reveal lesions, discharge, or discoloration that may suggest other pathologies.

❷ A microscopic examination of any vaginal secretions present under both saline and 10% KOH (potassium hydroxide) should be performed. Early or subclinical vaginitis may first present as mild or persistent vulvar itching.

❸ Skin scrapings from the vulva (obtained with a wooden spatula or the side of a scalpel blade) should be examined under 10% KOH solution. The presence of hyphae is diagnostic for cutaneous dermatophytes.

❹ Atrophic changes in the skin caused by the loss of estrogen stimulation (menopause) or lichen sclerosis often result in intense itching. If the diagnosis is in question, a dermal biopsy is indicated.

❺ A dusky or hyperpigmented appearance of the vulva may suggest chronic irritation (contact vulvitis) or the early stages of Bowen's disease. Once again, a biopsy will resolve the diagnosis.

❻ In the absence of irritants, behavioral and psychological interactions should be explored. Chronic urinary tract infections or vulvar human papilloma virus infection may cause itching with few other signs.

❼ Topical or systemic factors may be cause vulvar symptoms. Whenever possible, these should be identified and eliminated as a first line of therapy. If this fails, antihistamines, especially at night when itching is often intense, and sedation may be desirable. Crotamiton (Eurax) may be applied topically, twice daily, to suppress itching. Occasionally, the use of a topical anesthetic, such as 2% lidocaine jelly, may be required.

❽ Dermatologic conditions ranging from simple excoriation to cancer may present with vulvar symptoms and a visible lesion. Biopsy of the lesion is generally required to establish the diagnosis and should be performed liberally when the diagnosis is uncertain.

❾ Intense itching characterizes virtually all cases of lichen sclerosis. The vulva takes on a thinned, atrophic appearance, with linear scratch marks or fissures. The skin often has a "cigarette-paper" or parchment-like appearance. These changes frequently extend around the anus in a figure-eight configuration.

❿ Focal inflammation, punctation, and ulceration of the perineal and vaginal epithelium are generally found in patients with vulvar vestibulitis. Punctate areas (1 to 10) of inflammation 3 to 10 mm in size may be seen between the Bartholin glands, hymeneal ring, and mid-perineum in these patients (75% of cases). General reddening of the vulva skin without punctations may suggest hyperkeratosis or early dermatophye infection.

REFERENCES

American College of Obstetricians and Gynecologists. Vaginitis. ACOG Technical Bulletin 226. Washington, DC: ACOG, 1996.

American College of Obstetricians and Gynecologists. Vulvar Nonneoplastic Epithelial Disorders. ACOG Technical Bulletin 241. Washington, DC: ACOG, 1997.

McKay M. Vulvodynia versus pruritis vulvae. Clin Obstet Gynecol 1985;28:123.

McKay M. Vulvar dermatoses. Clin Obstet Gynecol 1991;34:614.

Nanda VS. Common dermatoses. Am J Obstet Gynecol 1995;173:488.

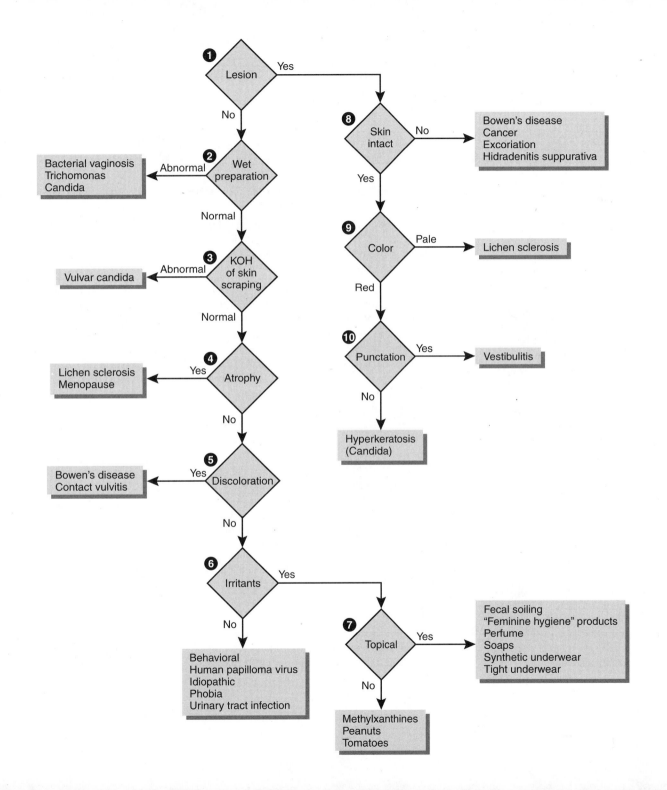

Puberty

Delayed

INTRODUCTION

Delayed puberty is a relatively uncommon problem in girls. When it occurs, the possibility of a genetic or hypothalamic–pituitary abnormality must be considered, along with a moderately large number of other possibilities. The objective is to evaluate patients who do not experience the normal events of puberty when expected and to provide reassurance when appropriate or timely diagnosis and intervention when more sinister processes are at work.

❶ Based on the average age and normal variation of puberty, any girl who has not exhibited breast budding by age 13 requires preliminary investigation. Similarly, girls who do not menstruate by age 15 or 16, regardless of other sexual development, should be evaluated. Patients should also be evaluated any time there is a disruption in the normal sequence of puberty, or there is patient or parental concern. Patients with significant abnormalities of either height or weight should be evaluated for chromosomal abnormalities or endocrinopathies.

❷ The evaluation of patients with delayed pubertal development must begin with a general history, including general health, weight and height records, and family history including the pubertal experience of others in the family. Physical examination should identify the type and degree of sexual development pressent. The presence of breast changes generally indicates the production of estrogen, while the development of pubic or axillary hair indicates the production of androgens. The pelvic examination will often identify a number of possible causes, including an imperforate hymen and other structural malformations.

❸ Measurement of gonadotropins will distinguish those patients who have hypergonadotropic hypogonadism (43%), hypogonadotropic hypogonadism (31%), and eugonadism (26%).

❹ Alkylating chemotherapy and radiation therapy may both cause the loss of ovarian follicles and premature ovarian failure, resulting in delayed or absent pubertal changes.

❺ Karyotypic abnormalities account for 26% of pubertal delays, though 17% of patients will have normal karyotypes with gonadal failure. One of the most common chromosomal causes is Turner syndrome (45, X). The absence of one X chromosome results in accelerated ovarian follicular atresia, to the extent that by the age of puberty, no functionally competent follicles remain. These patients are noteworthy for their short stature, webbed neck (pterygium colli), a shieldlike chest with widely spaced nipples, and an increased carrying angle of the arms (cubitus valgus). Buccal smears will not demonstrate Barr bodies and chromosomal analysis will confirm the diagnosis. Deletions of only a part of the long arm of the X chromosome have been shown to be associated with premature ovarian failure, with the earliest failures associated with the greatest deletions.

❻ Abnormalities of weight may be associated with hypogonadotropic hypogonadism.

❼ Pituitary and other tumors account for less than 3% of cases of delayed puberty.

❽ Cushing's disease and primary hypothyroidism are uncommon sources of pubertal delays and are often suggested by other symptoms or findings.

❾ Chronic marijuana use has been associated with delayed puberty in a number of published studies.

❿ The inability to detect odors is characteristic of Kallmann syndrome. Roughly 10% of patients with delayed puberty have a constitutional delay as the only cause found. Hormonal therapy for these patients will allow normal height and bone mass deposition to be achieved. Therapy usually begins with unopposed estrogen in the form of 0.3 mg of conjugated estrogen, 0.5 mg estradiol, or their equivalent daily. In 6 to 12 months, this dose is roughly doubled and medroxyprogesterone acetate (10 mg for the first 12 days of the month) is added. This will result in regular menstruation, but is insufficient for contraception. Normal pubertal development will generally proceed when the patient reaches a bone age of 13.

REFERENCES

American College of Obstetricians and Gynecologists. Pediatric Gynecologic Disorders. ACOG Technical Bulletin 201. Washington, DC: ACOG, 1995.

American College of Obstetricians and Gynecologists. The Adolescent Gynecologic Patient. ACOG Technical Bulletin 145, Washington, DC: ACOG, 1990.

Lee PA. Normal ages of pubertal events among American males and females. J Adolesc Health Care 1980;1:26.

Reindollar RH, Byrd JR, McDonough PG. Delayed sexual development: a study of 252 patients. Am J Obstet Gynecol 1981; 140:371–380.

Reindollar RH, McDonough PG. Pubertal aberrancy: etiology and clinical approach. J Reprod Med 1984; 29:391–398.

Zacharias L, Rand WM, Wurtman RJ. A prospective study of sexual development and growth in American girls: the statistics of menarch. Obstet Gynecol Surv 1976; 31:325.

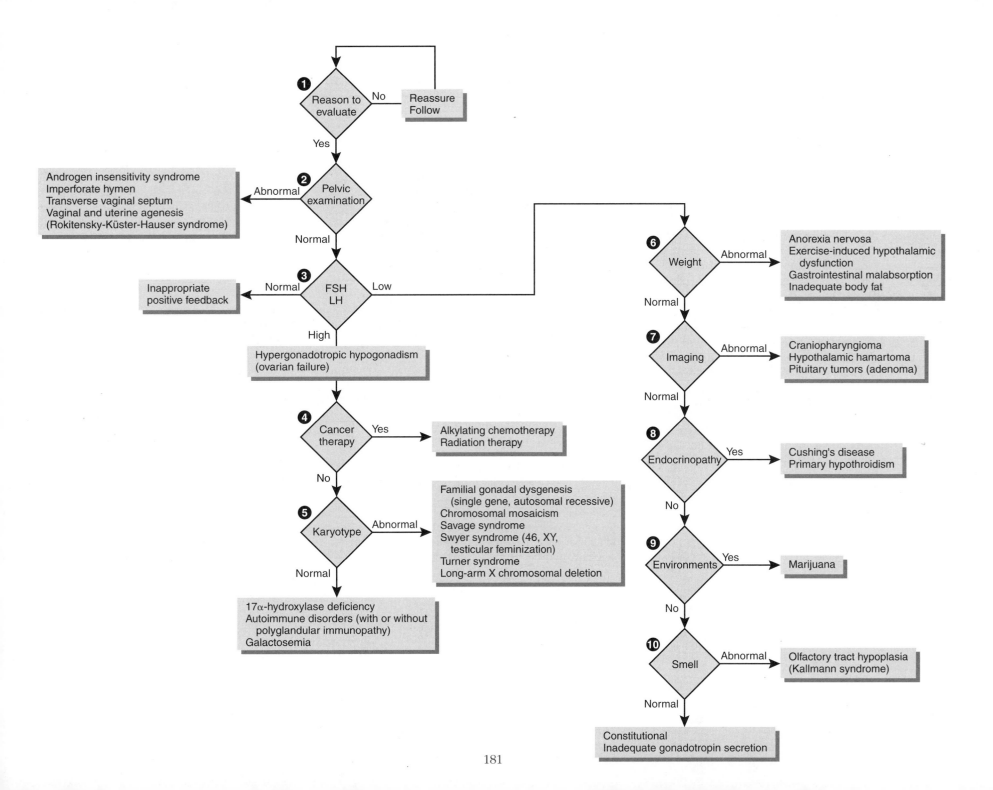

1 Reason to evaluate — No → Reassure Follow

Yes ↓

2 Pelvic examination — Abnormal → Androgen insensitivity syndrome
Imperforate hymen
Transverse vaginal septum
Vaginal and uterine agenesis
(Rokitensky-Küster-Hauser syndrome)

Normal ↓

3 FSH LH
— Normal → Inappropriate positive feedback
— Low →

High ↓

Hypergonadotropic hypogonadism (ovarian failure)

↓

4 Cancer therapy — Yes → Alkylating chemotherapy
Radiation therapy

No ↓

5 Karyotype — Abnormal → Familial gonadal dysgenesis
(single gene, autosomal recessive)
Chromosomal mosaicism
Savage syndrome
Swyer syndrome (46, XY,
testicular feminization)
Turner syndrome
Long-arm X chromosomal deletion

Normal ↓

17α-hydroxylase deficiency
Autoimmune disorders (with or without polyglandular immunopathy)
Galactosemia

6 Weight — Abnormal → Anorexia nervosa
Exercise-induced hypothalamic dysfunction
Gastrointestinal malabsorption
Inadequate body fat

Normal ↓

7 Imaging — Abnormal → Craniopharyngioma
Hypothalamic hamartoma
Pituitary tumors (adenoma)

Normal ↓

8 Endocrinopathy — Yes → Cushing's disease
Primary hypothroidism

No ↓

9 Environments — Yes → Marijuana

No ↓

10 Smell — Abnormal → Olfactory tract hypoplasia
(Kallmann syndrome)

Normal ↓

Constitutional
Inadequate gonadotropin secretion

181

Puberty

Premature

INTRODUCTION

While precocious puberty is most often heralded by the sequence of increased growth, thelarche, and adrenarche, these events may occur simultaneously, or menarche itself may be the first indication. True precocious puberty, also known as complete, isosexual, or central precocity, is related to early activation of the hypothalamic–pituitary–gonadal axis. In 75% of patients, there is no indication of how or why the normal processes of puberty are accelerated. In the remaining 25%, a central nervous system abnormality is to blame. A number of central nervous system pathologies may result in activation of gonadotropin-releasing hormone (GnRH) secretion and the early onset of pubertal changes.

Precocious pseudopuberty, also referred to as incomplete or peripheral puberty, may be isosexual or heterosexual. In these patients, there may be secretion of sex steroids or human chorionic gonadotropin from sources other than the pituitary.

❶ Many causes of premature puberty will be established or suggested by findings in the history or during the physical examination. Evaluations of percentiles for height, weight, Tanner stage, and growth rates should be measured and recorded.

Over 10% of girls with precocious puberty have an ovarian tumor. These tumors are palpable in 80% of cases, or may be readily detected by ultrasonography or tomographic studies. Bleeding is heavy and irregular in character, befitting their escape from the normal control mechanisms.

❷ Imaging of the head and/or abdomen and pelvis (as indicated by clinical findings or suspicions) can diagnose some of the more sinister causes of premature puberty. Organic brain disease accounts for approximately 7% of premature puberty. Ovarian tumors (most often detected during the physical examination) may be discovered in up to 11% of premature puberty patients.

❸ The laboratory evaluation of patients with premature puberty should include the measurement of serum follicle-stimulating hormone (FSH), luteinizing hormone (LH), and prolactin, a sensitive thyroid-stimulating hormone (TSH) and thyroxine (T_4 measurement, and an evaluation of steroids (dehydroepiandrosterone, testosterone, estradiol, progesterone, and 17α-hydroxyprogesterone).

❹ Idiopathic (constitutional) precocious puberty accounts for 74% of cases. When the diagnosis of true precocious puberty is established, generally by exclusion, treatment with GnRH agonists will usually halt the progression of change. This therapy is expensive and will only be effective if the observed changes are under central control. Suppression of GnRH may also be carried out using medroxyprogesterone acetate (Depo-Provera), in doses of 100 to 200 mg given intramuscularly every 2 to 4 weeks. This therapy is less likely to control bone-growth abnormalities than is GnRH agonist treatment.

REFERENCES

American College of Obstetricians and Gynecologists. Pediatric Gynecologic Disorders. ACOG Technical Bulletin 201. Washington, DC: ACOG, 1995.

American College of Obstetricians and Gyencologists. The Adolescent Gynecologic Patient. ACOG Technical Bulletin 145, Washington, DC: ACOG, 1990.

Lee PA. Normal ages of pubertal events among American males and females. J Adolesc Health Care 1980;1:26

Reindollar RH, McDonough PG. Pubertal aberrancy: etiology and clinical approach. J Reprod Med 1984;29:391–398.

Stein DT. New developments in the diagnosis and treatment of sexual precocity. Am J Med Sci 1992;303:53.

Wheeler MD, Styne DM. The treatment of precocious puberty. Endocrinol Metab Clin North Am 1991;20:183.

Zacharias L, Rand WM, Wurtman RJ. A prospective study of sexual development and growth in American girls: the statistics of menarch. Obstet Gynecol Surv 1976;31:325.

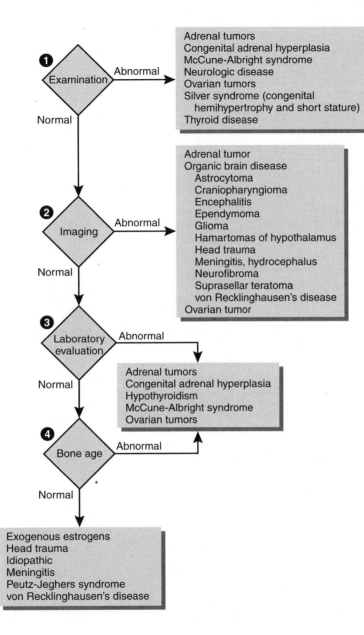

1 Examination —— Abnormal ——▶ Adrenal tumors
Congenital adrenal hyperplasia
McCune-Albright syndrome
Neurologic disease
Ovarian tumors
Silver syndrome (congenital
 hemihypertrophy and short stature)
Thyroid disease

Normal

2 Imaging —— Abnormal ——▶ Adrenal tumor
Organic brain disease
 Astrocytoma
 Craniopharyngioma
 Encephalitis
 Ependymoma
 Glioma
 Hamartomas of hypothalamus
 Head trauma
 Meningitis, hydrocephalus
 Neurofibroma
 Suprasellar teratoma
 von Recklinghausen's disease
Ovarian tumor

Normal

3 Laboratory
evaluation —— Abnormal ——▶

Normal

Adrenal tumors
Congenital adrenal hyperplasia
Hypothyroidism
McCune-Albright syndrome
Ovarian tumors

4 Bone age —— Abnormal ——▶

Normal

Exogenous estrogens
Head trauma
Idiopathic
Meningitis
Peutz-Jeghers syndrome
von Recklinghausen's disease

Rectal Bleeding

Frank

INTRODUCTION

The significance of rectal bleeding can span as wide a range of threat as the volume of bleeding itself: from the scant bleeding of external hemorrhoids to life-threatening losses due to lacerations or tumors. Prompt evaluation and treatment are required to protect the patient's health and to provide peace of mind.

❶ When faced with the acute evaluation of ongoing rectal bleeding, one of the first issues to ascertain is the volume of blood loss involved. Large-volume losses represent a different level of threat and etiology than do smaller bleeding episodes.

❷ At times, the blood loss associated with rectal bleeding can be so massive that resuscitation and surgical evaluation may be needed before any attempt at diagnosis can be finalized.

❸ Patients who are stable should undergo an examination of the perineum to look for lacerations, and a digital examination for tumors or polyps. When present, these may require surgical evaluation or treatment to control bleeding. Hemorrhoidal bleeding is common, but not commonly of large volume.

❹ Small-volume rectal bleeding that is associated with a bowel movement is most often caused by local conditions such as hemorrhoids, fissures, or small lacerations associated with constipation. Blood on the toilet tissue may also arise from perineal or vulvar lesions and be misattributed to a rectal origin. Pelvic and rectal examinations are generally sufficient to establish the diagnosis.

❺ When the diagnosis is not apparent by history and physical examination, sigmoidoscopy or colonoscopy will be necessary to establish a diagnosis.

REFERENCES

Bassford T. Treatment of common anorectal disorders (review). Am Fam Phys 1992;45:1787.

Bleday R, Pena JP, Rothenberger DA, et al. Symptomatic hemorrhoids: current incidence and complications of operative therapy. Dis Colon Rectum 1992;35:477–481.

Devine R, Ory S. Treatment of hemorrhoids in pregnancy. J Fam Pract 1992;17:65.

Guthri JF. The current management of hemorrhoid. Pract Gastroenterol 1987;11:56.

Mazier WP. Hemorrhoids, fissures, and pruritus ani (review). Surg Clin North Am 1994;74:1277.

Medich DS, Fazio VW. Hemorrhoids, anal fissure, and carcinoma of the colon, rectum, and anus during pregnancy. Surg Clin North Am 1995;75:77.

Schussman LC, Lutz LJ. Outpatient management of hemorrhoids. Prim Care 1986;13:527.

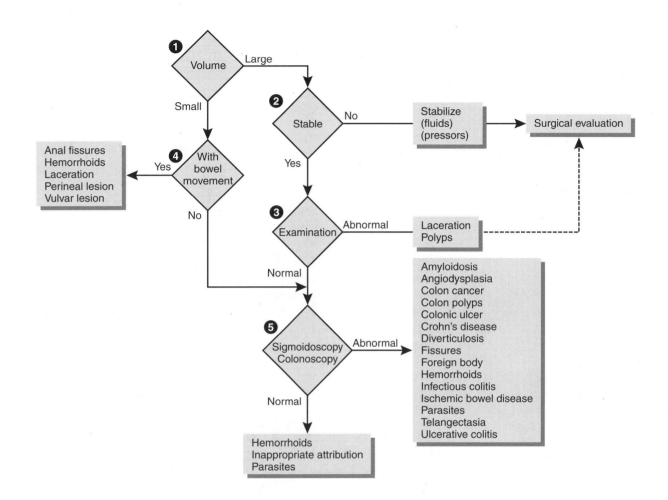

1 Volume
— Large
— Small

2 Stable
— No → Stabilize (fluids) (pressors) → Surgical evaluation
— Yes

4 With bowel movement
— Yes → Anal fissures / Hemorrhoids / Laceration / Perineal lesion / Vulvar lesion
— No

3 Examination
— Abnormal → Laceration / Polyps ⤑ Surgical evaluation
— Normal

5 Sigmoidoscopy Colonoscopy
— Abnormal → Amyloidosis / Angiodysplasia / Colon cancer / Colon polyps / Colonic ulcer / Crohn's disease / Diverticulosis / Fissures / Foreign body / Hemorrhoids / Infectious colitis / Ischemic bowel disease / Parasites / Telangectasia / Ulcerative colitis
— Normal → Hemorrhoids / Inappropriate attribution / Parasites

Rectal Bleeding

Occult

INTRODUCTION

Current guidelines for screening for colorectal cancer suggest that low-risk individuals have a digital rectal examination with a test for fecal occult blood performed annually after the age of 50. For high-risk individuals this testing may be begun earlier or performed more frequently. The result of this screening is often a positive test for occult blood in the absence of any clinically obvious cause. The evaluation of these patients must be balanced between cost effectiveness and appropriate vigilance.

❶ A number of factors can result in either false-positive or false-negative tests for fecal occult blood: Oral iron therapy can provide a false-positive, while large dose of vitamin C can result in a false-negative test. Obvious sources of confusion, including excessive meat intake, should be eliminated and the test repeated. (Some authors suggest 3 days of a meatless diet before testing.) A hematocrit should also be considered if significant acute or ongoing loss is suspected.

❷ Internal and external hemorrhoids are the most common source of fecal occult blood. These are readily detected by anorectal examination. If these are present and it is apparent that they are source of the bleeding, the evaluation may be suspended. In any case where the diagnosis is not apparent, or the patient is at higher risk for alimentary canal pathology, further evaluation is required.

❸ Colonoscopy (or sigmoidoscopy in select cases) provides the next step in the evaluation of the patient with occult blood loss.

❹ If colonoscopy does not provide an explanation of the occult blood loss, an evaluation of the upper gastrointestinal tract is warranted. If all of this evaluation is fruitless, most authors suggest carefully monitoring the patient with follow-up stool guaiac tests and rectal examinations (with or without sigmoidoscopy) at 6-month intervals until there have been three negative examinations (18 months). If no further explanation is found in this period, it is unlikely that the lesion is significant.

REFERENCES

Bassford T. Treatment of common anorectal disorders (review). Am Fam Phys 1992;45:1787

Bleday R, Pena JP, Rothenberger DA, et al. Symptomatic hemorrhoids: current incidence and complications of operative therapy. Dis Colon Rectum. 1992;35;477–481.

Devine R, Ory S. Treatment of hemorrhoids in pregnancy. J Fam Pract 1992;17:65.

Guthri JF. The current management of hemorrhoid. Pract Gastroenterol 1987;11:56.

Mazier WP. Hemorrhoids, fissures, and pruritus ani (review). Surg Clin North Am 1994;74:1277.

Medich DS, Fazio VW. Hemorrhoids, anal fissure, and carcinoma of the colon, rectum, and anus during pregnancy. Surg Clin North Am 1995;75:77.

Schussman LC, Lutz LJ. Outpatient management of hemorrhoids. Prim Care 1986;13:527.

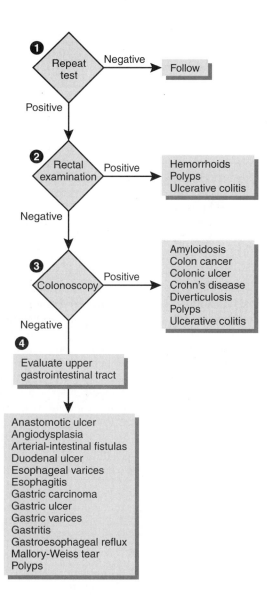

① Repeat test — Negative → Follow

Positive ↓

② Rectal examination — Positive → Hemorrhoids / Polyps / Ulcerative colitis

Negative ↓

③ Colonoscopy — Positive → Amyloidosis / Colon cancer / Colonic ulcer / Crohn's disease / Diverticulosis / Polyps / Ulcerative colitis

Negative ↓

④ Evaluate upper gastrointestinal tract

↓

Anastomotic ulcer
Angiodysplasia
Arterial-intestinal fistulas
Duodenal ulcer
Esophageal varices
Esophagitis
Gastric carcinoma
Gastric ulcer
Gastric varices
Gastritis
Gastroesophageal reflux
Mallory-Weiss tear
Polyps

Sexual Ambiguity

INTRODUCTION

Structural abnormalities present at birth may make the assignment of an appropriate sex of rearing (gender) difficult or impossible. The evaluation of these infants represents both a social and medical emergency because life-threatening conditions may be present. For example, in infants with congenital adrenal hyperplasia, symptoms of vomiting, diarrhea, dehydration, and shock may develop rapidly. Failure to establish a clear, unambiguous gender (sex of rearing) can result in life-long social and psychological problems and may limit future surgical reconstruction and sexual options. Therapy is medical and surgical: medical therapy to reverse the effects of enzyme defects, surgical therapy for cosmetics and sexual function. Surgery is often delayed until late infancy or adolescence (based on the type of reconstruction planned). If a Y-chromosome cell line is present, removal of the gonads is indicated.

❶ The evaluation must begin with a careful overall assessment, including a review of the patient's pregnancy history. In utero androgen exposure can result in signs that vary from mild clitoral hypertrophy from low levels of androgens late in fetal development, all the way to complete labioscrotal fold formation and a penile urethra. If a history of androgen exposure is present, and the severity of the abnormality, then either a karyotype or pelvic ultrasonography (to determine the presence or absence of a uterus) should be performed to determine genetic gender and guide future management.

❷ The newborn should be carefully examined for the presence of other anomalies that would suggest the wider problem of dysembryogenesis.

❸ When androgen exposure and other anomalies are absent, a karyotype (or buccal smears) should be performed. Ultrasonography may be used to determine the presence of a uterus, but this will not determine genetic gender because the internal genital tract will develop in the absence of müllerian-inhibiting factor. The genetic gender will class the infant as a male or female pseudohermaphrodite and guide the next step in testing.

❹ Genetic females should have levels of dehydroepiandrosterone sulfate (DHEAs), androstenedione, and 17α-hydroxyprogesterone (17α-OH-P) determined. This will identify the presence of enzyme defects or true hermaphroditism.

❺ Genetic males should have levels of testosterone measured following human chorionic gonadotropin (hCG) stimulation.

REFERENCES

Coran AG, Porley TZ. Surgical management of ambiguous genitalia in the infant and child. J Pediatr Surg 1991;26:812.

Donahue PK, Powell DM, Lee MK. Clinical management of intersex abnormalities. Curr Prob Surg 1992;28:515.

Myers-Seifer CH, Charest NJ. Diagnosis and management of patients with ambiguous genitalia. Sem Perinatol 1992;16:332.

New MI. Female pseudo-hermaphroditism. Sem Perinatol 1992;16:289.

Speroff L, Glass RH, Kase NG. Clinical Gynecologic Endocrinology and Infertility, 5th ed. Baltimore: Williams & Wilkins, 1994, p 350.

White PC, New MI, DuPont B. Congenital adrenal hyperplasia. N Engl J Med 1987;316:1519.

Wilson JD, Geroge FW, Griffin JE. The hormonal control of sexual development. Science 1981;211:1278.

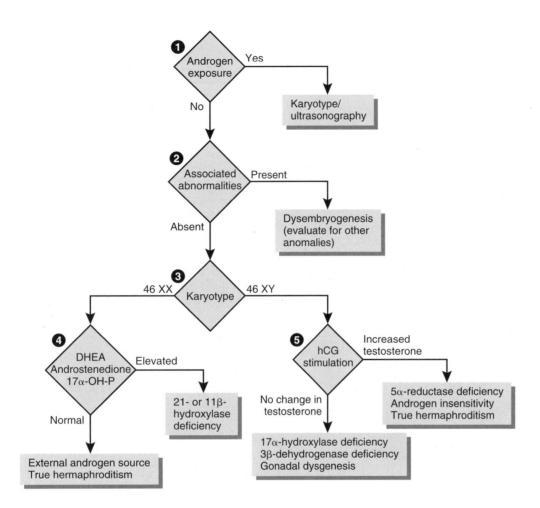

❶ Androgen exposure

Yes → Karyotype/ultrasonography

No ↓

❷ Associated abnormalities

Present → Dysembryogenesis (evaluate for other anomalies)

Absent ↓

❸ Karyotype

46 XX → **❹** DHEA Androstenedione 17α-OH-P

46 XY → **❺** hCG stimulation

❹ DHEA Androstenedione 17α-OH-P

Elevated → 21- or 11β-hydroxylase deficiency

Normal → External androgen source True hermaphroditism

❺ hCG stimulation

Increased testosterone → 5α-reductase deficiency Androgen insensitivity True hermaphroditism

No change in testosterone → 17α-hydroxylase deficiency 3β-dehydrogenase deficiency Gonadal dysgenesis

Sexual Counseling

INTRODUCTION

Sexual counseling by the nonspecalist is aimed at reducing anxiety and demands for performance, removing impediments to responsiveness, and providing guidance to the physical and psychological behaviors that will enhance sexual expression. The main objective of sexual counseling is to allow the couple to be comfortable with their sexual expressions and overcome any obstacles to satisfaction with this expression. These goals can be met in the context of a busy office practice.

❶ The first task is to determine if a problem exists. Frequently, a patient is uncertain about a behavior, feeling, or experience. As long as it does not pose a problem for the patient, involves no physical risk or coercion, and is not illegal, no problem exists and no intervention is required.

❷ The simplest and most effective initial intervention when a problem is found is simple permission. Just as in establishing the presence of a problem, if a given behavior or desire is not illegal, unsafe, or performed under duress, it is "OK". This reassurance that the patient is not abnormal is often sufficient to resolve the issue. Problems that are resolved at this level are often presented with "Is it OK to..." or "Is that OK?"

❸ When simple information is not enough, providing limited information is often sufficient to resolve the problem. This should not be an expansive medical lecture, but rather information to put in perspective the patient's concern. This may include medical information about sexual or reproductive function, or information about the prevalence of a behavior or activity. A number of resources are available for both the provider and patient that give this type of information.

❹ If permission and limited information are insufficient to resolve the problem, simple specific suggestions constitute the next step. For most providers this will be limited to common sense suggestions about mood, setting, timing, and alternate forms of sexual expression such as different forms of pleasuring or coital positions. Extensive suggestions and intensive interventions are rarely needed and are best left to specifically trained specialists.

REFERENCES

American College of Obstetricians and Gynecologists. Sexual Dysfunction. ACOG Technical Bulletin 211. Washington, DC: ACOG, 1995.

Duddle M, Brown ADG. The clinical management of sexual dysfunction. Clin Obstet Gynecol 1980;7(2):293.

Smith RP. Gynecology in Primary Care. Baltimore: Williams & Wilkins, 1997, pp 193–208, 517–536.

Wabrek AJ. Sex counseling in office practice. In Glass RH (ed): Office Gynecology, 4th ed. Baltimore: Williams & Wilkins, 1993, pp 189–210.

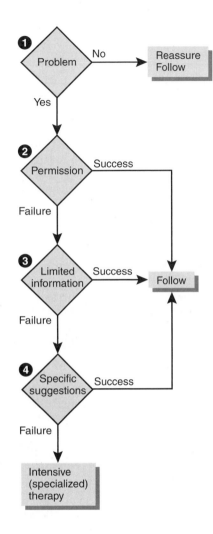

Sexual Dysfunction

Libidinal Dysfunction

INTRODUCTION

Libidinal dysfunction is a lack of interest in sexual expression or sexual contact. The most common causes of sexual dysfunction are relationship problems, intrapsychic factors, and medical factors. Relationship problems are an obvious source for sexual problems, but both the patient and her doctor often overlook them. Marital or relationship stresses may be acted out by sexual distancing, orgasmic failure, or exploitation. Anger, hidden agendas, lack of trust, or infidelity may be expressed through the withdrawal of intimacy. Libidinal mismatches are common, but when combined with poor communication, lead to dysfunction. Dual-income families may not realize the impact fatigue and a fast-paced lifestyle may be having on their ability to express warmth and be sexually expressive. Medical factors that influence sexual performance include drugs and alcohol, depression, anxiety, chronic illness, pregnancy, untreated menopause, and the effects of surgical therapies.

❶ It should be apparent that the patient's history is the most critical part of the evaluation of libidinal problems. Among the first aspects to explore are the characteristics of the lack of desire; do the patient's concerns represent a global lack of interest in sexual contact that has always been present and precludes any thoughts of sexual activity of any sort. Depression, physical or sexual abuse (current or past), or phobias may present in this manner.

❷ The loss of interest in sexual expression that had been established in the past may suggest the onset of depression or abuse, the effects of medical disease that alter the pleasure of sexual activities. Examples of the latter problems, are vulvodynia, and diabetic neuropathy, or in younger patients, multiple sclerosis.

❸ When the lack of sexual interest is episodic but longstanding, the symptoms may be manifestations of variable moods, inappropriate expectations by either or both partners, or a perceived problem resulting from a mismatch of sexual drives between partners. The loss of pleasure (or the failure to achieve it in the first place) may result in the loss of interest as well.

❹ The abrupt onset of libidinal dysfunction with a new partner should suggest the possibility, if not the probability, of sexual or physical abuse. A perceived mismatch of levels of interest may result in one or the other partner's believing that he or she is abnormal in his or her level of interest (either high or low). Painful intercourse, fears of pregnancy, depression over a change in life or lifestyle, or other factors may all present as a loss of sexual interest.

REFERENCES

Alexander B. Disorders of sexual desire: Diagnosis and treatment of decreased libido. Am Fam Phys 1993;47(4): 832–838.

American College of Obstetricians and Gynecologists. Sexual Dysfunction. ACOG Technical Bulletin 211. Washington, DC: ACOG, 1995.

Smith RP. Gynecology in Primary Care. Baltimore: Williams & Wilkins, 1997, pp 193–208, 517–536.

Wabrek AJ. Sex counseling in office practice. In Glass RH (ed): Office Gynecology, 4th ed. Baltimore: Williams & Wilkins, 1993, pp 189–210.

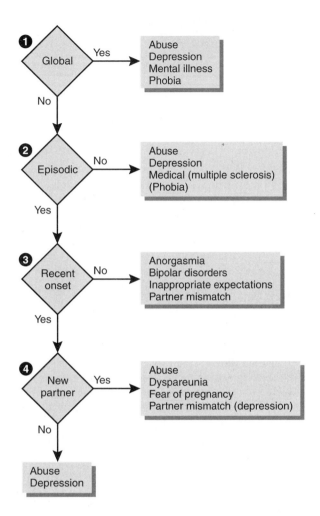

193

Sexual Dysfunction

Orgasmic Failure (Anorgasmia)

INTRODUCTION

Studies indicate that only 30% to 40% of women are able to experience orgasm during intercourse, and up to 15% of sexually active women have never experienced sexual release. Once proximation and arousal have occurred, orgasmic success requires effective stimulation, of a sufficient quality over a sufficient time, provided in a supportive environment. Failures in any of these areas may present as orgasmic problems. Medical factors that influence sexual performance include drugs and alcohol, depression, anxiety, chronic illness, pregnancy, untreated menopause, and the effects of surgical therapies. Many patients who do not achieve orgasm during intercourse are fully orgasmic with additional manual stimulation, oral–genital stimulation, use of a vibrator, or through masturbation. (About 30% to 40% of women require concurrent clitoral stimulation to achieve orgasm.) This is common enough that it should be viewed as a problem only if it is a source of concern for the patient or her partner.

❶ When evaluating patients with orgasmic difficulties, it is important to differentiate between situational dysfunction and complete orgasmic failure. This may help to differentiate those with relationship problems, intrapsychic factors, and medical factors.

❷ Popular media portrayals of orgasm are often unrealistic or glamorized. As a result, some orgasmic women may not realize that what they are experiencing is an orgasm. One very functional description of an orgasm is that it is like a sneeze: It is difficult to describe, but it was what was needed at the time.

❸ Women who have never been able to achieve orgasm may benefit from self-exploration. Popular rearing styles result in the majority of women viewing their genitalia as dirty, forbidding, and the source of embarrassment. Anatomic instruction and an opportunity to explore both the structure and sensations associated with their genitalia, in a nondemand setting, can often provide both the permission and the tools for sexual expression.

❹ The inability to perform self-exploration suggests a phobia or the possibility of past (or current) abuse. The possibility of depression, phobias, or mental illness should be carefully, and sensitively, considered for patients who do not benefit from self-exploration exercises. This should not be considered in a punitive manner, but only as the next step in the evaluation. When these factors have been ruled out, the possibility of a medical condition that affects the patient's ability to perform and respond sexually should be explored.

❺ Women who are unable to achieve success on an occasional basis should be questioned about the possibilities of a new partner, a change in sexual techniques or modes of expression, or the development of fears associated with intercourse (such as pregnancy or disease).

❻ Women who have previously been orgasmic but now find themselves unable to achieve success should be evaluated for the emergence of psychological or medical factors that are interfering with success. The unfolding of depression, phobias, or mental illness can lead to the loss of sexual responsiveness. Sleep disorders, with their attendant fatigue, myalgias, and common depressive symptoms may result in anorgasmia. Medical diseases, including many medications, can have a deleterious effect on sexual performance.

❼ Both systemic and local factors can adversely affect orgasmic ability. Pelvic examination may reveal vaginal atrophy, vulvar or vaginal lesions, infections, vulvodynia, or vestibulitis. History, physical examination, and limited, directed laboratory or other investigations, will identify systemic factors, not all of which can be successfully reversed.

REFERENCES

American College of Obstetricians and Gynecologists. Sexual Dysfunction. ACOG Technical Bulletin 211. Washington, DC: ACOG, 1995.

Duddle M, Brown ADG. The clinical management of sexual dysfunction. Clin Obstet Gynecol 1980;7(2):293.

Shen WW, Sata LS. Inhibited female orgasm resulting from psychotropic drugs. J Reprod Med 1983;28:497.

Smith RP. Gynecology in Primary Care. Baltimore: Williams & Wilkins, 1997, pp 193–208, 517–536.

Wabrek AJ. Sex counseling in office practice. In Glass RH (ed): Office Gynecology, 4th ed. Baltimore: Williams & Wilkins, 1993, pp 189–210.

Zeiss AM, Rosen GM, Zeiss RA. Orgasm during intercourse: a treatment strategy for women. J Consult Clin Psychol 1977;45:891.

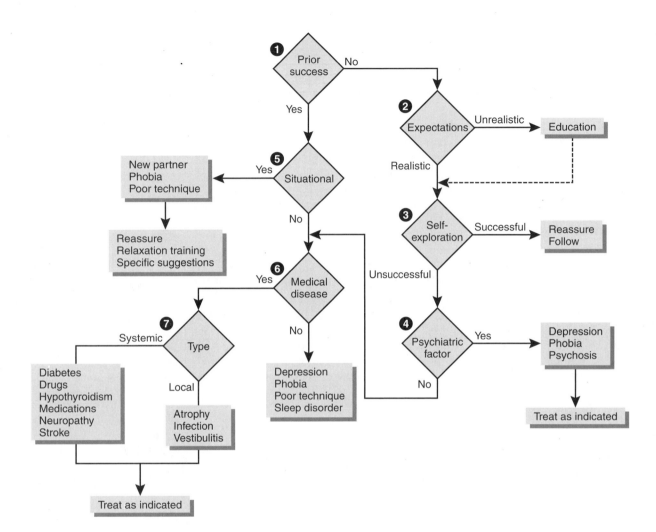

Syphilis

Positive Screening Test

INTRODUCTION

The VDRL (Venereal Disease Research Laboratory) and RPR (rapid plasma reagin) are nonspecific tests for syphilis that are good for screening because they are rapid and inexpensive. Unfortunately, as with most screening tests, the results obtained must be confirmed by other means to establish a diagnosis.

❶ When screening tests are positive, a follow-up with a treponemal-specific serologic test is indicated. The FTA-ABS (fluorescent treponemal antibody absorption) and MHA-TP (microhemagglutination assay—*Treponema pallidum*) tests are specific treponemal antibody tests that are confirmatory or diagnostic, but are not used for routine screening. These latter tests are useful to rule out "false-positive" screening tests caused by such diverse conditions are atypical pneumonia, malaria, and some vaccinations. They are also useful in early infections before antibodies have been elaborated.

❷ If treponemal-specific tests are negative, the original screening test may be presumed to represent a false-positive test. Patients who are at low risk for infection require no further evaluations, while those at high risk or test weakly positive (e.g., 1 : 8) should be rechecked periodically.

❸ If treponemal-specific tests are positive, it must be determined if the infection is new or old. If the patient has no history of previous infection, she is diagnosed as a new case and must undergo staging and appropriate therapy.

❹ It the patient has been previously diagnosed but has not received therapy, a lumbar puncture with a VDRL test performed on the cerebro-spinal fluid is required to stage the disease prior to beginning treatment.

❺ If the adequacy of treatment cannot be verified or was inadequate, staging (including a lumbar puncture) must be performed. If the treatment is determined to have been adequate, reinfection or treatment failure is presumed.

REFERENCES

Centers for Disease Control and Prevention, 1998. Guidelines for treatment of sexually transmitted diseases. MMWR 1998:47(RR-1):28.

EI-Zaatari MM, Martens MG, Anderson GD. Incidence of the prozone phenomenon in syphilis serology. Obstet Gynecol 1994;84:609–612.

Rolfs RT. Treatment of syphilis, 1993. Clin Infect Dis 1995;20(S1):S23.

Romanowski B, Sutherland R, Fick GH, et al. Serologic response to treatment of infectious syphilis. Ann Intern Med 1991;114:1005–1009.

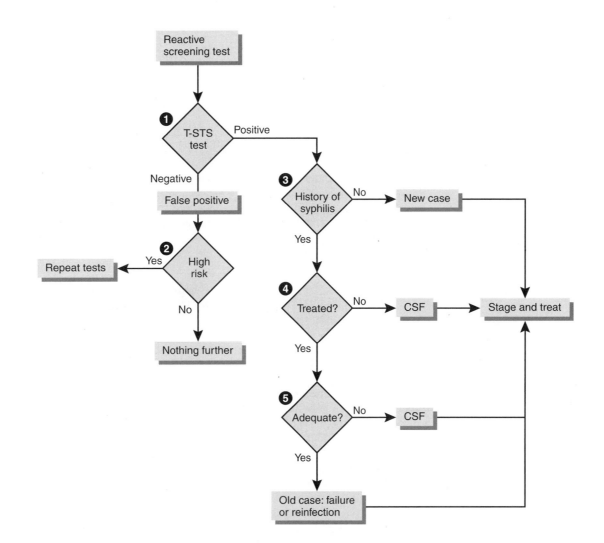

Toxic Shock Syndrome

INTRODUCTION

Toxic shock syndrome (TSS) is an acute, multisystem, life-threatening illness first identified in 1978. The disease most commonly affects menstruating women (95%) and is characterized by a dramatic onset of high fever, a "sunburn-like" rash, myalgia, nausea, vomiting, watery diarrhea, hypotension, vascular collapse, and multiorgan failure. Those patients who survive have desquamation of the skin of the hands and feet. Toxic shock syndrome is caused by toxins produced by an often asymptomatic infection with *Staphylococcus aureus.*

❶ Toxic shock syndrome (TSS) is a truly life-threatening syndrome that requires prompt recognition and aggressive intervention. This can only occur if the possibility of TSS is considered early in the clinical course of the disease. While many other illnesses can mimic TSS, it should be considered in any reproductive-age woman who presents with the rapid onset of a high fever around the time of menstruation.

❷ The patient with possible TSS is generally acutely ill and a working diagnosis must be established rapidly. Patients who meet the screening criteria (inset) should be managed as if they have TSS until another cause can be found. Patients who do not meet these criteria must be evaluated for a number of serious illnesses that may present with similar symptoms. Aggressive support is required in most cases while the diagnosis is being established.

❸ Patients meeting the screening critrion for TSS must be admitted to an intensive care setting. These patients require aggressive integrated monitoring of multiple organ systems and deteriorate rapidly, with little warning.

❹ The patient should be carefully examined for a possible site of infection. In menstruating women,

this may be a vaginal tampon. In others, it may be an infected cutaneous wound. These wounds may not be apparent on first examination, necessitating a meticulous search.

❺ If an infected cutaneous wound is found, it must be rapidly drained and debrided. This includes the removal of any packing or sutures that may be present. If a tampon is removed, some authors advocate vaginal irrigation. Cultures for staphylococcal or streptococcal infection should be obtained.

❻ Aggressive supportive and antibiotic therapy must be instituted rapidly. Vigorous fluid resuscitation is uniformly required, with careful monitoring of cardiac and renal function. A bladder catheter is required and a central venous catheter should be strongly considered to measure central venous pressure. Adult respiratory or cardiac failure common and should be anticipated. Broad-spectrum antibiotic therapy (including coverage for *Staphylococcus*) should be started until septicemia can be ruled out. If Rocky Mountain spotted fever is possible, tetracycline should be included in the treatment. Short-course corticosteroid therapy has been reported to hasten improvement. One study has used naloxone to reverse the hypotensive effects of endogenous endorphins.

❼ Patients with TSS are at great risk for cardiac, pulmonary, renal, or hepatic failure as a part of their illness. These possibilities, if not probabilities, should guide the surveillance and management of these patients. When organ failure occurs, specific and rigorous supportive measures must be instituted.

❽ Following recovery, patients who have experienced toxic shock should be counseled that recurrence rates of up to 30% have been reported for

menstrually related cases. These patient should be counseled to limit tampon use to only their heaviest days, avoid highly absorbent brands, and limit the duration each tampon is used. Tampons should not be used for mid-cycle bleeding or the control of vaginal discharge. Careful hand washing before handling tampons and separation of the vulva during insertion may further reduce the risk. Many prefer to counsel patients to avoid tampons completely. Some studies suggest reduced rates of TSS in women who use oral contraceptives or condoms with nonoxynol-9 spermicide.

REFERENCES

Broome CV. Epidemiology of toxic shock syndrome in the United States. Rev Infect Dis 1989;11:S14.

Chesney PJ, Davis JP, Purdy WK, et al. Clinical manifestations of toxic shock syndrome. JAMA 1981;246:741.

Davis JP, Vergernot JM, Amsterdam LE, et al. Long-term effects of toxic shock syndrome in women: sequelae, subsequent pregnancy, menstrual history, and long-term trends in catamenial product use. Rev Infect Dis 1989;11:S50.

Kain KC, Schulzer M, Chow AW. Clinical spectrum of nonmenstrual toxic shock syndrome (TSS): Comparison with menstrual TSS by multivariate discriminant analyses. Clin Infect Dis 1993;16:100.

Reingold AL. Toxic shock syndrome: An update. Am J Obstet Gynecol 1991;165(suppl):1236.

Reingold AL, Shards KN, Dan BB, Broome CV. Toxic-shock not associated with menstruation. A review of 54 cases. Lancet 1982;1:1.

Schauchat A, Broome CV. Toxic shock syndrome and tampons. Epidemiol Rev 1991;13:99.

Wiesenthal AM, Ressman M, Caston SA. Toxic shock syndrome. I. Clinical exclusion of other syndromes by strict screening definitions. Am J Epidemiol 1985;122:847.

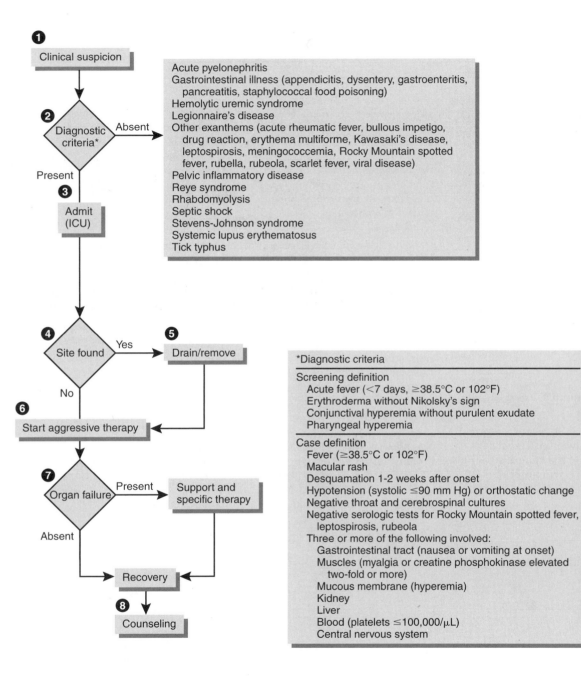

❶ Clinical suspicion

❷ Diagnostic criteria*

— Absent →

Acute pyelonephritis
Gastrointestinal illness (appendicitis, dysentery, gastroenteritis,
   pancreatitis, staphylococcal food poisoning)
Hemolytic uremic syndrome
Legionnaire's disease
Other exanthems (acute rheumatic fever, bullous impetigo,
   drug reaction, erythema multiforme, Kawasaki's disease,
   leptospirosis, meningococcemia, Rocky Mountain spotted
   fever, rubella, rubeola, scarlet fever, viral disease)
Pelvic inflammatory disease
Reye syndrome
Rhabdomyolysis
Septic shock
Stevens-Johnson syndrome
Systemic lupus erythematosus
Tick typhus

Present

❸ Admit (ICU)

❹ Site found — Yes → **❺** Drain/remove

No

❻ Start aggressive therapy

❼ Organ failure — Present → Support and specific therapy

Absent

Recovery

❽ Counseling

*Diagnostic criteria

Screening definition
   Acute fever (<7 days, ≥38.5°C or 102°F)
   Erythroderma without Nikolsky's sign
   Conjunctival hyperemia without purulent exudate
   Pharyngeal hyperemia

Case definition
   Fever (≥38.5°C or 102°F)
   Macular rash
   Desquamation 1-2 weeks after onset
   Hypotension (systolic ≤90 mm Hg) or orthostatic change
   Negative throat and cerebrospinal cultures
   Negative serologic tests for Rocky Mountain spotted fever,
      leptospirosis, rubeola
   Three or more of the following involved:
      Gastrointestinal tract (nausea or vomiting at onset)
      Muscles (myalgia or creatine phosphokinase elevated
         two-fold or more)
      Mucous membrane (hyperemia)
      Kidney
      Liver
      Blood (platelets ≤100,000/μL)
      Central nervous system

Urethritis

INTRODUCTION

For patients with urethritis, irritation or inflammation of the urethra leads to painful urination, discharge, dyspareunia, or pelvic pain. The short female urethra, with its opening near a rich bacterial flora and the risk of trauma during sexual activity, places women at increased risk for infectious and mechanical urethritis.

❶ The most common cause of urethral symptoms is infection. As a result, any patient suspected of having urethritis should have a urinalysis performed. The use of leukocyte esterase dipsticks is associated with a false-negative rate of up to 25% and may give false-positive tests if the sample is contaminated by vaginal white blood cells. Similarly, nitrate dipsticks fail to detect infections in 10% to 30% of patients. If the urinalysis is positive, a culture and sensitivity should be performed on the sample, though therapy should no be delayed pending the results.

❷ Empiric antibiotic therapy should be started while the results of the culture are awaited. The choice of antibiotic should be based on the clinical suspicion of cause. Patients who have symptoms of cystitis or upper urinary tract infection should have a broad-spectrum agent, while those with urethritis alone should receive an agent with good coverage for chlamydia and gonorrhea (the most common infections encountered in isolation). Other infections to be considered are those caused by *Ureaplasma urealyticum* and *Trichomonas*. Once culture results are available, the correctness of the diagnosis should be evaluated along with the choice of antibiotics.

❸ Patients who do not have an obvious urethral infection should undergo a careful examination of the urethra and surrounding tissues. Infection of the Skene's ducts, urinary diverticula, foreign bodies, and other potential causes of urethritis may be evident during this evaluation. Diffuse tenderness along and adjacent to the urethra is typical of chronic urethritis or Reiter or Stevens–Johnson syndrome. Reiter syndrome results from an immunologic response to chlamydial infection. When this syndrome is suspected, urethral cultures from the patient and her sexual partner(s) should be obtained to confirm eradication of the infection.

❹ A culture of the urethra should be performed. The most common urethral infections are *Chlamydia trachomatis* and *Neisseria gonorrhoeae*. When infection is documented, appropriate antibiotic therapy should be started. Patients with urethral atrophy due to uncorrected hypoestrogenism, those with acute or recurrent urethral trauma ("honeymoon cystitis"), and those who use or abuse some medications (such as amphetamines) may experience urethritis in the absence of specific findings. A careful history will suggest these in most cases.

❺ Because of the nature of the infections associated with urethritis and the emergence of increasingly resistant strains, a test of cure should be planned as part of the follow-up care of these patients.

REFERENCES

American College of Obstetricians and Gynecologists. Gonorrhea and Chalmydial Infections. ACOG Technical Bulletin 190. Washington, DC: ACOG, 1994.

Centers for Disease Control. Sexually transmitted diseases treatment guidelines. MMWR 1993; 42:56.

Centers for Disease Control and Surveillance. Decreased susceptibility of *Neisseria gonorrhoeae* to fluoroquinolones—Ohio and Hawaii, 1992–1994. MMWR 1994;43:325–327.

Hammerschlag MR, Golden NH, Oh MK, et al. Single dose of azithromycin for the treatment of genital chalmydial infections in adolescents. J Pediatr 1993;122(6):961–965.

Martin DH, Mroczkowski TF, Dalu ZA, et al. A controlled trial of a single dose of azithromycin for the treatment of chlamydial urethritis and cervicitis: the Azithromycin for Chlamydia Infections Study Group. N Engl J Med 1992;327:921–925.

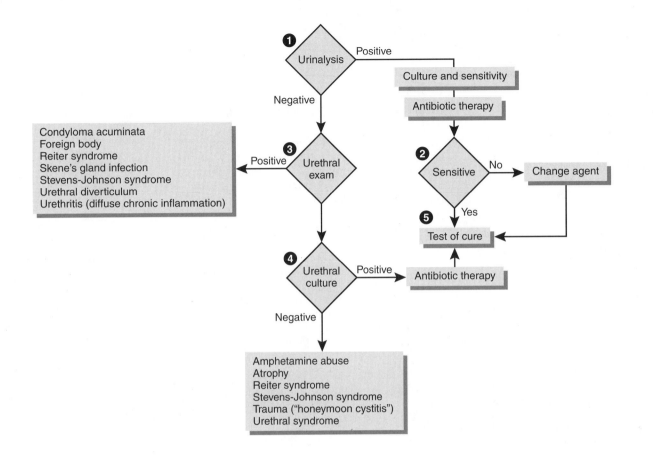

1 Urinalysis — Positive → Culture and sensitivity → Antibiotic therapy

1 Urinalysis — Negative ↓

2 Sensitive — No → Change agent

2 Sensitive — Yes ↓

3 Urethral exam — Positive →
Condyloma acuminata
Foreign body
Reiter syndrome
Skene's gland infection
Stevens-Johnson syndrome
Urethral diverticulum
Urethritis (diffuse chronic inflammation)

4 Urethral culture — Positive → Antibiotic therapy

5 Test of cure

4 Urethral culture — Negative ↓
Amphetamine abuse
Atrophy
Reiter syndrome
Stevens-Johnson syndrome
Trauma ("honeymoon cystitis")
Urethral syndrome

Urinary Frequency

INTRODUCTION

The frequent passage of urine may be an indication of pathologies affecting the bladder, the kidneys, or the body in general. As a result, the evaluation of this complaint must include the routine and ordinary (urinary tract infection) and the uncommon.

❶ Symptoms of urgency or dysuria should suggest the possibility, if not the probability, of a lower urinary tract infection.

❷ Patients who experience urinary frequency but have small voided volumes should be evaluated for a possible urinary tract infection even when symptoms of urgency and dysuria are absent. If this evaluation suggests infection, antibiotic therapy as outlined in No. 6 should be implemented. A negative urinalysis will be present in patients who have urinary frequency because of interstitial cystitis or bladder scarring, or have behavioral causes for their symptoms. Excessive caffeine intake may result in frequent small-volume voiding as may obsessive or psychotic emotional disturbances. A poorly enervated, overdistended bladder may also present with symptoms of small-volume frequent voiding.

❸ While interstitial cystitis is most often associated with small-volume voiding, relatively normal volumes may occur in the early stages of the disease or when fluid intake is above average. The use of diuretics or caffeine may result frequency as well.

❹ High-volume voiding that occurs with increased frequency imply a high output of urine. This is most common in patients who drink excessive volumes of fluid and must be considered in the differential diagnosis. Diabetes mellitus or insipidus may present in this manner.

❺ An effective, but optional, method of screening for urinary tract infection is the microscopic examination of urinary sediments. To perform this, approximately 10 ml of clean-catch mid-stream urine is centrifuged for 30 to 60 seconds in a table-top centrifuge, the fluid decanted, and the resulting button of sediment resuspended in the liquid that remains. This is then placed on a microscope slide, covered with a cover slip and examined under high power. The presence of more than 10 white blood cells per field suggests the presence of an infection. If a significant number of squamous cells are present, vaginal contamination is presumed and the evaluation is inconclusive.

❻ A formal urinalysis should be performed on any patient with the complaint of urinary frequency, urgency, and dysuria. The use of leukocyte esterase dipsticks is associated with a false-negative rate of up to 25% and may give false-positive results if the sample is contaminated by vaginal white blood cells. Similarly, nitrate dipsticks fail to detect infections in 10% to 30% of patients. If the urinalysis is positive, a culture and sensitivity should be performed on the sample, though therapy should not be delayed pending the results.

❼ If a urinary tract infection is suspected based on the results of a microscopic examination, urinalysis or other means, a culture and sensitivity should be performed. Uncomplicated patients with frank urinary tract infections may not require this step for an initial infection, but those patients generally will present with a different symptom pattern from those with isolated dysuria. Empiric antibiotic therapy should be started while the results of the culture are awaited. Once these results are available, the correctness of the diagnosis should be evaluated along with the choice of antibiotics. A test of cure is generally not required unless there have been frequent recurrences, the patient is at high risk, or sensitivity demonstrated on culture was marginal. The resolution of the patient's symptoms of frequency may also suggest a cure.

❽ Even when the urinalysis is negative, patients with urinary frequency and either urgency or dysuria should have a culture and sensitivity performed and, if positive, have antibiotic therapy started.

❾ Patients with a negative urinalysis and sterile urine cultures may have evidence of chronic inflammation of the urethra, body of the bladder, or trigone. The absence of physical findings is most common in patients with interstitial cystitis, though some patients with advanced involvement may have tenderness demonstrated over the body of the bladder. This tenderness will be greatest when the bladder is full. The possibility of traumatic trigonitis or cystitis ("honeymoon cystitis") should be suggested by history.

REFERENCES

Bump RC. Urinary tract infection in women. Current role of single-dose therapy. J Repro Med 1990;35:785.

Kunin CM. Urinary tract infections in females. Clin Infect Dis 1994;18:1.

Pappas P. Laboratory in the diagnosis and management of urinary tract infections. Med Clin North Am 1991;75:313–325.

Powers R. New directions in the diagnosis and therapy of urinary tract infections. Am J Obstet Gynecol 1991;164:1387–1389.

Smith RP. Gynecology in Primary Care. Baltimore: Williams & Wilkins, 1997, pp 577–602.

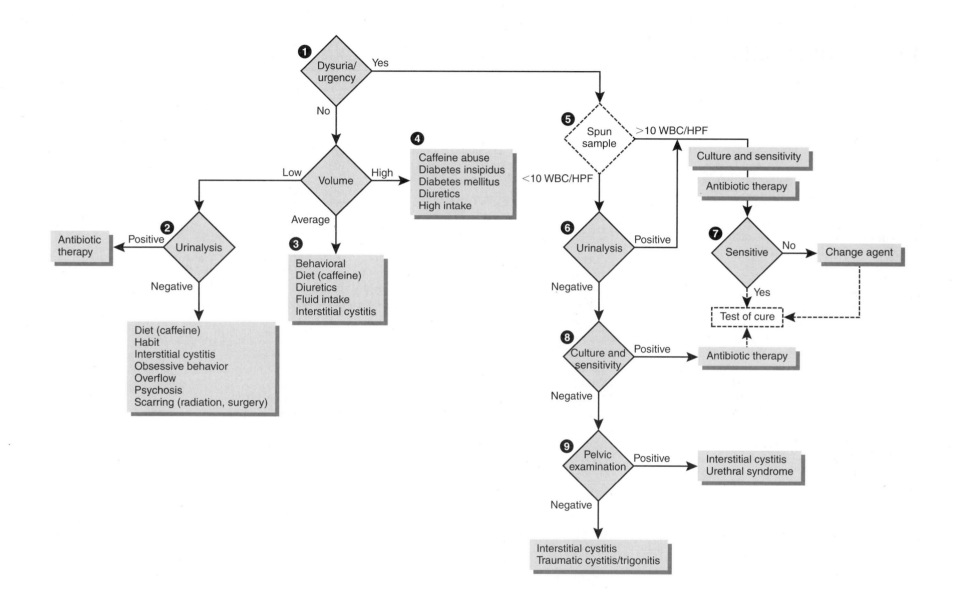

Urinary Incontinence

Bypass

INTRODUCTION

Continuous incontinence will occur when the normal continence mechanism is bypassed, as with fistulae from the vagina to the bladder (vesicovaginal), urethra (urethrovaginal), or ureter (ureterovaginal). Rarely, communication between the bladder and the uterus (vesicouterine) may also occur through the same mechanisms. Fistulae may result from surgical or obstetric trauma, irradiation, or malignancy, though the most common cause by far is unrecognized surgical trauma. Roughly, 75% of fistulae occur after abdominal hysterectomy. Though it is estimated that urinary tract injury occurs in about 8000 of the estimated 700,000 hysterectomies performed each year in the United States, fistulae occur in only about 0.05% of all hysterectomies. Signs of a urinary fistula (watery discharge) usually occur from 5 to 30 days after surgery, though they may be present in the immediate postoperative period.

❶ Fistulae between the urinary tract and the vagina will result in the continuous loss of urine. Patients who have an intermittent, but frequent, small-volume loss may be experiencing overflow or urgency incontinence instead.

❷ Pelvic examination may reveal the point of leakage if care is taken to inspect all portions of the vaginal wall, moving the speculum so that the blades do not hide any part. If a suspected communication between the bladder and the vagina is found, cystoscopy, with canalization of any fistulae to assist with their localization, should be performed. Intravenous pyelography may demonstrate the location of ureterovaginal communications.

❸ A simple office approach to fistula identification is the tampon test. This test makes use of oral phenazopyridine hydrochloride (Pyridium) and sterile saline tinted with methylene blue instilled into the bladder. Phenazopyridine hydrochloride (a urinary analgesic) will turn the urine an orange-red color. A tampon is placed in the vagina before ingesting the medication and then, at a later time, it is examined for the presence, location, and color of staining. Based on the findings, a fistula may be confirmed and its location suspected.

REFERENCES

American College of Obstetricians and Gynecologists. Genitourinary fistulas. ACOG Technical Bulletin 83. Washington, DC: ACOG, 1985.

American College of Obstetricians and Gynecologists. Lower Urinary Tract Operative Injuries. ACOG Technical Bulletin 238. Washington, DC: ACOG, 1997.

Diaz-Ball FL, Moore CA. A diagnostic aid for vesicovaginal fistula. J Urol 1969;102:424.

Holley RL, Kilgore LC. Urologic Complications. In Orr JW, Jr, Shingleton HM (eds): Complications in Gynecologic Surgery: Prevention, Recognition, and Management. Philadelphia: JB Lippincott, 1994, pp 149–151.

Sims JM. On the treatment of vesico- vaginal fistula. Am J Med Sci 1852;23:59.

Smith RP. Gynecology in Primary Care. Baltimore: Williams & Wilkins, 1997, pp 577–602.

Symmonds RE. Incontinence: Vesical and urethral fistulas. Clin Obstet Gynecol 1984;27:499–514.

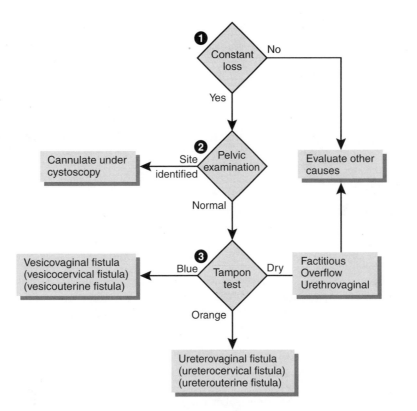

Urinary Incontinence

General Evaluation

INTRODUCTION

"Urinary incontinence" may be a sign, symptom, or condition. It is defined as a condition in which involuntary loss of urine may be objectively demonstrated, and the loss presents a social or hygienic problem. The volume of the loss in not as important as the impact it has on the patient and her life. Almost half of all women will have involuntary loss of a few drops of urine at some time in their lifetime, with 10% to 15% of women suffering significant, recurrent loss. It has been estimated that over one quarter of women of reproductive age suffer from some degree of urinary incontinence. This number increases to 30% to 40% of women after the age of menopause.

❶ Infrequent, small-volume urine loss may be tolerable to some patients. Because it is the impact of loss, not its presence, that determines the significance of incontinence, these patients need no treatment. Only if there is evidence that the incontinence reflects medical risk (recurrent infections) or an underlying condition that threatens the health of the patient should evaluation be pressed.

❷ The abrupt onset of either stress or urgency incontinence suggests either an infectious or allergic cause. If a urinary culture is positive, appropriate treatment should be instituted. If the incontinence persists, a formal evaluation is indicated.

❸ A voiding log, which chronicles intake and voided volumes and times, is an inexpensive and rapidly achieved screening test of urinary function. This log should be recorded over a period of 3 days. While it is preferable that these be consecutive, they do not have to be to provide the needed information.

❹ Low-volume voids may be symptomatic of bladder scarring or dysfunction. Poor collections and behavioral problems may also present in this manner. Frequent voiding may be seen in patients with urinary urgency or neurogenic bladders. Very high-volume voids are typically seen in patients with excessive fluid intake. These patients may consume 15 or more liters of fluid a day through habit, delusion, or misinformation.

❺ Patients who have a normal voiding log should be evaluated by a postvoiding residual. Elevated residuals may result from outflow obstruction or poor detrusor function. The evaluation of overflow incontinence is shown separately.

❻ Office cystometrics can be easily performed using only a straight catheter, catheter-tipped syringe, and sterile saline. Fluctuations in the fluid meniscus suggest detrusor instability. Most centers offer sophisticated evaluation of bladder compliance and contractility, cystoscopy, and evaluations of the voiding process itself. Pressure profiles of the bladder and urethra, electromyography, and fluoroscopic examinations may also be included. These tests are useful in the evaluation of patients in whom "mixed" causes are suspected. They should also be performed before any invasive therapy. The evaluation or urgency incontinence is shown separately.

❼ Cystourethroceles may be quantitated using the Q-Tip test. To perform this test a sterile cotton swab, dipped in 2% lidocaine, is placed in the urethra (up to the urethrovesical junction) and the angle of upward rotation present when the patient strains is measured. Rotation of greater than 30° from the starting point is generally associated with stress incontinence. Normal examinations suggest the possibility of urinary losses that bypass the normal control mechanism. The evaluations of stress and bypass incontinence are shown separately.

REFERENCES

Abrams P, Blaivas JG, Stanton SL, Andersen JT. The standardization of terminology of lower urinary tract function produced by the International Continence Society Committee on Standardization of Terminiology. Scand J Urol Nephrol 1988;114:5.

American College of Obstetricians and Gyneologists. Urinary incontinence. ACOG Technical Bulletin 213. Washington, DC: ACOG, 1995.

Consensus Conference. Urinary incontinence in adults. JAMA 1989;261:2685.

Crystle CD, Charme LS, Copeland WE. Q-tip test in stress urinary incontinence. Obstet Gyencol 1971;38:313.

Norton PA (ed). Urinary incontinence. Clin Obstet Gynecol 1990;33:293.

Urinary Incontinence Guideline Panel. Urinary Incontinence in Adults: Clinical Practice Guidelines. Rockville, Maryland: Agency for Health Care Policy and Research, Public Health Service, U.W. Department of Health and Human Services, 1992; AHCPR Publication No. 92-0038.

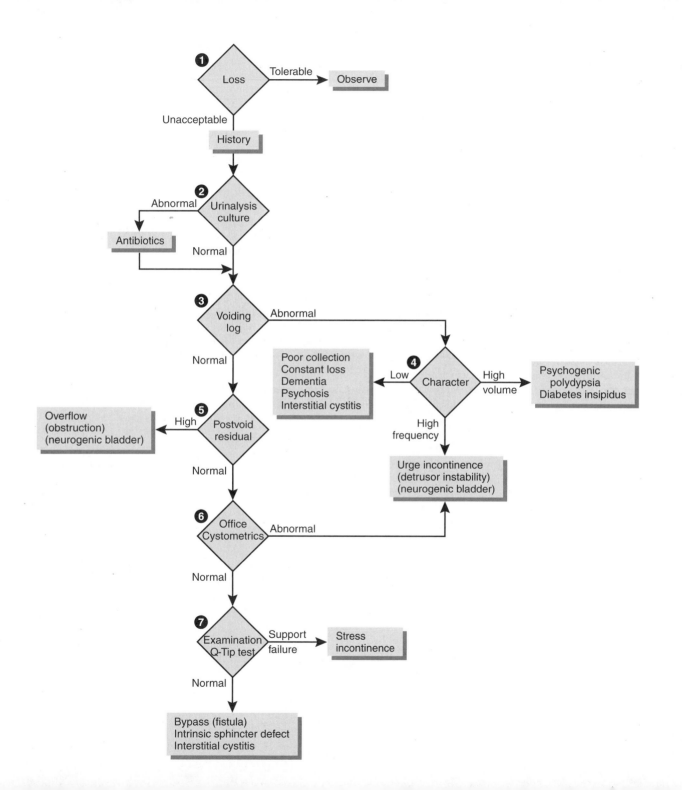

1 Loss
— Tolerable → Observe
— Unacceptable → History

2 Urinalysis culture
— Abnormal → Antibiotics
— Normal →

3 Voiding log
— Abnormal →
— Normal →

4 Character
— Low → Poor collection / Constant loss / Dementia / Psychosis / Interstitial cystitis
— High volume → Psychogenic polydypsia / Diabetes insipidus
— High frequency → Urge incontinence (detrusor instability) (neurogenic bladder)

5 Postvoid residual
— High → Overflow (obstruction) (neurogenic bladder)
— Normal →

6 Office Cystometrics
— Abnormal → Urge incontinence (detrusor instability) (neurogenic bladder)
— Normal →

7 Examination Q-Tip test
— Support failure → Stress incontinence
— Normal → Bypass (fistula) / Intrinsic sphincter defect / Interstitial cystitis

Urinary Incontinence

Overflow

INTRODUCTION

Overflow incontinence may occur when the bladder becomes massively overdistended and unable to empty, yielding constant uncontrollable urinary leakage.

❶ The acute onset of overflow incontinence may occur because of an abrupt change in bladder function brought on by surgery, medication, infection, or the deterioration of a pre-existing condition.

❷ Abdominal or pelvic surgical procedures, especially those performed under regional anesthesia, may result in the acute retention of urine, leading to symptoms of overflow incontinence. These patients generally require catheter drainage for 24 to 48 hours, but no further treatment or evaluation.

❸ Medical conditions can result in reduced bladder function ("neurogenic bladder"), leading to poor emptying, urinary retention, and overflow loss. This can also occur in those with outlet obstruction, who develop a distended, atonic bladder that may overflow episodically. Overflow loss may be exacerbated by intra-abdominal pressure change, mimicking stress incontinence. Patients suspected of having a neurogenic bladder require a thorough neurologic evaluation. Pharmacologic therapy for these patients is often unsatisfactory and many require long-term catheter drainage, or intermittent self-catheterization, to manage their problem. In young patients, the possibility of multiple sclerosis must seriously considered.

❹ Medications that directly, or indirectly, affect bladder function may lead to poor emptying and overflow incontinence. These agents will have an exaggerated effect when an outflow obstruction is present. Obstruction of the urethra can, by itself, produce the same symptoms.

REFERENCES

American College of Obstetricians and Gynecologists. Urinary Incontinence. Technical Bulletin 213. Washington, DC:ACOG, 1995.

Mishell DR, Stenchever MA, Droegemueller W, Herbst AL. Comprehensive Gynecology, 3rd ed. St Louis: CV Mosby, 1997, p 592.

Ostergard DR, Bent AE. Urogynecology and Urodynamics, 3rd ed. Baltimore: Williams & Wilkins, 1991, pp 346–351, 478–480.

Smith RP. Gynecology in Primary Care. Baltimore: Williams & Wilkins, 1997, pp 577–602.

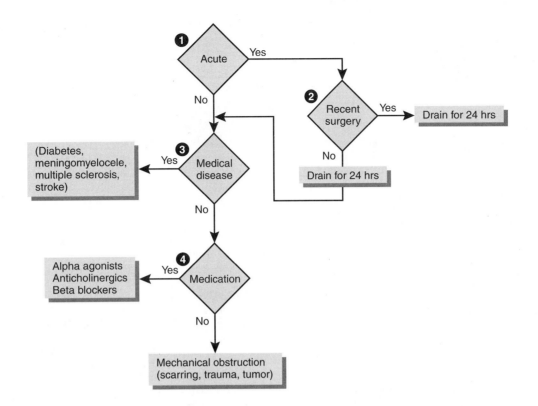

Urinary Incontinence

Stress

INTRODUCTION

Urine will pass from the body any time the pressure inside the bladder exceeds the pressure in the urethra. This is the physiologic mechanism of voluntary voiding, when urethral relaxation and bladder contraction occur. Involuntary urinary loss may take place when there is unequal transmission of intra-abdominal pressure to the bladder and urethra. Stress incontinence is a passive loss and therefore is notable for urine loss in the absence of bladder muscle contraction. This may happen with the loss of pelvic support, therefore stress incontinence is a common complaint of patients with a cystocele or urethrocele. In stress incontinence, the loss of urine is small, directly proportional to the pressure generated and limited to the time of maximal pressure.

❶ The patient should be carefully questioned about the volume of urinary loss. Because of the mechanics of stress incontinence, the volume lost is directly proportional to the degree and duration of the provoking stress and is generally small. Large-volume loss suggests other causes, including detrusor instability.

❷ Despite the beguiling simplicity of a history of urine loss with a cough or sneeze, history alone is only 75% accurate in establishing the diagnosis. Careful physical examination should include an evaluation of pelvic support with emphasis on the bladder trigone, and urethra. Stress incontinence is almost always associated with support defects, and when these are absent, a referral should be strongly considered.

❸ Cystoscopy and urethroscopy are required, along with multichannel urodynamics testing, to evaluate the possibility of an intrinsic sphincter defect, or the so-called stovepipe urethra, both of which present with stress incontinence and normal pelvic support.

❹ Some authors advocate the Q-Tip test to evaluate the degree of urethral support loss. To perform this test a sterile cotton swab, dipped in 2% lidocaine, is placed in the urethra (up to the urethrovesical junction) and the angle of upward rotation present when the patient strains is measured. Rotation of greater than 30° from the starting point is generally associated with stress incontinence.

❺ A rough indication of the functional significance of a cystourethrocele may be gauged by elevating the bladder neck (using fingers or an instrument) and asking the patient to strain (referred to as the Bonney or Marshall–Marchetti test). If the patient is rendered continent (with at least 200 ml of urine or saline in the bladder), this test may suggest the effect of a pessary or surgical repair. Care must be taken that the results accurately reflect the effects of elevation of the structures and not mechanical obstruction of the urethra. Because of this uncertainty, this test should not provide the sole means of evaluation or the selection of therapy. Some centers have abandoned its use completely.

❻ Pessaries may provide mechanical support for the pelvic organs. The most commonly used forms of pessary for pelvic relaxation are the ring (or donut), the ball, and the cube. Pessaries offer an excellent alternative to surgical repair, but the use of a pessary requires the cooperation and involvement of the patient. Patients who are unable, or unwilling, to manage the periodic insertion and removal of the device are poor candidates for their use. Pessaries will not be well tolerated or provide optimal support in the poorly estrogenized patient. For this reason, many suggest a minimum of 30 days of topical estrogen therapy (for those not already on estrogen replacement) before a trial of pessary therapy. Surgical therapy, in many forms, is often chosen for these patients.

REFERENCES

Abrams P, Blaivas JG, Stanton SL, Andersen JT. The standardization of terminology of lower urinary tract function produced by the International Continence Society Committee on Standardization of Terminology. Scand J Urol Nephrol 1988;114:5–19.

American College of Obstetricians and Gynecologists. Pelvic organ prolapse. ACOG Technical Bulletin 214. Washington, DC: ACOG, 1995.

American College of Obstetricians and Gynecologists. Urinary Incontinence. ACOG Technical Bulletin 213. Washington, DC: ACOG, 1995.

Federkiw DM, Sand PK, Retzky SS, Johnson DC. The cotton swab test. Receiver-operating characteristics curves. J Reprod Med 1995;40:42–46.

Kinn AC, Lindskog M. Estrogens and phenylpropanolamine in combination for stress urinary incontinence in postmenopausal women. Urology 1988;32:273–280.

Videla FLG, Wall LL. Diagnosing stress incontinence without multichannel urodynamic studies. Obstet Gynecol 1998;91:965.

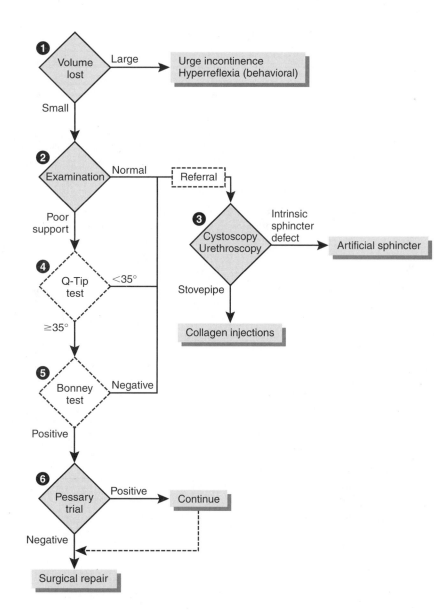

Urinary Incontinence

Urgency

INTRODUCTION

In urgency urinary incontinence the volume of loss is often large, including complete emptying of the bladder. The loss follows the sensation or provoking event by a slight delay. Therefore, a cough may lead to loss, but the loss occurs after, not during, the cough. Urgency incontinence occurs in approximately 35% of patients with incontinence. For most of these patients, no specific cause for their bladder irritability is found and they are referred to as having "idiopathic detrusor instability." Neurologic disease must be considered as a possible cause, with multiple sclerosis a major concern for younger patients. Trauma, spinal cord tumors, radical pelvic surgery, stroke, radiation therapy, chronic irritation, and the effects of diabetes may also affect bladder sensation and motor control.

❶ Roughly, 5% of urinary tract infections are asymptomatic, lacking the frequency, urgency, and dysuria usually seen. Because subclinical infections may cause urgency incontinence, the first step in the evaluation of these patients is a urine culture. Some would even suggest an empiric trial of antibiotic therapy before beginning any evaluation.

❷ Patients with sterile urine should have measurements of their residual urine and bladder capacity made. This can easily be carried out in the office as a part of office cystometrics performed to assist the differential diagnosis. (See Urinary Incontinence: General Evaluation.)

❸ Scarring of the bladder can follow radiation therapy or chronic inflammation, such as with interstitial cystitis. The severity of scarring that follows radiation generally requires surgical correction, while milder forms of scarring and stenosis may respond to hydrodistention therapy.

❹ Cystoscopy should be the next step in the evaluation of those patients with normal- or low-capacity bladders. Trigonitis or interstitial cystitis may be evident during the examination. Interstitial cystitis should be confirmed by bladder biopsy.

❺ Behavioral modification is often helpful, if not completely successful, in resolving the patient's symptoms. This consists of caffeine reduction, fluid intake management, and timed voiding. The fluid and voiding history will often identify those with excessive caffeine or fluid intake or inappropriate voiding intervals. Getting the patient to change these behaviors, however, can be difficult. Bladder training is directed toward increasing the patient's bladder control and capacity by gradually increasing the amount of time between voidings. Patients are asked to void on a set schedule based on their shortest normal voiding interval. Once this has been practiced for several days, the interval is lengthened by 10 to 15 minutes each day or two until times of 1 1/2 to 2 1/2 hours are attained. Often successful by itself (up to 80%), bladder training may be augmented by biofeedback (when available).

❻ Beta-sympathetic activity in the body and dome of the bladder leads to muscle relaxation, while alpha-adrenergic activity causes urethral contraction. The pharmacologic treatment of urgency incontinence may take many forms, such as anticholinergic drugs (Pro-Banthine, Ditropan), beta-sympathomimetic agonists (Alupent), musculotropic drugs (Urispas, Valium), antidepressants (Tofranil), and dopamine agonists (Parlodel). Because the bladder is parasympathetically innervated, anticholinergic drugs are most commonly used to treat bladder instability of any cause. When complete failure with medical therapy occurs, long-term catheter drainage may be required.

REFERENCES

Abrams P, Blaivas JG, Stanton SL, Andersen JT. The standardization of terminology of lower urinary tract function produced by the International Continence Society Committee on Standardization of Terminology. Scand J Urol Nephrol 1988;114:5–19.

American College of Obstetricians and Gynecologists. Urinary Incontinence. ACOG Technical Bulletin 213. Washington, DC: ACOG, 1995.

Consensus Conference. Urinary incontinence in adults. JAMA 1989;261:2685–2690.

Norton PA (ed). Urinary incontinence. Clin Obstet Gynecol 1990;33:293–399.

Urinary Incontinence Guideline Panel. Urinary incontinence in adults: clinical practice guidelines. Rockville, Maryland: Agency for Health Care Policy and Research, Public Health Service, U.W. Department of Health and Human Services, 1992; AHCPR Publication No. 92-0038.

Wall LL. Diagnosis and management of urinary incontinence due to detrusor instability. Obstet Gynecol Surv 1990;45:1s.

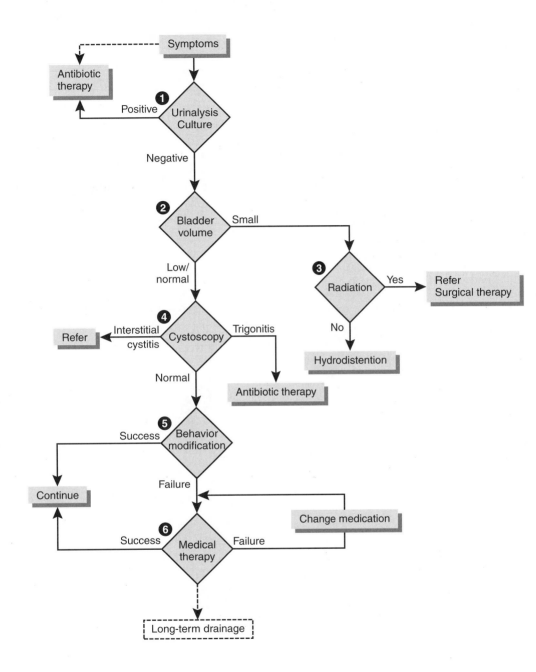

Urinary Retention

INTRODUCTION

Acute urinary retention and bladder distention may follow surgery, epidural or general anesthesia, trauma, and herpetic vulvitis, and rarely may occur with pelvic masses, marked prolapse of the bladder, and retroversion of the uterus (causing pressure on the base of the bladder). Acute urinary retention requires prompt and continuous drainage for 24 to 48 hours.

❶ Acute urinary retention may occur because of an abrupt change in bladder function brought on by surgery, medication, infection, or the deterioration of a pre-existing condition.

❷ Abdominal or pelvic surgical procedures, especially those performed under regional anesthesia, may result in the acute retention of urine. These patients generally require catheter drainage for 24 to 48 hours, but no further treatment or evaluation.

❸ Medical conditions can result in reduced bladder function ("neurogenic bladder"), leading to poor emptying, and urinary retention. This can also occur to those with outlet obstruction, who develop a distended, atonic bladder, resulting in retention. Patients suspected of having a neurogenic bladder require a thorough neurologic evaluation. Pharmacologic therapy for these patients is often unsatisfactory, and many require long-term catheter drainage, or intermittent self-catheterization, to manage their problem. In young patients, the possibility of multiple sclerosis must seriously considered.

❹ Medications that directly, or indirectly, affect bladder function may lead to poor emptying and urinary retention. These agents will have an exaggerated effect when an outflow obstruction is present. Obstruction of the urethra can, by itself, produce the same symptoms.

REFERENCES

American College of Obstetricians and Gynecologists. Urinary Incontinence. Technical Bulletin 213. Washington, DC:ACOG, 1995.

Mishell DR, Stenchever MA, Droegemueller W, Herbst AL. Comprehensive Gynecology, 3rd ed. St Louis: CV Mosby, 1997, p 2592.

Ostergard DR, Bent AE. Urogynecology and Urodynamics, 3rd ed. Baltimore: Williams & Wilkins, 1991, pp 346–351, 478–480.

Smith RP. Gynecology in Primary Care. Baltimore: Williams & Wilkins, 1997, pp 577–602.

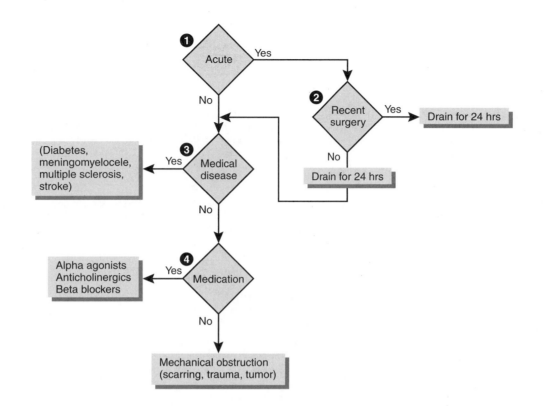

Urinary Tract Infection

INTRODUCTION

Urinary tract infections are much more common in women because of their shortened urethral length and exposure of the urinary tract to trauma and pathogens during sexual activity. The prevalence is estimated to be 3% to 8%, with roughly 45% of women aged 15 to 60 experiencing at least one urinary tract infection. Most urinary tract infections in women ascend from contamination of the urethra, acquired via instrumentation, trauma, or sexual intercourse (within the preceding 24 to 48 hours in up to 75% of cases of acute infection). Coliform organisms, especially *Escherichia coli,* are the most common organisms responsible for asymptomatic bacteriuria, cystitis, and pyelonephritis. Ninety percent of first infections and 80% of recurrent infections are caused by *E. coli,* with between 10% and 20% due to *Staphylococcus saprophyticus.*

❶ While roughly 5% of urinary tract infections are asymptomatic, most present with frequency, urgency, and dysuria. Some authors suggest that if the symptoms are consistent and the patient has not had previous infections or is at risk for complications, empiric treatment with a urinary tract antibiotic is acceptable. Pregnant patients should not be treated empirically.

❷ When empiric treatment is chosen, the patient must be monitored for prompt and complete relief of symptoms within the first 48 to 72 hours of treatment. If resolution of symptoms is not achieved, a culture of the urine is required.

❸ Many clinicians have the facilities to centrifuge a clean-catch urine sample and examine it directly in the office setting. This is an effective, but optional, method of screening for urinary tract infection. To perform this, approximately 10 ml of clean-catch midstream urine is centrifuged for 30 to 60 seconds in a table-top centrifuge, the fluid decanted, and the resulting button of sediment resuspended in the liquid that remains. This is then placed on a microscope slide, covered with a cover slip, and examined under high power. The presence of more than 10 white blood cells per field suggests the presence of an infection. If a significant number of squamous cells are present, vaginal contamination is presumed and the evaluation is inconclusive.

❹ A formal urinalysis should be performed on any patient suspected of infection for whom empiric therapy has not been chosen or is inappropriate. The use of leukocyte esterase dipsticks is associated with a false-negative rate of up to 25% and may give false-positive tests if the sample is contaminated by vaginal white blood cells. Similarly, nitrate dipsticks fail to detect infections in 10% to 30% of patients. If the urinalysis is positive, a culture and sensitivity should be performed on the sample, though therapy should not be delayed pending the results.

❺ If a urinary tract infection is suspected based on the results of a microscopic examination, urinalysis, or other means, a culture and sensitivity should be performed. Uncomplicated patients with frank urinary tract infections may not require this step for an initial infection, but those patients generally will present with a different symptom pattern than isolated dysuria. Empiric antibiotic therapy should be started while the results of the culture are awaited.

Once these results are available, the correctness of the diagnosis should be evaluated along with the choice of antibiotics. A test of cure is generally not required unless there have been frequent recurrences, the patient is at high risk, or sensitivity demonstrated on culture was marginal.

❻ Pregnant patients and those with recurrent infections should be strongly considered for a follow-up urinalysis or culture as a test of cure. Frequent recurrences should prompt an investigation for risk factors such as metabolic changes, stones, or anomalies.

❼ A number of conditions ranging from mechanical trauma due to intercourse ("honeymoon cystitis") to amphetamine abuse can cause symptoms that mimic an infection but result in a normal urinalysis.

REFERENCES

American College of Obstetricians and Gyneologists. Antimicrobial Therapy for Obstetric Patients. ACOG Technical Bulletin 117. Washington, DC: ACOG, 1988.

Bump RC. Urinary tract infection in women. Current role of single-dose therapy. J Reprod Med 1990;35:785.

Greenberg RN, Reilly PM, Luppen KL, et al. Randomized study of single-dose, three-day, and seven-day treatment of cystitis in women. J Infect Dis 1986;153:277.

Kunin CM. Urinary tract infections in females. Clin Infect Dis 1994;18:1.

Pappas P. Laboratory in the diagnosis and management of urinary tract infections. Med Clin North Am 1991;75:313–325.

Powers R. New directions in the diagnosis and therapy of urinary tract infections. Am J Obstet Gynecol 1991;164:1387–1389.

Smith RP. Gynecology in Primary Care. Baltimore: Williams & Wilkins, 1997, pp 577–602.

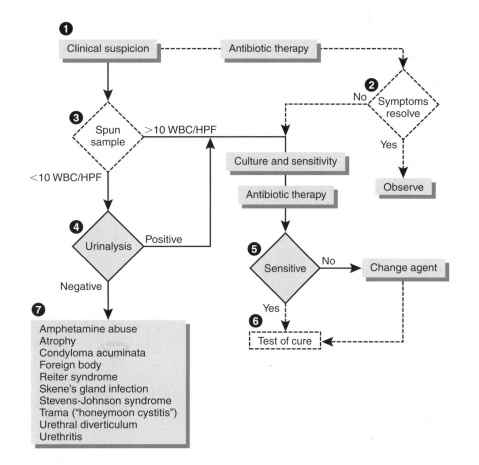

❶ Clinical suspicion - - - - - - - - Antibiotic therapy - - - - - - - - →

❷ Symptoms resolve

No

Yes

Observe

❸ Spun sample

>10 WBC/HPF

<10 WBC/HPF

Culture and sensitivity

Antibiotic therapy

❹ Urinalysis

Positive

Negative

❺ Sensitive

No → Change agent

Yes

❻ Test of cure

❼
Amphetamine abuse
Atrophy
Condyloma acuminata
Foreign body
Reiter syndrome
Skene's gland infection
Stevens-Johnson syndrome
Trama ("honeymoon cystitis")
Urethral diverticulum
Urethritis

Uterine Leiomyomata

Management Strategies

INTRODUCTION

Uterine leiomyomata (fibroids) are benign connective tissue tumors found in or around the uterus, which may be disseminated in rare cases. Fibroids represent the most common pelvic tumor in nonpregnant women. Up to 30% of hysterectomies performed in the United States, and almost half of those performed on women between the ages of 35 and 50 years, are performed for "fibroids." Clinically identifiable fibroids occur in one fourth of white and one half of black women, reaching their peak incidence in the fifth decade of life, when they are found in roughly 40% of all patients. Fibroids are more common in nulliparous women and those with early menarche. They vary in size from microscopic to over 100 pounds in weight. Up to one half of women with fibroids will have symptoms, most commonly pelvic pain and abnormal bleeding, which occur in approximately 30% of cases. Uterine fibroids are extremely rare before the age of 20. As a result, other diagnoses should be entertained in these patients.

❶ The need for, and type of, therapy indicated for patients with uterine leiomyomata are based on the presence of symptoms and the size of the tumors in asymptomatic patients.

❷ In the case of bleeding or dysmenorrhea, therapies such as nonsteroidal anti-inflammatory drugs (NSAIDs) or oral contraceptives may give satisfactory results. Medical therapy with medroxyprogesterone acetate usually resolves symptoms of pain or bleeding, but the uterine fibroids generally remain unchanged. Danazol sodium may be used to reduce estrogen levels, but is associated with a number of side effects, making it less desirable.

❸ When satisfactory relief is obtained, the therapy may be continued and the size of the fibroids monitored.

❹ At one time, uterine fibroids of greater than 12 cm were an automatic indication for surgery. The management of patients with uterine leiomyomata has changed somewhat over the past decade. Improved imaging techniques have allowed more conservative therapy to be available for the majority of patients.

❺ Large fibroids may cause symptoms of pelvic heaviness, fullness, pressure, or reduced bladder capacity. If these are absent, the fibroids may followed in the same manner as smaller tumors.

❻ Small fibroids, and asymptomatic larger fibroids, may be followed conservatively. Those that show little or no growth may safely be followed for prolonged periods. Those that enlarge significantly or rapidly require further evaluation or therapy.

❼ When symptoms cannot be controlled through simple symptomatic therapies or the fibroids produce pressure symptoms, the therapeutic decision is driven by the patient's desire for fertility. Those desiring fertility may be considered for gonadotropin-releasing hormone (GnRH) agonist therapy. Excellent but relatively short-term results may be obtained using GnRH agonists. Reductions of 50% to 60% in overall uterine volume and 50% in the size of largest uterine fibroids are not uncommon. Maximal uterine response is achieved in 3 months of therapy, but a return to pretreatment levels is often seen within 6 months of discontinuing treatment. Therapy is generally restricted to attempts to increase the possibility of myomectomy, to enable endoscopic or vaginal approaches to therapy, to improve the patient's preoperative condition, and to reduce the operative blood loss and chance of intraoperative transfusion.

REFERENCES

American College of Obstetricians and Gynecologists. Uterine Leiomyomata. ACOG Technical Bulletin 192. Washington, DC: ACOG, 1994.

American Fertility Society. Myomas and Reproductive Dysfunction: Guideline for Practice. Birmingham, Alabama: AFS, 1992.

Cramer SF, Horiszny JA, Leppert P. Epidemiology of uterine leiomyomas. J Reprod Med 1995;40:595–600.

Reiter RC, Wagner PL, Gambone JC. Routine hysterectomy for large asymptomatic uterine leiomyomata: A reappraisal. Obstet Gynecol 1992;79:481–484.

Vollenhoven BJ, Lawrence AS, Healy DL. Uterine fibroids: A clinical review. Br J Obstet Gynaecol 1990;97:285–298.

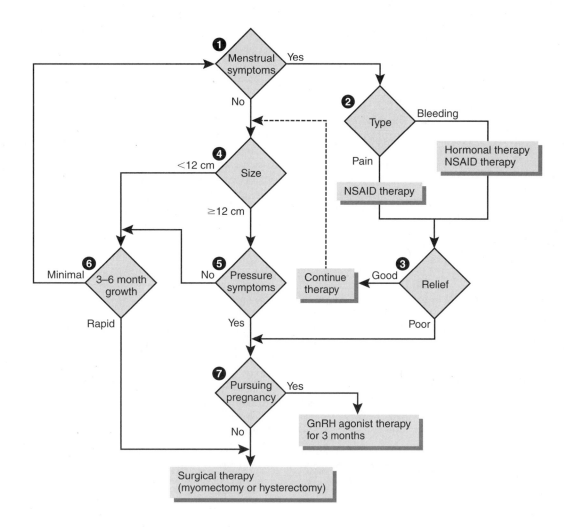

Uterine Prolapse

INTRODUCTION

Uterine prolapse occurs through the loss of the normal support mechanism with the consequent descent of the uterus down the vaginal canal. In the extreme, this may result in the uterus descending beyond the vulva to a position outside the body (procidentia). The loss of normal structural support may be due to trauma (childbirth), surgery, chronic intra-abdominal pressure elevation (such as occurs in obesity, chronic coughing, or heavy lifting), or intrinsic weakness. Most common causes are injury to the cardinal and uterosacral ligaments, and relaxation or rupture of the levator ani muscles that form the pelvic floor. Rarely, increased intra-abdominal pressure from a pelvic mass or ascites may weaken pelvic support and result in prolapse. Injury to, or neuropathy of, the S1 to S4 nerve roots may also result in decreased muscle tone and pelvic relaxation. The degree of prolapse is often quantitated in three steps: in first degree prolapse the cervix descends into the upper vagina, in second degree prolapse the cervix is in the lower vagina near the introitus, and in third degree (or total) prolapse part or all of the uterus is beyond the introitus.

❶ Asymptomatic uterine prolapse demands no therapy and can be followed for prolonged periods.

❷ Therapeutic approaches to patients with symptomatic uterine prolapse are often driven by the degree of descent present. Patients with mild prolapse may obtain some relief through pelvic muscle strengthening (Kegel's exercises) and lifestyle changes. Lifestyle changes include weight reduction, modification of activity (lifting), and address of factors such as chronic cough. Moderated uterine descent is often treated by a trial of pessary therapy, while severe prolapse may be treated by surgery or pessary therapy.

❸ Pessaries offer an excellent alternative to surgical repair, but the use of a pessary requires the cooperation and involvement of the patient. Patients who are unable, or unwilling, to manage the periodic insertion and removal of the device are poor candidates for their use. Pessaries will not be well tolerated or provide optimal support in the poorly estrogenized patient. For this reason, many suggest a minimum of 30 days of topical estrogen therapy (for those not already on estrogen replacement) before a trial of pessary therapy.

❹ The choice of surgical or pessary therapy is based on a number of factors. Surgery brings the hope of long-term relief and the possibility of addressing a number of problems at one time, but carries specific risks and the possibility of failure or complications. Pessaries may be used as a test of cure or a definitive therapy. The fill choice between these two must be individualized for each patient.

❺ Surgical therapy may include colpoclysis.

REFERENCES

American College of Obstetricians and Gynecologists. Pelvic Organ Prolapse. ACOG Technical Bulletin 214. Washington, DC: ACOG, 1995.

Beecham CT. Classification of vaginal relaxation. Am J Obstet Gynecol 1980;136:957.

Miller DC. Contemporary use of the pessary. In Sciarra JJ (ed): Gynecology and Obstetrics. Philadelphia: JB Lippincott, 1991;(1)39:1.

Porges RF. Abnormalities of pelvic support. In Sciarra JJ (ed): Gynecology and Obstetrics. Philadelphia: JB Lippincott, 1993;(1)61:1.

Thomas AG, Brodman ML, Dottino PR, et al. Manchester procedure vs vaginal hysterectomy for uterine prolapse: a comparison. J Reprod Med 1995;40:299.

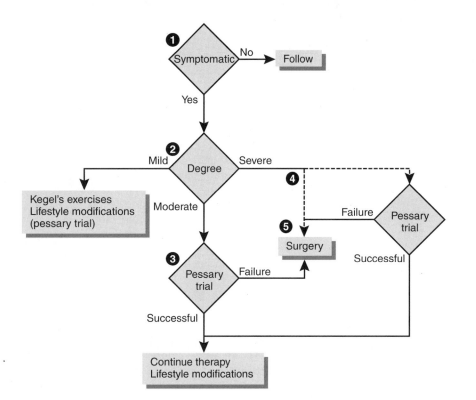

❶ Symptomatic — No → Follow

Yes

❷ Degree

Mild → Kegel's exercises
Lifestyle modifications
(pessary trial)

Moderate

❸ Pessary trial — Failure → Surgery **❺**

Successful → Continue therapy
Lifestyle modifications

Severe **❹** → Pessary trial

Failure → Surgery

Successful → Continue therapy
Lifestyle modifications

Vaginal Cysts

INTRODUCTION

Cystic masses in the vaginal wall are uncommon and may arise from either congenital (Gartner's duct cysts) or acquired processes (epithelial inclusion cysts, >50% of cases). While they are generally asymptomatic, they may be associated with a sense of fullness, difficulty with tampon insertion or retention, or, uncommonly, dyspareunia. Surgical excision is indicated if the mass is symptomatic or its cause is uncertain, otherwise not therapy is required.

❶ The location of the cyst often suggests its origin. The location may be identified by inspection or by careful palpation during pelvic examination. Congenital cysts (Gartner's duct cyst or remnants) are generally found in lateral vaginal wall, often slightly anterior of the mid-lateral line. Nests of adenomatous cells found in the vaginal wall (vaginal adenosis) are generally congenital rests and are more common in women exposed to diethylstilbestrol while in utero.

❷ Cystic masses in the upper anterior vaginal wall may arise from epithelial inclusions (generally at the time of delivery) or, less commonly, from urethral diverticula. While an isolated urethrocele could be mistaken for a cystic mass, these are most commonly associated with a cystocele and other signs of pelvic support loss. Skene's gland cysts will be located in the outer portion of the anterior vaginal wall, near the urethral meatus.

❸ Inclusion cysts result when a portion of vaginal epithelium becomes tucked under itself following an obstetric laceration or episiotomy. These are most common in the outer portions of the vagina but may be found through out its length. Hymeneal carruncles may take on a cystic character but will be easily identified by their location in the hymeneal ring. Rectovaginal abscesses may present as a midline posterior vaginal mass similar to a rectocele in character.

REFERENCES

Delmore JE, Horbelt DV. Benign neoplasma of the vagina. In Sciarra JJ (ed): Gynecology and Obstetrics. Philadelphia: JB Lippincott, 1995;(1)10:1.

Deppisch LM. Cysts of the vagina. Obstet Gynecol 1975;45:623.

Dmochowski RR, Ganabathi K, Zimmern PE, Leach GE. Benign female periurethral masses. J Urol 1994;152:1943.

Hillard PA. Benign diseases of the female reproductive tract: Symptoms and signs. In Berek JS, Adashi EY, Hillard PA (eds): Novak's Gynecology, 12th ed. Baltimore: Williams & Wilkins, 1996, p 390.

Junaid TA, Thomas SM. Cysts of the vulva and vagina: a comparative study. Int J Gynaecol Obstet 1981;19:239.

Robboy SJ, Ross JS, Prat J, et al. Urogenital sinus origin of mucinous and ciliated cysts of the vulva. Obstet Gynecol 1978;51:347.

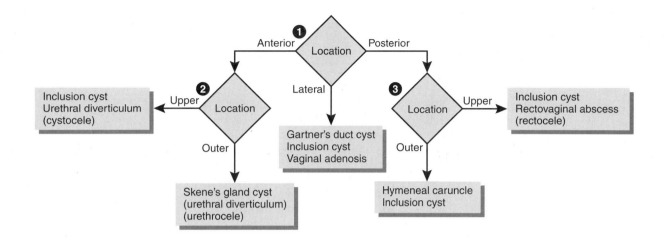

Vaginal Discharge

INTRODUCTION

The clinical evaluation of vaginal discharges is critical to the diagnosis of vaginal complaints and infection. The diagnosis is established using several readily available modalities.

❶ The gross character of the vaginal discharge present may be used to separate the possible causes. Initially, they may be divided based on the thickness or thinness of the secretions. Those that are of a viscosity that is similar to or less than that of normal should be differentiated from those with a thicker character.

❷ If the viscosity of the secretions present appears to be normal or increased, microscopic examination of the material mixed with a few drops of 10% potassium hydroxide (KOH) should differentiate between thickened secretions due to dehydration or other factors and those due to a monilial infection.

❸ Thin, runny secretions with a foamy or frothy nature are characteristic of *Trichomonas* infections.

These secretions often have a gray-green or yellow color and carry a musty odor.

❹ Thin, runny secretions without a foamy or frothy nature may be either physiologic or the result of a shift in bacterial flora typical of bacterial vaginosis or vaginitis. The addition of a few drops of 10% KOH solution to a sample of the vaginal secretions ("whiff" test) will liberate amines that carry a "fishy" odor if bacterial vaginosis is present.

❺ Because the amine test in not always positive in cases of bacterial vaginosis, additional confirmatory tests are indicated. These may include either the microscopic evaluation of the secretions mixed with normal saline or the measurement of pH. The latter is easily done using pH paper of an appropriate pH range. If the microscopic approach is chosen, clue cells are sought, but are only diagnostic of bacterial vaginosis if they represent greater than 20% of the cells present. This diagnostic criteria is often difficult to achieve, making the measurement of pH faster and more reliable. (The use of pH as a diagnostic tool by itself is discussed separately.)

REFERENCES

American College of Obstetricians and Gynecologists. Vaginitis. ACOG Technical Bulletin 226. Washington, DC: ACOG, 1996.

Faro S. Bacterial vaginitis. Clin Obstet Gynecol 1991;34:582.

Horowitz BJ. Candidiasis: Specification and therapy. Curr Probl Obstet Gynecol Fertil 1990;8:233.

Ledger WJ. Historical review of the treatment of bacterial vaginosis. Am J Obstet Gynecol 1993;169:474–478.

MacDermott RIJ. Bacterial vaginosis. Br J Obstet Gynaecol 1995;102:92.

McLellan R, Spence MR, Brockman M, et al. The clinical diagnosis of trichomoniasis. Obstet Gynecol 1982;60:30–34.

Smith RP. Gynecology in Primary Care. Baltimore: Williams & Wilkins, 1997, pp 603–632.

Spiegel CA. Bacterial vaginosis. Clin Microbiol Rev 1991;4:485.

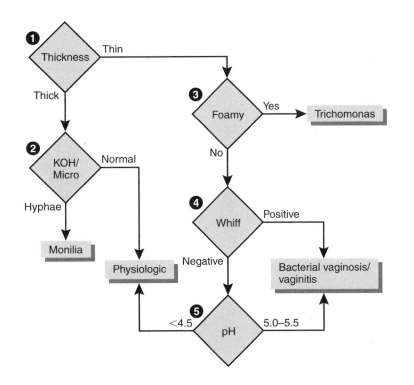

Vaginal Discharge

Evaluation by pH

INTRODUCTION

The pH of vaginal secretions may be used to diagnose vaginal infections in most cases. The most common forms of infection produce or thrive in different ranges of pH, making this possible.

❶ The use of pH to establish a diagnosis is predicated on distinguishing the pH changes caused by infection from that of the normal physiology. As a result, patients who are premenarchal or postmenopausal should be examined by microscopic techniques because of their more neutral natural pH.

❷ The microscopic examination of vaginal secretions from premenarchal and postmenopausal women is unchanged by the altered pH typical of these women.

❸ Women who are breastfeeding may be relatively hypoestrogenic. This results in vaginal atrophy and a pH that mimics that of a postmenopausal woman. Microscopic techniques, and not pH alone, should be used to evaluate these women.

❹ The pH of the vaginal secretions may be measured by a pH meter or by the use of suitable pH paper chosen to indicate pHs in the range of 4.5 to 6.0 or greater. When a pH of 6.0 or greater is found, the presence of *Trichomonas* may be presumed. Vaginal secretions with a pH of 5.0 to 5.5 suggest changes in the normal bacterial flora typical of bacterial vaginosis or vaginitis. When the pH is 4.5 or below, the patient may have either a physiologic discharge or a monilial infection. In this case, additional characteristics help to differentiate these two possibilities.

❺ While both physiologic and monilial discharges share a similar pH, the gross characteristics of these discharges are sufficiently different to augment the diagnostic process. A thick, curdlike discharge, especially when associated with itching, suggests a monilial infection.

REFERENCES

American College of Obstetricians and Gynecologists. Vaginitis. ACOG Technical Bulletin 226. Washington, DC: ACOG, 1996.

Faro S. Bacterial vaginitis. Clin Obstet Gynecol 1991;34:582.

Horowitz BJ. Candidiasis: Specification and therapy. Curr Probl Obstet Gynecol Fertil 1990;8:233.

Ledger WJ. Historical review of the treatment of bacterial vaginosis. Am J Obstet Gynecol 1993;169:474–478.

MacDermott RIJ. Bacterial vaginosis. Br J Obstet Gynaecol 1995;102:92.

McLellan R, Spence MR, Brockman M, et al. The clinical diagnosis of trichomoniasis. Obstet Gynecol 1982;60:30–34.

Smith RP. Gynecology in Primary Care. Baltimore: Williams & Wilkins, 1997, pp 603–632.

Spiegel CA. Bacterial vaginosis. Clin Microbiol Rev 1991;4:485.

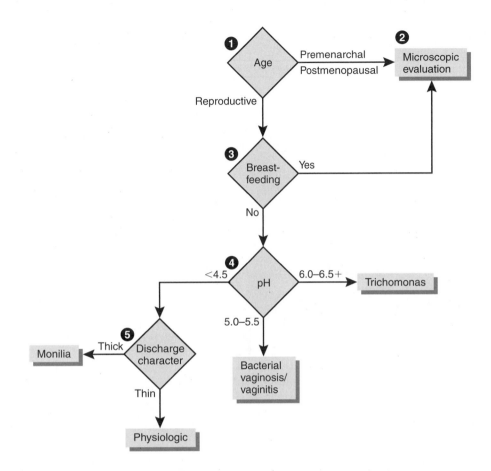

Vaginal Dryness

INTRODUCTION

Symptoms of vaginal dryness affect most women at some point in their lives. These symptoms may range from mild irritation or itching to painful intercourse and vaginal cracking or lacerations. Simple interventions will be successful in most cases.

❶ The first issue to be determined is whether the patient's symptoms are constant or recurrent (episodic). Symptoms that are present most of the time have different origins from those that are coitally related or cyclic.

❷ The most common cause of continuous symptoms of vaginal dryness are the atrophic changes brought on by the loss of ovarian steroids associated with natural or surgical menopause.

❸ The most effective treatment for genital atrophy is estrogen replacement therapy. This may be systemic or topical, or a combination of both. Systemic therapy provides the additional benefits attributed to estrogen replacement therapy, while local therapy provides a slightly more rapid effect and higher local tissue levels. Topically applied estrogen is absorbed into the systemic circulation. This absorption amounts to approximately 25% of the dose given, though that percentage is much higher when the tissues are thinned by atrophy. Complete reversal of symptoms may take up to 6 months to achieve. Adjunctive lubricants and moisturizing agents are appropriate whereas estrogen therapy is instituted or for those patients who choose to or should not use estrogen.

❹ Women who are not menopausal should be investigated for the presence of clinically apparent causes, such as a chronic vaginitis, or hygiene practices such as inappropriate douching or chronic tampon use (which deplete normal moisture). The tissues should be inspected for estrogen effects and the degree of moisture and suppleness present. Occasionally, the complaint of vaginal dryness is incongruent with the physical findings, suggesting other agendas such as sexual dysfunction, vaginismus, or abuse.

❺ Episodic vaginal dryness that is not related to intercourse may be the result of normal physiologic variations related to the menstrual cycle, recurrent infections, or episodic hygiene habits that deplete normal moisture. Menstrually related changes may be exacerbated by the use of hormonally based contraceptives.

❻ Coitally related vaginal dryness may reflect poor coital technique or an emotional response to the specific circumstances. Prolonged foreplay or coital thrusting may exhaust vaginal moisture, while inadequate foreplay or arousal provokes an insufficient evolution of moisture even when the tissues are capable of a normal response. Reassurance, exploration of the situations that result in symptoms, and the use of adjunctive lubricants will generally result in a satisfactory resolution of symptoms.

❼ When coitally related symptom of dryness do not appear to be related to technique or the situations surrounding sexual expression, the possibility of vaginismus must be considered. Additional history and the physical examination will confirm this diagnosis, and specific, often prolonged, therapy is required.

❽ Vaginal dryness or perceived dryness may be the result of, or a surrogate for, libidinal dysfunction. A careful history should reveal these concerns and suggest a course of therapy (discussed elsewhere).

REFERENCES

Bygdeman M, Swahn ML. Replens versus dienoestrol cream in the symptomatic treatment of vaginal atrophy in postmenopausal women. Maturitas 1996;23:259.

Coope J. Hormonal and non-hormonal interventions for menopausal symptoms. Maturitas 1996;23:159.

Lamont JA. Dyspareunia and vaginismus. In Sciarra JJ (ed): Gynecology and Obstetrics. Philadelphia: JB Lippincott, 1998;(6)102:2.

Loprinzi CL, Abu-Ghazaleh S, Sloan JA, et al. Phase III randomized double-blind study to evaluate the efficacy of a polycarbophil-based vaginal moisturizer in women with breast cancer. J Clin Oncol 1997;15:969.

Mishell DR. Menopause. In Mishell DR, Stenchever MA, Droegemueller W, Herbst AL (eds): Comprehensive Gyencology, 3rd ed. St. Louis: CV Mosby, 1997, p 1163.

Smith RP. Gynecology in Primay Care. Baltimore: Williams & Wilkins, 1997, pp 197, 522.

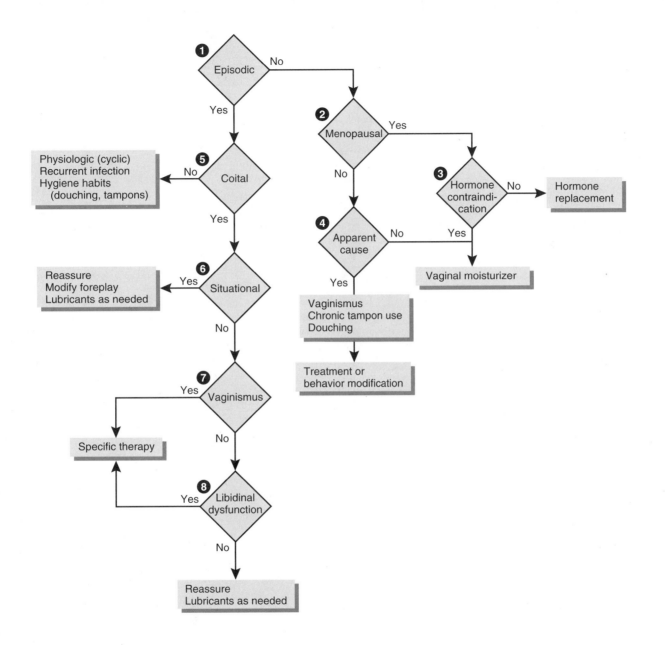

Vaginal Lacerations

INTRODUCTION

Direct trauma to the vulva or vagina may occur through many activities, including falls, abuse, and sexual intercourse (consensual or otherwise) (80%). Tears of the hymen or vaginal wall are more likely when the tissues are stiff, scarred, or atrophic. Impairment of judgment, through drugs or alcohol, is commonly a factor. The most commonly encountered tear is a transverse rent of the posterior fornix, followed by lacerations of the lateral fonices. Laceration of the apex of the vagina after hysterectomy is most common in the first few weeks after hysterectomy, but has been reported many years later. Rarely, tears secondary to the use of tampons or contraceptive devices have been reported.

❶ Bleeding from vaginal lacerations may be scant or massive, depending on the depth and extent of tissues damaged. Because the extent of bleeding may be difficult to assess and the location or source of injury a cause of embarrassment, care may delayed, resulting in hemodynamic instability. Penetrating injuries to other surrounding tissues, including the intra-abdominal organs, may result in profound risk to life. Vaginal evisceration may occur. Rapid stabilization and immediate surgical exploration and repair may be required.

❷ Lacerations of the vulva or vagina may extend into deep tissues or the peritoneal cavity and are uniformly deeper than anticipated on initial inspec-

tion. Even deep lacerations may be surprisingly asymptomatic, making a careful assessment mandatory. General anesthesia may be required to evaluate fully the extent and significance of the damage.

❸ Lacerations that extend into the peritoneal cavity require immediate surgical exploration, including laparotomy, to assess the possibility of intra-abdominal damage. Because of the need to evaluate the full extent of the bowel, laparoscopy does not provide an adequate evaluation. The integrity the bladder must also be evaluated; hematuria indicates the need for cystoscopy.

❹ Bleeding to any extent must be treated by surgical repair. The loose tissues and lack of tissue planes present in the vulva and vagina results in bleeding that is not self-limited when trauma occurs. When ever possible, ligatures should be placed only on bleeding vessels or to close a deep space. Fine, delayed absorbable sutures may then be used to close the vaginal epithelium. Antibiotic coverage for the flora of the vulva, vagina, and rectum, as well as possible sexually transmitted diseases, should be instituted.

❺ Particularly deep lacerations, or those of moderate size, require surgical assessment and repair. Repair should consist of exploration of the defect to identify unrecognized injuries, removal of necrotic tissue or foreign bodies, and copious irrigation. Clo-

sure of the tissues should be made in a tension-free manner with fine, delayed absorbable suture materials. Small lesions may not require closure and will spontaneously heal without intervention. Topical or systemic antibiosis, along with analgesia as needed, should be instituted. Tetanus prophylaxis should be provided for any patient who has not received a booster in the preceding 5 years.

REFERENCES

American College of Obstetricians and Gynecologists. Operative Vaginal Delivery. ACOG Technical Bulletin 196. Washington, DC: ACOG, 1994.

Ahnaimugan S, Asuen MI. Coital laceration of the vagina. Aust N Z J Obstet Gynaecol 1980;20:180.

Barret KF, Bledsoe S, Greer BE, et al. Tampon-induced vaginal or cervical ulceration. Am J Obstet Gynecol 1977;127:332.

Friedel W, Kaiser IH. Vaginal evisceration. Obstet Gynecol 1975;45:315.

Haefner HK, Andersen F, Johnson MP. Vaginal laceration following a jet-ski accident. Obstet Gynecol 1991;78:986.

Niv J, Lessing JB, Hartuv J, Peyser MR. Vaginal injury resulting from sliding down a water chute. Am J Obstet Gynecol 1992;166:930.

Rafla N. Vaginismus and vaginal tears. Am J Obstet Gynecol 1988;158:1043.

Smith NC, Van Coeverden de Groot HA, Gunston KD. Coital injuries of the vagina in nonvirginal patients. S Afr Med J 1983;64:746.

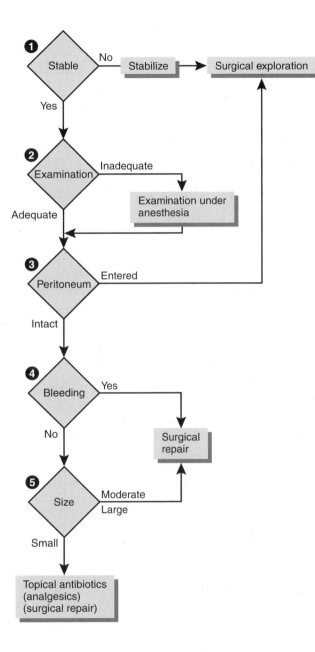

Vaginal Odors

INTRODUCTION

A certain amount of "aroma" is normal for the vaginal secretions of reproductive-age women. These come from aliphatic (cheesy odor) and lactic (sour milk odor) acids found in these fluids. The relative amounts present, determine the predominant odor. An "odor" is often a sign of the change in vaginal flora associated with a vaginal infection, though as a complaint it may originate from a variety of sources. Amine salts are converted into volatile free bases in an alkaline environment such as that provided by semen, menstrual blood, alkaline douches (e.g., baking soda) or the potassium hydroxide solutions used in the "whiff" test. The presence of such amines is not normal.

❶ The acute onset of offensive vaginal odors suggests an equally abrupt cause.

❷ Patients with an acute onset of a malodorous discharge should be examined for the presence of a foreign body. Retained tampons, condoms, pessaries, and other items may be in advertently left in the vagina, resulting in a change in vaginal flora and an acute inflammatory reaction. The makeup of the resulting secretions closely mimics those of a draining abscess. If this is the cause of the odor, the foreign body must be removed. The use of topical antibiotic preparations may speed the resolution of symptoms but is generally not necessary.

❸ Lesions on the exterior portions of the genital tract may result in aerobic bacterial overgrowth and the development of a "vaginal" odor. Secondary infections or necrotic lesions are most likely to be the cause. These will usually be grossly evident on inspection of the vulva. Treatment will be dictated by the nature of the lesion present.

❹ The character of the vaginal discharge present, if any, may suggest the organism responsible when a vaginal infection is the basis of the odor. A frothy discharge suggests a trichomonal infection, while a thin homogeneous discharge that coats the tissues suggests bacterial vaginosis or vaginitis. (Intense itching, but generally without a change in odor, characterizes monilial infections.) These clinical suspicions should be confirmed by other methods, such as vaginal pH and a microscopic evaluation of the secretions.

❺ The presence of apparently normal secretions should prompt a microscopic evaluation. Clue cells or trichomonads will confirm the diagnosis.

❻ Patients with microscopically normal vaginal secretions should be evaluated for other potential sources of "odor." A common cause of a change in odor is urinary or fecal incontinence. While the odor itself may suggest this source, it is an easily overlooked possibility. When this source is absent, the perception itself should be evaluated. The complaint of odor may represent an obsessive focus on normal aromas, the effects of inadequate or overly compulsive perineal hygiene, or a surrogate ("hidden agenda") for other concerns.

REFERENCES

American College of Obstetricians and Gynecologists. Vaginitis: ACOG Technical Bulletin 226. Washington, DC: ACOG, 1996.

Faro S. Bacterial vaginitis. Clin Obstet Gynecol 1991;34:582.

Horowitz BJ. Candidiasis: Specification and therapy. Curr Probl Obstet Gynecol Fertil 1990;8:233.

Ledger WJ. Historical review of the treatment of bacterial vaginosis. Am J Obstet Gynecol 1993;169:474–478.

MacDermott RIJ. Bacterial vaginosis. Br J Obstet Gynaecol 1995;102:92.

McLellan R, Spence MR, Brockman M, et al. The clinical diagnosis of trichomoniasis. Obstet Gynecol 1982;60:30–34.

Smith RP. Gynecology in Primary Care. Baltimore: Williams & Wilkins, 1997, pp 603–632.

Spiegel CA. Bacterial vaginosis. Clin Microbiol Rev 1991;4:485.

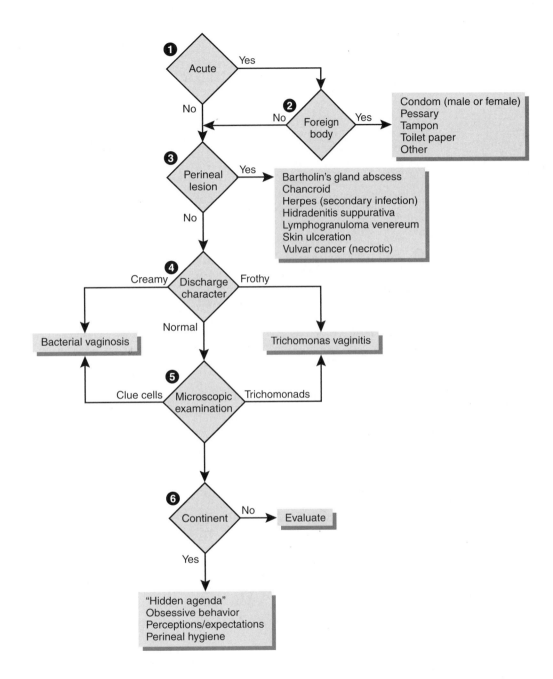

Vaginal Prolapse

INTRODUCTION

Vaginal prolapse occurs through the loss of the normal support mechanisms. Vaginal prolapse is generally found only following hysterectomy. In the extreme, this may result in the vagina becoming everted beyond the vulva to a position outside the body.

❶ Asymptomatic vaginal prolapse demands no therapy and can be followed for prolonged periods.

❷ Therapeutic approaches to patients with symptomatic vaginal prolapse is often driven by the degree of descent present. Patients with mild prolapse may obtain some relief through pelvic muscle strengthening (Kegel's exercises) and lifestyle changes. Lifestyle changes include weight reduction, modification of activity (lifting), and addressing factors such as chronic cough. Moderated descent is often treated by a trial of pessary therapy, while severe prolapse may be treated by surgery or pessary therapy.

❸ Pessaries offer an excellent alternative to surgical repair, but the use of a pessary requires the cooperation and involvement of the patient. Patients who are unable, or unwilling, to manage the periodic insertion and removal of the device are poor candidates for their use. Pessaries will not be well tolerated or provide optimal support in the poorly estrogenized patient. For this reason, many suggest a minimum of 30 days of topical estrogen therapy (for those not already on estrogen replacement) before a trial of pessary therapy.

❹ The choice of surgical or pessary therapy is based on a number of factors. Surgery brings the hope of long-term relief the possibility of addressing a number of problems at one time, but carries specific risks and the possibility of failure or complications. Pessaries may be used as a test of cure or a definitive therapy. The fill choice between these two must be individualized for each patient.

❺ Surgical therapy may include culdoplasty, plication of the uterosacral ligaments, sacrospinous ligament fixation, or colpoclysis.

REFERENCES

American College of Obstetricians and Gynecologists. Pelvic Organ Prolapse. ACOG Technical Bulletin 214. Washington, DC: ACOG, 1995.

Birnbaum SJ. Rational therapy for the prolapsed vagina. Am J Obstet Gynecol 1973;115:411.

Delancey JOL. Anatomic aspects of vaginal eversion after hysterectomy. Am J Obstet Gynecol 1992;166:1717.

Miller DC. Contemporary use of the pessary. In Sciarra JJ (ed): Gynecology and Obstetrics. Philadelphia: JB Lippincott, 1991;(1)39:1.

Morley GW, Delancey JOL. Sacrospinous ligament fixation for eversion of vagina. Am J Obstet Gynecol 1988;158:872.

Nichols DH. Sacrospinous fixation for massive eversion of vagina. Am J Obstet Gynecol 1982;142:901.

Percy NM, Perl JI. Total colpectomy. Surg Gynecol Obstet 1961;113:174.

Porges RF. Abnormalities of pelvic support. In Sciarra JJ (ed): Gynecology and Obstetrics. Philadelphia: JB Lippincott, 1993;(1)61:14.

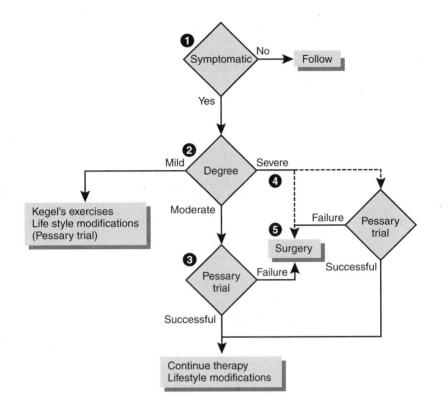

Vaginismus

INTRODUCTION

Vaginismus is a special case of insertional dyspareunia in which intense vaginal muscle spasms in the pelvic floor and vaginal wall virtually prevent intromission. Vaginismus occurs in less than 1% of sexually active women, but for those women it can have a devastating effect on their lives and relationships. Despite the intense pain associated with vaginal penetration, these patients may be fully orgasmic by other means.

❶ Vulvar or vestibular disease may mimic true vaginismus. This possibility is easily evaluated by history and physical examinations.

❷ There is no evidence that the vaginal canal is structurally different in these women; rather, a spasm of the pelvic floor results in functional narrowing. Vaginismus has been described as a manifestation of significant phobic reactions, anxiety, hostility, hysteria, or aversion. In severe cases this may be the case, but in milder forms it may also be a learned behavior or protective reaction based on previous negative experiences. Some authors report that up to 80% of vaginismus is situational, suggesting the latter explanations are more common.

❸ Vaginal pathology as well as vaginal and introital muscle tone should be evaluated by gentle vaginal examination. Vaginismus may be present even if there is no sign of muscular spasm during pelvic examination. In mild forms, vaginal spasms occur only in the setting of attempted penile penetration. Clinical examination, tampon insertion, masturbation, and occasionally digital insertion by a partner may be tolerated. Obvious vaginal lesions or pathology should be ruled out before a diagnosis of vaginismus can be supported.

❹ The possibility of psychiatric disease must be explored in a sensitive manner. Obvious pathology should be addressed specifically. Some authors suggest the judicious use of anxiolytics or antidepressant medications for selected patients may be appropriate, for short periods of time only, even in the absence of a specific psychiatric diagnosis.

❺ Therapy generally takes a three-pronged approach consisting of behavior modification, vaginal dilatation, and emotional counseling. These should be applied in a graduated sequence and care must be maintained to watch for the emergence of phobias or depression. Self-exploration and training to allow vaginal containment without pain should be encouraged. Delaying penetration until maximal arousal has been achieved improves vaginal lubrication, ensures vaginal apex expansion, and provides an element of control for the female partner. Sexual positions that allow the woman to control the direction and depth of penetration (such as woman astride) may also be of help.

REFERENCES

Fordney DS. Dyspareunia and vaginismus. Clin Obstet Gynecol 1978;21(1):205.

Fuchs K. Therapy of vaginismus by hypnotic desensitization. Am J Obstet Gynecol 1980;137:1.

Lamont JA. Vaginismus. Am J Obstet Gynecol 1978;131:632.

Rafla N. Vaginismus and vaginal tears. Am J Obstet Gynecol 1988;158:1043.

Reamy K. The treatment of vaginismus by the gynecologists: An eclectic approach. Obstet Gynecol 1982;59:58.

Steege JF. Dyspareunia and vaginismus. Clin Obstet Gynecol 1984;27(3):750–759.

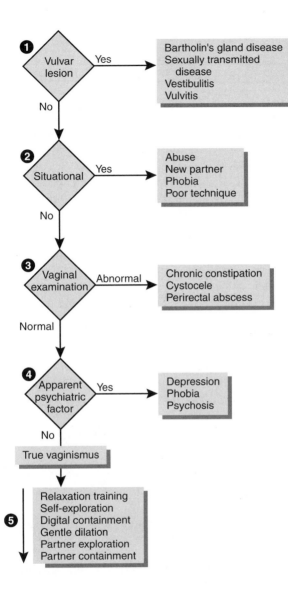

1 Vulvar lesion — Yes →
Bartholin's gland disease
Sexually transmitted
  disease
Vestibulitis
Vulvitis

No ↓

2 Situational — Yes →
Abuse
New partner
Phobia
Poor technique

No ↓

3 Vaginal examination — Abnormal →
Chronic constipation
Cystocele
Perirectal abscess

Normal ↓

4 Apparent psychiatric factor — Yes →
Depression
Phobia
Psychosis

No ↓

True vaginismus

↓

5 Relaxation training
Self-exploration
Digital containment
Gentle dilation
Partner exploration
Partner containment

Virilization

INTRODUCTION

Virilization refers to the loss of female sexual characteristics such as body contour and the acquisition of masculine qualities such as increased muscle mass, temporal balding, deepening of the voice, and clitoromegaly (discussed separately). Virilization generally indicates the presence of increased levels of androgens, though it does not indicate the source. When virilization occurs over a short period of time or after the age of 25, it is presumed to indicate the presence of a hormonally active tumor.

❶ It is important to distinguish between true virilization and the presence of some masculine features such as excessive hair growth. When excessive hair growth is not associated with signs of true virilization (such as clitoromegaly, loss of breast mass, change in voice, or amenorrhea), it should be classed a hirsutism (discussed separately).

❷ The patient should be carefully questioned about the use of medications, diet supplements, and over-the-counter health or nutritional supplements. Many medications have androgenic side effects or can alter sex binding globulin levels sufficiently to result in hirsutism or virilization. Examples include phenytoin, diazoxide, minoxidil, cyclosporine, glucocorticoids, penicillamine, and psoralens. Hirsutism has been reported by patients using danazol, metyrapone, some 19-nortestosterone derivatives used in oral contraceptives, and androgens (including topical androgens used for vulvar conditions).

❸ Patients who are pregnant and show signs of virilization may have a luteoma or hyperreactio luteinalis. Ultrasonography of the adnexa may suggest the diagnosis.

❹ The laboratory evaluation of virilization includes the measurement of serum testosterone, dehydroepiandrosterone sulfate (DHEA-s) and 3α-androstanediol glucuronide (3α-AG). Other tests such as measurements of follicle-stimulating hormone (FSH), luteinizing hormone (LH), or thyroid function should be dictated by clinical indications.

❺ If serum testosterone levels are above 2 ng/mL, a hormonally active ovarian tumor must be presumed.

❻ Measurement of serum LH will generally separate those patients with polycystic ovaries from those with stromal hyperthecosis or early tumor.

❼ The measurement of 3α-AG has been somewhat controversial because of a high rate of both false positives and false negatives. Elevations suggest an abnormality of the peripheral conversion of precursors into 5α-dihydrotestosterone (DHT) by the enzyme 5α-reductase. This abnormal conversion rate is typical in cases of idiopathic hirsutism.

❽ If serum DHEA-s levels are greater than 8 μg/mL a renal adenoma should be presumed as the source of androgen excess.

❾ Elevations of DHEA-s less than 8 μg/mL suggest an adrenal source but do not differentiate between possible causes. The measurement of serum cortisol after an overnight dexamethasone suppression test (1 mg po at 11 PM with 8 AM measurement of serum cortisol) may be used to separate patients with adult-onset congenital adrenal hyperplasia (CAHD) and those with Cushing's disease. Morning measurement of the 17α-hydroxyprogesterone urinary metabolite, pregnanetriol, can help to differentiate between CAHD and polycystic ovary disease. Computed tomography or magnetic resonance imaging should be performed if a tumor is suspected.

❿ Plasma cortisol levels above 5 μg/dL are nonspecific and require a formal Liddle's test to make the final diagnosis.

REFERENCES

Bakri YN, Bakhashwain M, Hugosson C. Massive theca-lutein cysts, virilization, and hypothyroidism associated with normal pregnancy. Acta Obstet Gynecol Scand 1994;73:153.

Hall JE. Polycystic ovarian disease as a neuroendocrine disorder of the female reproductive axis. Endocrinol Metab Clin North Am 1993;22:75.

Ireland K, Woodruff JD. Masculinizing ovarian tumors. Obstet Gynecol Surv 1976;31:83.

Tagitz GE, Kopher RA, Nagel TC, Okagaki T. The clitoral index: A bioassay of androgenic stimulation. Obstet Gynecol 1979;54:562–564.

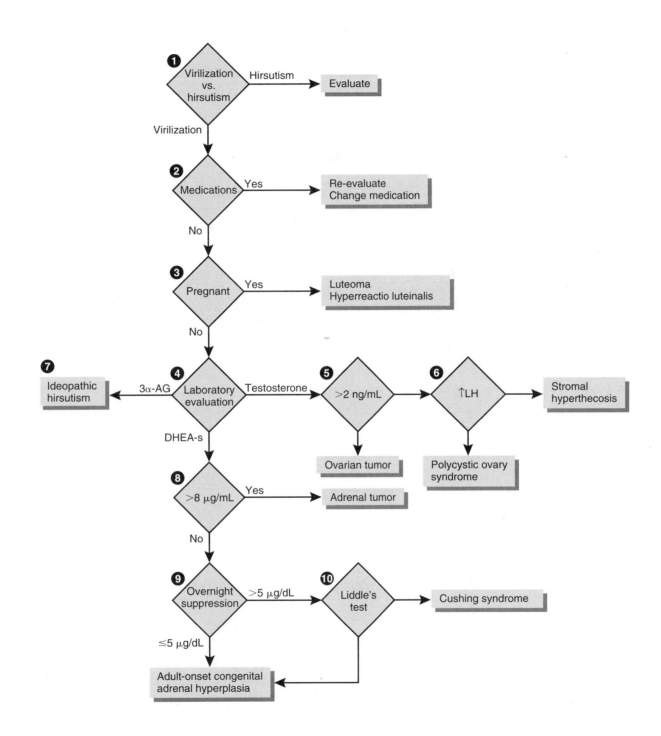

Vulvar Cancer Staging

INTRODUCTION

Squamous cell cancer of the vulva generally presents as an exophytic ulcer or hyperkeratotic plaque. It may arise as a solitary lesion or develop hidden within hypertrophic or other vulvar skin changes, making diagnosis difficult and often delayed.

1 Vulvar cancer that is limited to in situ disease is classified as stage 0 disease. The degree of invasion of a vulvar cancer cannot be determined unless the entire lesion is available for study. It cannot be evaluated by biopsy alone.

2 Stage I and II vulvar cancers are confined to the vulva and/or perineum, with no palpable lymph node involvement.

3 The distinction between stage I and II vulvar cancer is made on the basis of tumor size measured in greatest dimension. Tumors less than or equal to 2 cm in size are stage I, while larger tumors (confined to the vulva and/or perineum) are stage II.

4 Tumors that are limited to the lower urethra, vagina, or anus and those with a unilateral regional lymph node metastasis are stage III disease regardless of the size of the lesion.

5 Disease that involves the upper urethra, bladder or rectal mucosa, pelvic bone, or regional lymph nodes bilaterally is stage IVA. If there is any distant metastasis, including the pelvic lymph nodes, the tumor is classed as stage IVB. The latter may occur with lesions arising in the anterior third of the vulva, which may bypass the superficial lymph nodes and spread directly to deep pelvic nodes.

REFERENCES

American College of Obstetricians and Gynecologists. Vulvar Dystrophies. ACOG Technical Bulletin 139. Washington, DC: ACOG, 1990.

American College of Obstetricians and Gynecologists. Classification and Staging of Gynecologic Malignancies. ACOG Technical Bulletin 155. Washington, DC: ACOG, 1991.

American College of Obstetricians and Gynecologists. Vulvar Cancer. ACOG Technical Bulletin 186. Washington, DC: ACOG, 1993.

DiSaia PJ. Management of superficially invasive vulvar carcinoma. Clin Obstet Gynecol 1985;28:196.

Hacker NF, Van der Velden J. Conservative management of early vulvar cancer. Cancer 1993;71(Suppl):1673.

Kurman RJ, Norris HJ, Wilkinson EJ. In Rosai J (ed): Atlas of Tumor Pathology: Tumors of the Cervix, Vagina and Vulva, Vol 4. Washington, DC: AFIP, 1992.

Wilkinson EJ, Stone IK. Atlas of Vulvar Disease. Baltimore: Williams & Wilkins, 1995, p 162.

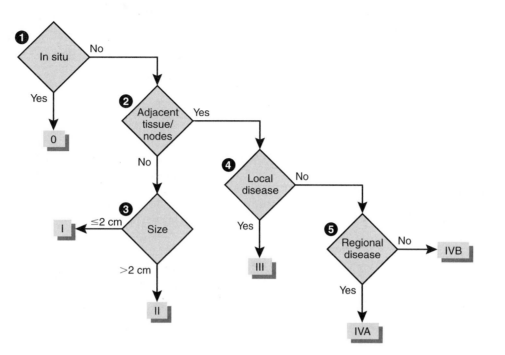

Vulvar Hematoma

INTRODUCTION

A vulvar hematoma presents as a swelling of one or both labia due to interstitial bleeding, most often following blunt trauma. Vulvar hematomas may result from blunt or sharp injuries, though 75% of cases result from a straddle injury. A vulvar wound may conceal deeper injuries, including vaginal lacerations, urethral compromise, pelvic fracture, or penetrating wounds. Vulvar injuries may result from rape or abuse. Children and adults who have not had a tetanus booster in the past 5 years should receive a booster.

❶ The first obligation in the evaluation of a patient with a vulvar hematoma is to ensure her medical stability. Because the extent of trauma cannot be immediately ascertained, internal injuries or excessive blood loss may not be apparent; to presume that the injury is minor risks peril. Unstable patients must be rapidly stabilized and surgically explored.

❷ The management of simple hematomas is based on the size of the lesion. While the distinction of small and large is subjective, a cutoff of 10 cm is often used in the literature; small lesions are treated with ice and pressure, while larger lesions may require intervention.

❸ Ice and pressure are the first line of treatment for most patients. These usually result in compression and vasospasm that arrest the bleeding within the damaged tissue. If this fails, drainage, with the placement of sutures or packing (as discussed in No. 7), may be required.

❹ If ice and pressure stop further bleeding and the skin of the vulva is intact, mild analgesics and observation complete the management. If the skin is broken, antibiotic prophylaxis should be instituted and the possibility of a penetrating injury to the vagina or intra-abdominal structures must be considered.

❺ When a large hematoma is encountered, the patency of the urethra must be evaluated. This is most easily accomplished with a small catheter; if extensive resistance to passage is encountered or there is hematuria, the catheter may be left in place.

❻ Many large hematomas may have already stabilized in response to increased tissue pressure, resulting in self-limited bleeding. Patients who appear stable may be treated with analgesics, ice, and pressure while the hematoma is assessed. Rapidly growing lesions and those that progress despite simple intervention will require surgical intervention.

❼ The loose character of the tissue and the lack of tissue planes to limit the dissection of the bleeding hamper incision and drainage of a vulvar hematoma. Any bleeding points should be ligated or cauterized. Packing may be required, but should be avoided if possible because of the discomfort created, the need to eventually remove the hematoma, and the increased risk of infection.

❽ Large hematomas with a breach of the vulvar skin suggest the possibility, if not probability, of more serious underlying injuries. Antibiotic prophylaxis is required and careful evaluation for other injuries should be carried out.

❾ While most hematomas will spontaneously resolve, some may persist or remain symptomatic. These may be drained, but drainage should be delayed for 4 to 5 days to allow the hematoma to liquefy. Rarely, a hematoma may persist, going through periods of stability, resolution and recurrence. These requires surgical management.

REFERENCES

Naumann RO, Droegemueller W. Unusual etiology of vulvar hematomas. Am J Obstet Gynecol 1982;142:357.

Huddock JJ, Dupayne N, McGeary JA. Traumatic vulvar hematomas. Am J Obstet Gynecol 1955;70:1064.

Mishell DR, Stenchever MA, Droegemueller W, Herbst AL. Comprehensive Gynecology, 3rd ed. St Louis: CV Mosby, 1997, pp 270, 474.

Niv J, Lessing JB, Hartuv J, Peyser MR. Vaginal injury resulting from sliding down a water chute. Am J Obstet Gynecol 1992;166:930.

Ridgeway LE. Puerperal emergency: vaginal and vulvar hematomas. Obstet Gynecol Clin North Am 1995;22:275.

Smith RP. Gynecology in Primary Care. Baltimore: Williams & Wilkins, 1997, pp 603–632.

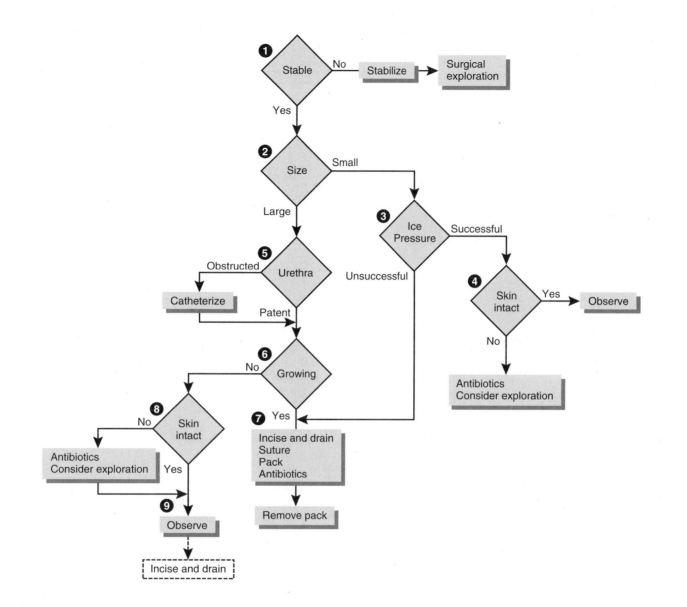

Vulvar Lesions

Deep

INTRODUCTION

The evaluation of vulvar lesions is based on the character and extent of the lesion present. Many other possible diagnoses, ranging from skin freckles (ephelides) to vulvar amyloidosis, are not represented. Those presented here are the most likely and suggest pathways for further investigation. Processes that result in lesions that occupy a superficial location are very different from those that cause processes deep within the tissues of the vulva. When cystic structures are encountered, the possibility of congenital remnants such as mesothelial cysts (cysts of the canal of Nuck), wolffian duct remnants, and periurethral cysts must be considered. Lipomas, neurofibromas, rhabdomyomas, schwannomas, and leiomyomas may present as fleshy tumors of the vulva.

Of special importance are those lesions that involve significant necrosis: necrotizing fasciitis and pyoderma gangrenosum. Both of these processes represent a significant threat to the life and health of the patient and require prompt and aggressive treatment.

❶ Deep vulvar and perineal lesions may be sorted based on their character: solid, cystic, or ulcerated. The most commonly encountered cystic lesions are the epithelial inclusion cysts and cystic dilatations of the Bartholin gland or duct. (Vaginal cystic lesions are discussed separately.)

❷ Solid tumor located on the perineum should be evaluated in the same manner at solid cutaneous tumors elsewhere on the body.

❸ Limpomas of the labia majora or minora are the most commonly encountered of the uncommon solid masses. Other tumors are possible and must be ultimately diagnoses by biopsy.

❹ Deep ulcerations of the vulva may arise as a result of infection (sexual or otherwise) or tumor. A number of deep vulvar ulcerative lesions must be diagnosed by biopsy.

❺ When herpes simplex or chancroid are suspected, a culture is indicated.

❻ Serologic testing can provide the final diagnosis for a number of deep vulvar ulcerative lesions.

REFERENCES

American College of Obstetricians and Gynecologists. Vulvar Dystrophies. ACOG Technical Bulletin 139. Washington, DC: ACOG, 1990.

American College of Obstetricians and Gynecologists. Genital Human Papillomavirus Infections. ACOG Technical Bulletin 193. Washington, DC: ACOG, 1994.

McKay M. Vulvar dermatoses. Clin Obstet Gynecol 1991;34:614.

Nanda VS. Common dermatoses. Am J Obstet Gynecol 1995;173:488.

Pecknam EM, Maki DG, Patterson JJ, et al. Focal vulvitis: a characteristic syndrome and cause of dyspareunia. Am J Obstet Gynecol 1986;154:855.

Wilkinson EJ, Stone IK. Atlas of Vulvar Disease. Baltimore: Wiliams & Wilkins, 1995.

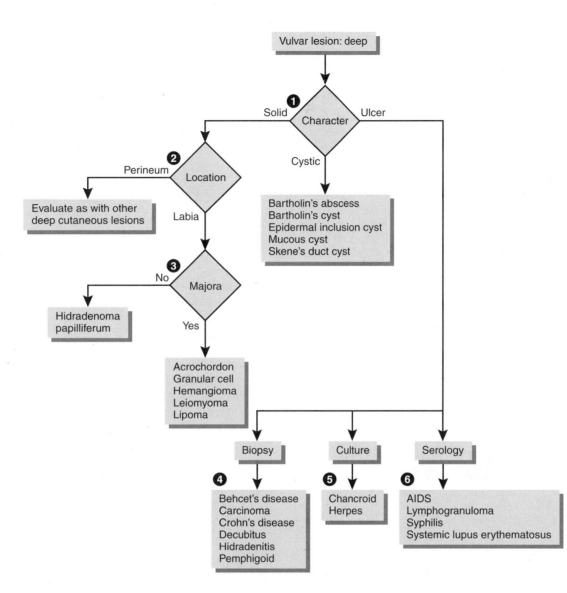

Vulvar lesion: deep

❶ Character

Solid · Cystic · Ulcer

❷ Location

Perineum · Labia

Evaluate as with other deep cutaneous lesions

❸ Majora

No · Yes

Hidradenoma papilliferum

Bartholin's abscess
Bartholin's cyst
Epidermal inclusion cyst
Mucous cyst
Skene's duct cyst

Acrochordon
Granular cell
Hemangioma
Leiomyoma
Lipoma

Biopsy

Culture

Serology

❹
Behcet's disease
Carcinoma
Crohn's disease
Decubitus
Hidradenitis
Pemphigoid

❺
Chancroid
Herpes

❻
AIDS
Lymphogranuloma
Syphilis
Systemic lupus erythematosus

Vulvar Lesions

Sexually Transmitted Diseases

INTRODUCTION

In the United States there are approximately 13 million cases of sexually transmitted diseases annually, excluding human immunodeficiency virus infections. For many sexually transmitted infections, the most common sites of entry are those directly exposed to infected semen; the vulva, vagina, and cervix. It is in these tissues that the first signs of infection may occur.

❶ While many possible ways exist to begin the differentiation of the lesions of sexually transmitted diseases, the contour of the lesion is one of the first attributes perceived when the lesion is first seen. Several sexually transmissible infections may take on more than one appearance depending on the stage of the disease or the duration that the lesion has been present.

❷ Raised lesions may be vesicular or papular, with intact or broken surfaces. Each of these characteristics can be suggestive of a specific infection.

❸ Multiple vesicular lesions with a regular shape, flat margins, and a red smooth base are typical of herpes simplex infections. The vesicles of lymphogranuloma venereum (LGV) tend to be single, painless, and regular in shape. They are superficial but are associated with tender, suppurative lymph nodes.

❹ Raised lesions that do not have a vesicular character may be papillary or broad and warty.

❺ Warty or pustular lesions with a broken surface may be found in chancroid. These lesions are few in number (one to three) and often painful. They have an irregular shape with red, undermined edges and an excavated, yellow-gray center that belies their initial raised appearance. Purulent or hemorrhagic secretions and tender nodes are common. Raised warty lesions with intact surfaces are typical of condyloma acuminata and of secondary syphilis (condyloma lata).

❻ Papillary lesions with intact, slightly umbillicated lesions with a waxy core are the hallmark of molluscum contagiosum. Early in the course of secondary syphilis mucous patches may form that become papillary before coalescing into the flattened shape of condyloma lata.

❼ Painless single or multiple papillary lesions with elevated rolled and regular margins are often seen in cases of granuloma inguinale. These lesions have a rough, red base with firm induration. Painless lesions with raised margins and a central, red, smooth base and serous secretions may be the chancre of primary syphilis.

❽ Flat lesions with a pale edge occur in cases of condyloma acuminata and lata, especially when they occur on the cervix or vaginal wall. Flat, itchy areas with red tracts or edges may signal the presence of scabes.

❾ Lesions that appear excavated because of the loss of surface epithelium appear painful but may be completely asymptomatic.

❿ Painful excavated lesions are found in herpes and in chancroid, with the latter characterized by fewer lesions and an undermined appearance.

⓫ Painless lesions occur in both syphilis (primary chancre) and granuloma inguinale. These two may be distinguished on physical examination by the rolled flat edge and raised center of granuloma inguinale, which is different from the flat, superficial lesions of syphilis.

REFERENCES

Abeck D, Freinkel AL, Korting HC, et al. Immunohistochemical investigations of genital ulcers caused by Haemophilus ducreyi. Int J STD & AIDS. 1997;8:585.

American College of Obstetricians and Gynecologists. Genital Human Papillomavirus Infections. ACOG Technical Bulletin 193. Washington, DC: ACOG, 1994.

American College of Obstetricians and Gynecologists. Genital Human Papillomavirus Infections. ACOG Technical Bulletin 193. Washington, DC: ACOG, 1994.

American College of Obstetricians and Gynecologists. Gynecologic Herpes Simplex Virus Infections. ACOG Technical Bulletin 119. Washington, DC: ACOG, 1988.

Faber BM. The diagnosis and treatment of scabies and pubic lice. Prim Care Update Ob/Gyns 1996;3:20.

Maccato ML, Kaufman RH. Herpes genitalis. Dermatol Clin 1992;10:415.

Morse SA. Atlas of Sexually Transmitted Diseases. Philadelphia: JB Lippincott, 1990.

Smith RP. Gynecology in Primary Care. Baltimore: Williams & Wilkins, 1997.

Wilkinson EJ, Stone IK. Atlas of Vulvar Disease. Baltimore: Williams & Wilkins, 1995.

Wong TY, Mihm MC Jr. Primary syphilis. N Engl J Med 1994;331:1492.

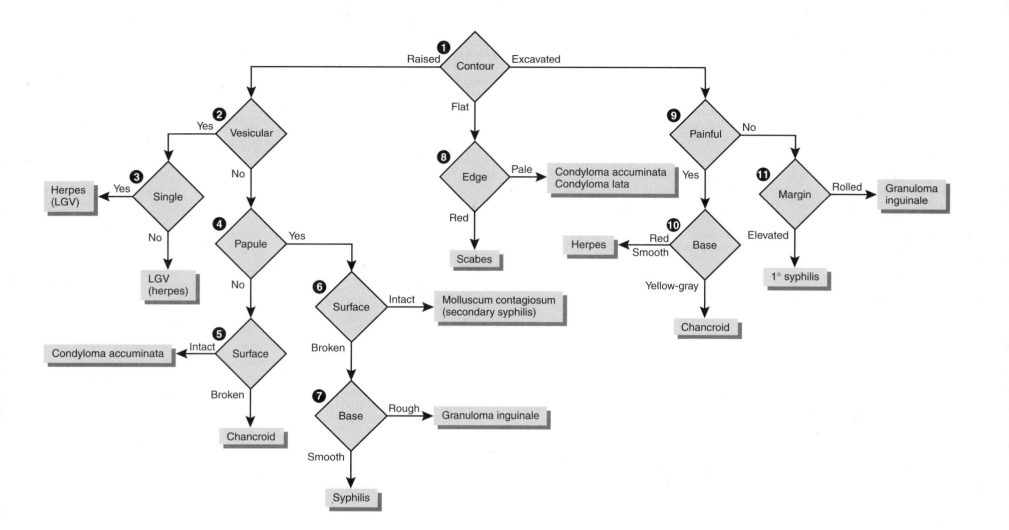

Vulvar Lesions

Superficial

INTRODUCTION

The evaluation of vulvar lesions is based on the character and extent of the lesion present. Many other possible diagnoses, ranging from skin freckles (ephelides) to vulvar amyloidosis, are not represented. Those presented here are the most likely and suggest pathways for further investigation. Processes that result in lesions that occupy a superficial location are very different from those that cause processes deep within the tissues of the vulva. It is important to keep in mind the fact that many conditions that cause vulvar lesions may present in several forms. Therefore, in any decision tree based on lesion morphology some diagnoses may be represented at the end of more than one branch (e.g., seborrheic kerotosis or nevus). Because symptoms and findings may overlap, no algorithm will apply in all cases. (Sexually transmitted diseases presenting as vulvar lesions are discussed separately.)

❶ Vulvar lesions that are limited to the surface epithelium may take on a number of forms. Those that are flat and do not rise above the skin surface may be classified by their color.

❷ Lichen planus and vestibulitis may both present are red, flat vulvar lesions. Lichen sclerosis and vitiligo both are characterized by the loss of pigment. Nevi may be found on the vulva but should be carefully monitored because of their higher rate of malignancy.

❸ Raised lesions that have a plaquelike character may also be subclassified on the basis of color.

❹ Inflammatory processes often take on a red or erythematous look. Typical of this type of plaque lesion are those of candidiasis or contact dermatitis. The application of 4% acetic acid will demonstrate the acetowhite changes associated with a number of cutaneous conditions. When applying acetic acid to the vulva, it must be left in place for several minutes for the acetowhite changes to develop owing to the thicker epithelium of the tissues.

❺ The most common vesicular vulvar lesions are those of herpes simplex. Other vesicular processes include chickenpox and lymphangioma circumscriptum.

❻ Condyloma acuminata (and lata) and seborrheic keratosis are the most common rough raised lesions.

❼ Condyloma acuminata may present as a smooth raised lesion in its earliest phases. This can make the differentiation between the results of human papilloma virus and syphilis (condyloma lata). In many cases, the presence of multiple lesions will suggest a different set of possible causes than those of solitary lesions.

REFERENCES

American College of Obstetricians and Gynecologists. Vulvar Dystrophies. ACOG Technical Bulletin 139. Washington, DC: ACOG, 1990.

American College of Obstetricians and Gynecologists. Genital Human Papillomavirus Infections. ACOG Technical Bulletin 193. Washington, DC: ACOG, 1994.

McKay M. Vulvar dermatoses. Clin Obstet Gynecol 1991;34:614.

Nanda VS. Common dermatoses. Am J Obstet Gynecol 1995;173:488.

Pecknam EM, Maki DG, Patterson JJ, et al. Focal vulvitis: a characteristic syndrome and cause of dyspareunia. Am J Obstet Gynecol 1986;154:855.

Wilkinson EJ, Stone IK. Atlas of Vulvar Disease. Baltimore: Williams & Wilkins, 1995.

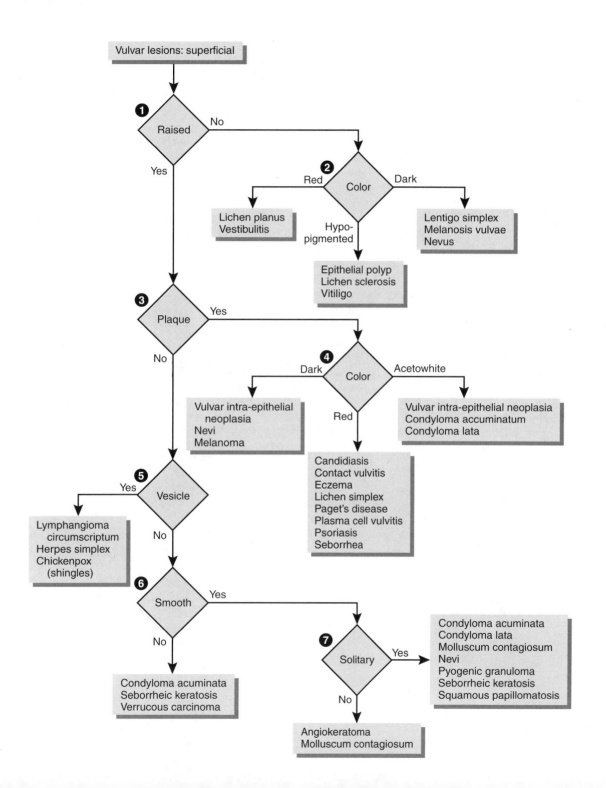

Vulvar lesions: superficial

1 Raised
- No
- Yes

2 Color
- Red → Lichen planus / Vestibulitis
- Hypo-pigmented → Epithelial polyp / Lichen sclerosis / Vitiligo
- Dark → Lentigo simplex / Melanosis vulvae / Nevus

3 Plaque
- Yes
- No

4 Color
- Dark → Vulvar intra-epithelial neoplasia / Nevi / Melanoma
- Red → Candidiasis / Contact vulvitis / Eczema / Lichen simplex / Paget's disease / Plasma cell vulvitis / Psoriasis / Seborrhea
- Acetowhite → Vulvar intra-epithelial neoplasia / Condyloma accuminatum / Condyloma lata

5 Vesicle
- Yes → Lymphangioma circumscriptum / Herpes simplex / Chickenpox (shingles)
- No

6 Smooth
- Yes
- No → Condyloma acuminata / Seborrheic keratosis / Verrucous carcinoma

7 Solitary
- Yes → Condyloma acuminata / Condyloma lata / Molluscum contagiosum / Nevi / Pyogenic granuloma / Seborrheic keratosis / Squamous papillomatosis
- No → Angiokeratoma / Molluscum contagiosum

Vulvar Vestibulitis

INTRODUCTION

Vulvar vestibulitis is an uncommon syndrome of intense sensitivity of the skin of the posterior vaginal introitus and vulvar vestibule that progressively worsens, leading to loss of function (inability to use tampons (33%) or have intercourse (entry dyspareunia, 100%)). While it has been reported in patients from 18 to 81, the median age is 36. These patients experience intense pain and tenderness at the posterior introitus and vestibule, with these symptoms present for an average of 2 to 5 years. Examination may reveal focal inflammation, punctation, and ulceration of the perineal and vaginal epithelium. Punctate areas (1 to 10) of inflammation 3 to 10 mm in size may be seen between the Bartholin's glands (75%), hymeneal ring, and mid-perineum.

❶ The most important aspect of the treatment of vulvar vestibulities is the establishment of a correct diagnosis. Dyspareunia and introital pain during tampon insertion are typical presenting symptoms, but these are nonspecific and may be caused by other pathologies. The changes of vestibulitis (flat, nonulcerated areas of erythema 2 to 8 mm in size) are generally restricted to the posterior fourchette, the introitus, and the area between the Bartholin's glands. The possibility of other vulvar skin conditions must be considered, with colposcopy or biopsies used as needed to establish a diagnosis. Nonvulvar causes such as vaginitis, vaginismus, and depression must be considered.

❷ Once the working diagnosis is established (or confirmed by biopsy), simple interventions such as perineal hygiene, cool sitz baths, moist soaks, and the application of soothing solutions such as Burow's solution are good initial therapies. Patients should be advised to wear loose-fitting clothing and keep the area dry and well ventilated. The use of topical anesthetics (2% lidocaine jelly (or 5% cream) topically as needed) may improve functionality, though sexual dysfunction due to loss of sensation may be a side effect of treatment. Some authors recommended the withdrawal of oral contraceptives (if used), though evidence of causation or efficacy is limited.

❸ As with some cases of vulvar dystrophy, selective use of antidepressant therapy has been effective. Antidepressants (amitriptyline hydrochloride (Elavil) 25 mg po qhs or 10 mg po tid) may be sufficient to reduce symptoms to a tolerable level. If this therapy is chosen, an assessment of its efficacy should be delayed until 6 or more weeks of treatment.

❹ Interferon injections 3 times weekly for 4 weeks introducing 1 million units at each of 12 areas (clock face) by the completion of the course has been shown to be effective for some patients. The need for frequent visits, the, the cost, and the availability of treatment have limited the use of this approach. This option is still less invasive than surgical excision, making it worthy of consideration. Low-dose 5-fluorouracil has also been reported to be effective.

❺ Surgical excision or laser ablation of the vestibule is associated with improvement rates of up to 90%. Secondary scarring, resulting in iatrogenic dyspareunia, must be considered by both the patient and the surgeon before proceeding with treatment. For this reason, some authors suggest delaying the choice of these options until 6 months or more of symptoms or alternative therapies have elapsed. If improvement is not obtained following ablation or excision, some authors suggest either re-excision or a complete re-evaluation with a return to conservative therapy prior to additional surgery.

❻ Critical to success is long-term follow-up of even symptom-free individuals. The possibility of recurrence, or other types of dyspareunia or sexual dysfunction emerging as a result of the prolonged symptoms and treatments involved, must be considered.

REFERENCES

Baggish MS, Miklos JR. Vulvar pain syndrome: A review, Obstet Gynecol Surv 1995;50:618–627.

Bornstein J, Goldik Z, Stolar Z, et al. Predicting the outcome of surgical treatment of vulvar vestibulitis. Obstet Gynecol 1997;89:695–698.

Bornstein J, Pascal B, Abramovici H. Intramuscular β-interferon treatment for severe vulvar vestibulitis. J Reprod Med 1993;38:117.

David GD. The management of vulvar vestibulitis syndrome with the carbon dioxide laser. J Gynecol Surg 1989;5:87.

Fischer G, Spurrett B, Fischer A. The chronically symptomatic vulva: aetiology and management. Br J Obstet Gynaecol 1995;102:773.

Friedrich EG, Jr. Vulvar vestibulitis syndrome. J Reprod Med 1987;32:110–114.

Goetsch MF. Vulvar vestibulitis: Prevalence and histologic features in a general gynecologic practice population. Am J Obstet Gynecol 1991;164:1609.

Marinoff SC, Turner MLC. Vulvar vestibulitis syndrome: an overview. Am J Obstet Gynecol 1991;165:228.

Pecknam EM, Maki DG, Patterson JJ, et al. Focal vulvitis: a characteristic syndrome and cause of dyspareunia. Am J Obstet Gynecol 1986;154:855.

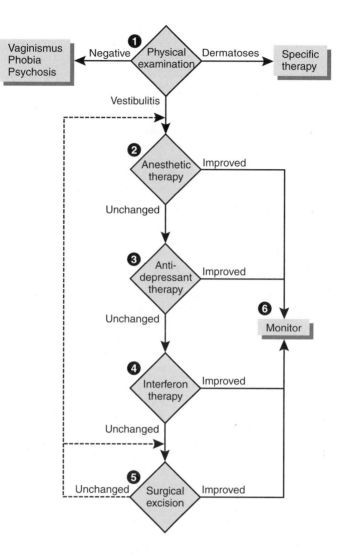

Vulvodynia

INTRODUCTION

Intense pain, insertional dyspareunia, itching, and irritation of the vulva can be debilitating. In most cases, a cause may be determined and effective therapy rendered.

❶ A careful history will frequently reveal one or more possible causes of vulvar pain. Gentle pelvic examination follows. Inspection of the vulva may reveal lesions, discharges, or discoloration that may suggest other pathologies. Careful palpation with a saline-moistened cotton-tipped applicator can help to map the area of pain.

❷ A microscopic examination of any vaginal secretions present under both saline and 10% KOH (potassium hydroxide) should be performed. Early or subclinical vaginitis may first present as mild or persistent vulvar irritation and pain.

❸ Skin scrapings from the vulva (obtained with a wooden spatula or the side of a scalpel blade) should be examined under 10% KOH solution. The presence of hyphae is diagnostic for cutaneous dermatophytes.

❹ Atrophic changes in the skin caused by the loss of estrogen stimulation (menopause) or lichen sclerosis often result in intense burning or pain. If the diagnosis is in question, a dermal biopsy is indicated.

❺ A dusky or hyperpigmented appearance of the vulva may suggest chronic irritation (contact vulvitis) or the early stages of Bowen's disease. Once again, a biopsy will resolve the diagnosis.

❻ In the absence of irritants, behavioral and psychological interactions should be explored. Chronic urinary tract infections or vulvar human papilloma virus infection may cause pain with few other signs. Herniation of the pudendal nerve through Alcock's canal may occur with pelvic floor relaxation. Scarring after surgery (episiotomy or other) or trauma, including straddle or back injuries, may result in persistent vulvar pain.

❼ Topical or systemic factors may cause vulvar symptoms. Whenever possible, these should be identified and eliminated as a first line of therapy. If this fails, antidepressants, especially at night when pain is often intense, and sedation may be desirable. When itching is prominent, crotamiton (Eurax) may be applied topically, twice daily, to suppress itching. Occasionally, the use of a topical anesthetic, such as 2% lidocaine jelly, may be required.

❽ Dermatologic conditions ranging from simple excoriation to cancer may present with vulvar symptoms and a visible lesion. Biopsy of the lesion is generally required to establish the diagnosis and should be performed liberally when the diagnosis is uncertain.

❾ Intense pain and itching characterizes virtually all cases of lichen sclerosis. The vulva takes on a thinned, atrophic appearance, with linear scratch marks or fissures. The skin often has a "cigarette-paper" or parchment-like appearance. These changes frequently extend around the anus in a figure-eight configuration.

❿ Focal inflammation, punctation, and ulceration of the perineal and vaginal epithelium are generally found in patients with vulvar vestibulitis. Punctate areas (1 to 10) of inflammation 3 to 10 mm in size may be seen between the Bartholin's glands, hymeneal ring, and mid-perineum in these patients (75% of cases). General readdening of the vulva skin without puncatations may suggest hyperkeratosis or early dermatophye infection.

REFERENCES

American College of Obstetricians and Gynecologists. Vulvar Nonneoplastic Epithelial Disorders. ACOG Technical Bulletin 241. Washington, DC: ACOG, 1997.

Baggish MS, Miklos JR. Vulvar pain syndrome: a review. Obstet Gynecol Survey 1995;50:618.

Fischer G, Spurrett B, Fischer A. The chonically symptomatic vulva: etiology and management. Br J Obstet Gynaecol 1995;102:773.

Goetsch MF. Vulvar vestibulitis: Prevalence and histologic features in a general gynecologic practice population. Am J Obstet Gynecol 1991;164:1609.

McKay M. Subsets of vulvodynia. J Reprod Med 1988;33:695.

McKay M. Vulvodynia versus pruitis vulvae. Clin Obstet Gynecol 1985;28:123.

Paavonen J. Diagnosis and treatment of vulvodynia. Ann Med 1995;27:175.

Paavonen J. Vulvodynia—a complex syndrome of vulvar pain. Acta Obstet Gynecol Scand 1995;74:243.

Stewart DE, Reicher AE, Gerulath AH, Boydel K. Vulvodynia and psychological distress. Obstet Gynecol 1994;84:587.

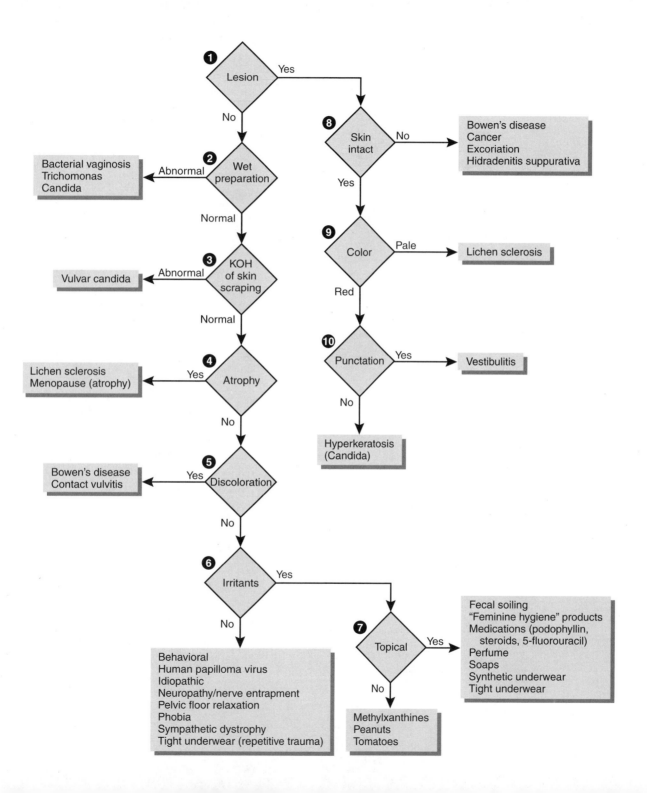

1 Lesion — Yes →

No ↓

2 Wet preparation — Abnormal → Bacterial vaginosis / Trichomonas / Candida

Normal ↓

3 KOH of skin scraping — Abnormal → Vulvar candida

Normal ↓

4 Atrophy — Yes → Lichen sclerosis / Menopause (atrophy)

No ↓

5 Discoloration — Yes → Bowen's disease / Contact vulvitis

No ↓

6 Irritants — Yes →

No ↓

Behavioral
Human papilloma virus
Idiopathic
Neuropathy/nerve entrapment
Pelvic floor relaxation
Phobia
Sympathetic dystrophy
Tight underwear (repetitive trauma)

7 Topical — Yes → Fecal soiling / "Feminine hygiene" products / Medications (podophyllin, steroids, 5-fluorouracil) / Perfume / Soaps / Synthetic underwear / Tight underwear

No ↓

Methylxanthines
Peanuts
Tomatoes

8 Skin intact — No → Bowen's disease / Cancer / Excoriation / Hidradenitis suppurativa

Yes ↓

9 Color — Pale → Lichen sclerosis

Red ↓

10 Punctation — Yes → Vestibulitis

No ↓

Hyperkeratosis (Candida)

Index

Note: Page numbers in *italics* refer to algorithms.